Study Guide to Accompany

Drug Therapy in Nursing

Diane S. Aschenbrenner, RN, CS, MS

Course Coordinator
Johns Hopkins University
School of Nursing
Baltimore, Maryland

Samantha J. Venable, RN, MS, FNP

Professor
Saddleback College
Mission Viejo, California

LIPPINCOTT WILLIAMS & WILKINS
A **Wolters Kluwer** Company

Philadelphia • Baltimore • New York • London
Buenos Aires • Hong Kong • Sydney • Tokyo

Managing Editor: Doris S. Wray
Production Managing Editor: Erika Kors
Senior Production Manager: Helen Ewan
Compositor: Peirce Graphic Services
Printer/Binder: Victor Graphics

ISBN: 0-7817-3270-0
Any procedure or practice described in this book should be applied by the health care practitioner under appropriate supervision in accordance with professional standards of care used with regard to the unique circumstances that apply in each practice situation. Care has been taken to confirm the accuracy of information presented and to describe generally accepted practices. However, the authors, editors, and publisher cannot accept any responsibility for errors or omissions or for any consequences from application of the information in this book and make no warranty, express or implied, with respect to the contents of the book.

Introduction

This study guide has been carefully designed to complement *Drug Therapy in Nursing*. Each chapter in the study guide opens with the Top Ten Things to Know about the drugs in the chapter. This is a synthesis of the most important points that were made in the chapter. You will note that each of the other headings in the study guide focuses on one type of knowledge presented in each chapter, not on each drug presented. Thus, Key Terms are the key terms identified at the beginning of each chapter. Physiology and Pathophysiology: The Body Human represents pertinent physiology and pathophysiology relevant to the drugs presented in the chapter. Core Drug Knowledge: Just the Facts details the facts that comprise the core drug knowledge about each drug. Core Patient Variables: Patients, Please highlights the core patient variables relevant to each drug. Nursing Management: Every Good Nurse Should. . . , Case Study, and Critical Thinking Challenge are opportunities to apply knowledge to patient scenarios and practice integrating the core drug knowledge with the core patient variables.

The study guide is also organized around how students learn a new, complex subject; that is, by starting to learn the basics and then moving on to harder material. In nursing, students start by memorizing some key points and then moving to understanding those points. As students become comfortable with this new knowledge, they begin to see how these new facts may have a bearing on or relationship with other facts they have learned. Students begin to realize that these two pieces of knowledge, which previously stood alone, mean something different when considered together. Students then continue to piece other facts together to draw conclusions. This is much like doing a jigsaw puzzle. At first it may seem that the 500 pieces have no relationship to each other, but as you sort them out you begin to see similarities. "These pieces together make the sky. These pieces together make the tree top." Eventually, it no longer looks like pieces of a puzzle, but one big picture.

Students advance from remembering facts to applying knowledge. They must be able to do this if they are to be competent nurses and care for patients. In drug therapy, the facts about the drug remain the same for every patient who takes that drug. But the relevancy of those facts depends on factors that are unique to that patient.

To help the student advance through these tiers of learning, each chapter in the study guide is arranged from the easiest to the most difficult learning tasks. The sections of Key Terms, Physiology, and Pathophysiology: The Body Human essentially require memorization, recognition, and understanding of some facts. Matching, essays, and word searches make up this level of learning, which may be time-consuming, but is not complex. The sections on Core Drug Knowledge: Just the Facts, and Core Patient Variables: Patients, Please are somewhat harder. Multiple choice questions are offered which encourage students to begin to compare and make basic judgments. The section Nursing Management: Every Good Nurse Should . . . asks students to recognize what the nurse does specific to the drug therapy. Some application of knowledge is needed here. This is a somewhat more complex process. Multiple choice and decision trees make up this level of learning. Finally, the Case Study and the Critical Thinking Challenge require students to synthesize the knowledge presented and apply it to patient scenarios. To do so, students must be able to interpret the possible interaction of core drug knowledge and core patient variables presented in the case. Short answers are asked for the problems posed. This requires a much higher level of thinking than simple memorization. Some students will have great difficulty doing this. If you are having trouble with this level of thinking, don't despair, don't give up, and don't stop trying to do the case studies. The way you get proficient at a new task is to practice, practice, practice. Critical Thinking Challenge is designed to require the most thinking. Here, additional questions related to the case study are posed. To answer the question, students may need to apply knowledge not necessarily from this chapter or from the text. Some of the information may not be strictly "pharmacology" information. It may be knowledge learned from other fields of study. This is because in the practice of nursing, patients are multidimensional, and to meet their needs you will need to know varied types of information.

We hope this study guide is helpful to you in your quest to master facts about pharmacology and to learn how to apply those facts in nursing management. And we hope we have helped you to "see the whole picture."

Diane S. Aschenbrenner
Samantha J. Venable

Contents

UNIT I

Principles and Process of Nursing Management in Drug Therapy

CHAPTER 1

Nursing Management in Drug Therapy

TOP TEN THINGS TO KNOW ABOUT NURSING MANAGEMENT IN DRUG THERAPY

1. Core drug knowledge consists of pharmacotherapeutics, pharmacokinetics, pharmacodynamics, contraindications and precautions, adverse effects, and drug interactions.
2. Core patient variables consist of health status; life span and gender; lifestyle, diet, and habits; environment; and culture.
3. Nursing management in drug therapy identifies potential interactions between core drug knowledge and core patient variables.
4. The nurse uses the nursing process and interactions of core drug knowledge and core patient variables to maximize therapeutic effects, minimize adverse effects, provide patient and family education, and evaluate effectiveness of the drug therapy.
5. *Pharmacotherapeutics* is why the drug is prescribed; *pharmacokinetics* is what the body does to the drug; and *pharmacodynamics* is what the drug does to the body.
6. *Contraindications and precautions* indicate restrictions in use or need for close monitoring during therapy; *adverse effects* are undesired effects of the drug, which range from minor to severe; *drug interactions* are effects that may occur when a drug is coadministered with another drug, food, or substance.
7. Health status includes assessment of acute and chronic conditions, potential organ dysfunction, allergies, drug history, and diminished memory or mental status.
8. Life span and gender are age, physiologic development, reproductive stage, ability to read and write, and sex; lifestyle, diet, and habits are the amount of activity and exercise, sleep–wake patterns, occupation, ability to pay for drug therapy, use or abuse of substances, use of over-the-counter drugs, use of alternative health practices, and eating preferences and patterns.
9. Environment includes the setting where drug therapy will be administered, the physical factors that may influence aspects of drug therapy, exposure to potentially harmful substances, and cost of the drug; culture is the religious, ethnic, and racial background of the patient.
10. Nursing assessment in drug therapy includes a health and drug history, physical assessment, and examination of the medical record, including current laboratory and other diagnostic findings.

KEY TERMS

Essay

Define the following terms.

1. pharmacotherapeutics
2. pharmacokinetics
3. pharmacodynamics
4. contraindications and precautions
5. adverse effects
6. drug interactions
7. core drug knowledge
8. core patient variables
9. health status
10. life span and gender
11. lifestyle, diet, and habits
12. environment
13. culture
14. drug response
15. nursing management in drug therapy
16. prototype drug
17. prototype approach

CORE DRUG KNOWLEDGE: JUST THE FACTS

Multiple choice

Circle the option that best answers the question or completes the statement.

1. Administration of aminophylline to a patient with acute asthma is an example of
   a. pharmacodynamics.
   b. pharmacokinetics.
   c. pharmacotherapeutics.
   d. adverse effects.

2. Mr. Jones has hypertension and is administered minoxidil (Loniten), an antihypertensive drug. Three months later, he notices an increase in the growth of his hair, which is an expected effect of the drug. This is an example of the _____ of minoxidil.
   a. pharmacodynamics
   b. pharmacokinetics
   c. pharmacotherapeutics
   d. adverse effects

3. Mrs. Queens, who is two months' pregnant, has just been diagnosed with pneumonia. Which of the following areas of core drug knowledge would be most relevant to selection of drug therapy for Mrs. Queens?
   a. pharmacodynamics
   b. contraindications and precautions
   c. pharmacotherapeutics
   d. adverse effects

4. Which of the following is an example of an adverse effect of a drug?
   a. lowered white blood cell count after drug therapy for cancer
   b. lowered blood pressure after drug therapy for hypertension
   c. increased urinary output after drug therapy for edema
   d. increased cardiac output after drug therapy for congestive heart failure

CORE PATIENT VARIABLES: PATIENTS, PLEASE

Multiple choice

Circle the option that best answers the question or completes the statement.

1. Which of the following statements/questions would be included in the nurse's assessment of health status?
   a. "Have you ever had any reactions to medications in the past?"
   b. "Will your insurance cover the cost of this prescription?"
   c. "When is your baby due?"
   d. "Tell me about your diet."

2. Mr. Cannon works from midnight to 8 AM and experiences insomnia during the day. This is an example of which of the following core patient variables?
   a. health status
   b. environment
   c. life span and gender
   d. lifestyle, diet, and habits

3. A history of smoking cigarettes is included in which of the following core patient variables?
   a. health status
   b. environment
   c. life span and gender
   d. lifestyle, diet, and habits

4. In assessing the patient care variable of environment, the nurse might include
   a. where the patient keeps his or her medication at home.
   b. what is the patient's diet.
   c. the last time the patient had a chest x-ray.
   d. the allergies of the patient.

NURSING MANAGEMENT: EVERY GOOD NURSE SHOULD . . .

Students may use grids like the ones below and on the next page to help them see the relationship between the core drug knowledge and the core patient variables. Use them as you wish to meet your learning needs. Some suggestions: base the map on each prototype or each class; use different colors to fill the blocks if there is an interaction that occurs (e.g., if the pharmacotherapeutics of the drug include use for congestive heart failure, the block under pharmacotherapeutics and next to health status would be filled in because the nurse would need to assess the cardiovascular system), or use words in the blocks. To compare multiple drugs in a class, use the second chart. These tools can be used in every drug chapter if so desired.

NURSING MANAGEMENT: CORE DRUG KNOWLEDGE

Drug Name_____

	Pharmaco-therapeutics	Pharmaco-kinetics	Pharmaco-dynamics	Contraindications/ Precautions	Adverse Effects	Drug Interactions
Health status						
Life span and gender						
Lifestyle, diet, and habits						
Culture						
Environment						

Drug Class_____

	Pharmaco-therapeutics	Pharmaco-kinetics	Pharmaco-dynamics	Contraindications/Precautions	Adverse Effects	Drug Interactions
Drug #1						
Drug #2						
Drug #3						
Drug #4						
Drug #5						
Drug #6						

CASE STUDY

1. Mrs. Newberry, a 60-year-old retired schoolteacher, has just started drug therapy with sulfamethoxazole-trimethoprim (Bactrim, Septra) for a urinary tract infection. List the questions you would ask to assess her patient care variables.

   health status

   life span and gender

   lifestyle, diet, and habits

   environment

   culture

2. Your assessment of Mrs. Newberry indicates that she has normal renal and liver function, has no chronic diseases, and does not take any other medications. Another nurse walks by, recognizes Mrs. Newberry, and asks about her garden. This information would lead you to further assess Mrs. Newberry's environment.
   What questions might you ask? (Are you lost? Go to Chapter 51 for information concerning the importance of environment with this drug.)

CRITICAL THINKING CHALLENGE

Essay

How would your assessment of Mrs. Newberry's environment influence your nursing interventions?

How can you minimize potential adverse effects?

CHAPTER 2

Pharmaceuticals: Development, Safeguards, and Delivery

TOP TEN THINGS TO KNOW ABOUT PHARMACEUTICALS, DEVELOPMENT, SAFEGUARDS, AND DELIVERY

1. Sources of drugs include plants, animals, synthetic chemicals, and genetically engineered chemicals.
2. Drugs have three names: chemical, generic, and trade.
3. A drug's chemical name describes the drug using exact chemical nomenclature to show atomic and molecular structure.
4. A drug's generic name is derived from the chemical name; the first letter of the generic name is not normally capitalized.
5. A drug's trade name, provided by the drug manufacturer, is usually easy to say and remember. It is protected by trademark, and the first letter is normally capitalized.
6. Drugs that are grouped by similar characteristics are called a drug class, or classification. Classification may be chemical, physiologic, or therapeutic. Drugs may belong to more than one class.
7. Drug regulations and legislation have been developed to control drug use and promote consumer safety from drug products.
8. The approval process for a new drug is lengthy and expensive.
9. The FDA MedWatch program and the USP Practitioners Reporting Network rely on all health care providers to report all problems or suspected problems with drug products to provide postmarketing surveillance of drugs.
10. Nurses administer drugs to patients, assess response to therapy, monitor for effectiveness, educate patients and families about all aspects of drug therapy, and, in some settings, adjust drug regimens according to protocols. Nurse practitioners may prescribe drug therapy. Nursing management in drug therapy may be considered an applied science.

KEY TERMS

Matching

Match the following key terms with their definitions.

1. _____ pharmacology
2. _____ toxicology
3. _____ pharmacotherapeutic
4. _____ pharmacokinetics
5. _____ pharmacodynamics
6. _____ chemical name
7. _____ generic name
8. _____ trade name
9. _____ drug classification
10. _____ chemical classification
11. _____ physiologic classification
12. _____ therapeutic classification
13. _____ *National Formulary*

a. Use of medicinal agents for managing and curing illness
b. What the drug does to the body
c. Exact chemical language of a drug
d. Brand name of the drug
e. Group of drugs that share similar characteristics
f. Classifies the drug by its use in therapy
g. Classifies the drug by its effects on a body system
h. Study of drugs
i. Classifies the drug by its chemical base
j. Nonproprietary name of the drug
k. What the body does to the drug
l. Study of poisons
m. Document that contains the official name for each drug

Match the following key terms with their definitions.

1. _____ Canadian Food and Drug Act
2. _____ clinical trials
3. _____ controlled substance
4. _____ drug classification
5. _____ legend drugs
6. _____ Federal Food, Drug, and Cosmetics Act of 1938
7. _____ pharmacogenetics
8. _____ pharmacognosy
9. _____ placebo response
10. _____ Practitioners Reporting Network
11. _____ Pure Food and Drug Act of 1906
12. _____ *United States Pharmacopoeia*
13. _____ United States Adopted Names Council

a. Study of natural elements as drug sources
b. Group established to ensure uniform drug nomenclature
c. Group of similar drugs
d. Established the Food and Drug Administration (FDA) as the agency for monitoring and controlling drug manufacture and marketing
e. Drug listed according to its abuse potential
f. Document that contains the official name for each drug
g. Positive response to any therapeutic intervention
h. Designated the USP and NF as the official standards
i. Postmarketing forum to report problems with prescribed drugs
j. System that allows testing of potential new drugs
k. Another term for a prescription drug
l. Laws maintained by the Health Protection Branch of government
m. Study of genetically inherited conditions that affect the way drugs act on the body and modify the way the body acts on drugs

CHAPTER 3

Drug Preparations and Administration

TOP TEN THINGS TO KNOW ABOUT DRUG PREPARATIONS AND ADMINISTRATION ROUTES

1. The three routes of drug administration are enteral, parenteral, and topical.
2. Oral administration is the most frequently used method for the enteral route.
3. Coatings on oral drugs, food, fluids, and other drugs may affect the absorption and onset of action of oral drugs.
4. Oral drugs are easy to administer, may be self-administered, and are less expensive than other forms of drug administration.
5. Parenteral drug administration methods are intramuscular (IM), subcutaneous (SC), and intravenous (IV).
6. Onset of action is more rapid with parenteral than enteral route.
7. Consider the patient and drug characteristics when selecting a needle, syringe, and intramuscular site.
8. Intravenous administration of drugs may be through continuous drip, intermittent infusion, or intravenous push methods.
9. Topical drugs are applied to skin and mucous membranes.
10. Topical drugs may produce local or systemic effects.

KEY TERMS

Fill in the blanks

Read each statement carefully and, using the chapter's key terms, write your answer in the space provided.

1. Drugs administered into the GI tract are given by way of the _____ route.

2. A good example of an _____ injection is a PPD test.

3. The _____ route circumvents the GI tract.

4. Drugs applied directly on the skin is known as the _____ route.

5. Drugs applied topically to the skin or mucous membranes exert a _____ .

6. Drugs that distribute throughout the body exert a _____ .

7. Drugs that come as an _____ must be shaken well before administration.

8. An _____ resists the acid environment of the stomach.

9. A solid drug dispersed within a liquid is called a _____ .

10. Administration of a drug into the cerebrospinal fluid is known as the _____ route.

11. _____ tablets are placed underneath the tongue.

12. A tablet placed between the cheek and gum in the mouth is known as _____ administration.

13. A _____ is also known as a pastilles or lozenge.

14. A drug compressed or molded into a specific shape is called a _____ .

15. An _____ drug is administered directly into the bloodstream.

16. A _____ tablet is formulated to release a drug slowly over an extended period.

17. A drug encased in a hard or soft gelatin container is known as a _____ .

18. A _____ is a concentrated solution of sugar in water.

19. Instillation of drugs into a muscle is known as the _____ route.

20. An _____ is a clear hydroalcoholic mixture that is usually sweetened.

21. An _____ medication is administered over a few minutes while a _____ medication is administered over 20–60 minutes.

22. _____ drugs are administered under the skin into the fat and connective tissues.

23. Drugs administered into a joint space are called _____ .

24. An _____ drug is administered directly into an artery.

CORE DRUG KNOWLEDGE: JUST THE FACTS

Multiple choice

Circle the option that best answers the question or completes the statement.

1. Absorption of enteral drugs occurs most frequently in the
   a. mouth.
   b. stomach.
   c. esophagus.
   d. small intestine.

2. What type of enteral medications should be avoided in children?
   a. syrups
   b. elixirs
   c. capsules
   d. tablets

3. The onset of action is rapid after IM administration because
   a. the drug is always in solution.
   b. the drug bypasses the vasculature.
   c. the muscle has a good blood supply.
   d. the drug reaches the gastrointestinal (GI) system quickly.

4. A saline lock is an example of
   a. subcutaneous administration.
   b. intradermal administration.
   c. peripheral access device.
   d. central access.

5. Which of the following would be affected if an enteric-coated tablet were cut in half?
   a. absorption
   b. drug interactions
   c. adverse effects
   d. elimination

Essay

1. List the pros and cons of IV administration of drugs.
2. List three parenteral delivery routes.
3. What is the purpose of an enteric coating on a drug?
4. How do sustained-release capsules slow the delivery of medication?
5. Name five types of topical drugs.

CORE PATIENT VARIABLES: PATIENTS, PLEASE

Essay

1. Which is the preferred site for IM administration of drugs to an infant?
2. List five reasons enteral drugs may be contraindicated for a patient.
3. Mrs. Timely, an 83-year-old woman, is admitted to your unit after having a cerebrovascular accident (CVA; stroke). She has difficulty swallowing. Develop three strategies to administer enteral medications to Mrs. Timely.
4. Jessica Peters has a nasogastric (NG) tube inserted. Describe the administration of medication into Jessica's NG tube.
5. List three reasons topical absorption of a drug may occur.
6. List three nursing interventions to maximize therapeutic effects and minimize adverse effects when administering topical drugs.
7. List the six rights of medication administration.
8. Mrs. Jones is admitted to the hospital for an exacerbation of asthma. She has been receiving theophylline syrup for 9 months at home. Name three assessments the nurse should make.
9. How would the nurse position a patient to administer an IM injection in the right vastus lateralis?
10. Mr. Kirth has been diagnosed with leukemia. He will be receiving chemotherapy for the next 6 months. What type of medication administration would be most appropriate for Mr. Kirth?

NURSING MANAGEMENT: EVERY GOOD NURSE SHOULD...

State the appropriate injection site based on the following situations.

SITUATIONS

a. Thin, 24-year-old male requiring 3 cc of a viscous drug (antibiotic) IM

b. Average, 60-year-old female requiring 0.5 cc of thin drug (vaccine) IM

c. Obese, 40-year-old male requiring 2.5 cc of thin drug (narcotic) IM

d. Newborn requiring 0.5 cc of thin drug (vitamin K) IM

e. Average, 16-year-old female requiring 0.2 cc thin solution (insulin) SC

CASE STUDY

Daryl Johnson is 63 years old and has dysphagia (trouble eating and swallowing) due to muscle weakness in his mouth and throat from a neuromuscular disorder. He is receiving oral drug therapy for his neuromuscular disorder, hypertension, gastric ulcer, and an infection in his chest. The drug therapy he receives is administered in the following oral drug forms: tablets, enteric-coated tablets, capsules, sustained-release capsules, and suspension.

1. What assessment is indicated for Mr. Johnson?

2. What questions regarding drug preparations might you discuss with the pharmacist and the prescriber of the drug therapy?

3. What teaching might be indicated for Mr. Johnson?

CRITICAL THINKING CHALLENGE

Mr. Johnson's dysphagia progresses until he can no longer swallow food, fluids, or his drug therapy. A gastroscopy tube is placed. Describe the (*a*) assessments and (*b*) teaching that might be needed now regarding administration of his drug therapies.

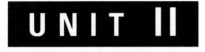

UNIT II

Core Drug Knowledge

CHAPTER 4

Pharmacotherapeutics and Pharmacokinetics

TOP TEN THINGS TO KNOW ABOUT PHARMACOTHERAPEUTICS AND PHARMACOKINETICS

1. *Pharmacotherapeutics* are the therapeutic or desired effects of the drug. *Pharmacokinetics* are the effects of the body on the drug.

2. There are four phases of pharmacokinetics: absorption, distribution, metabolism (biotransformation), and elimination. Pharmacokinetics are influenced by health status, life span, gender, and culture.

3. Drug absorption depends on route of administration, solubility and concentration of the drug, circulation, surface conditions, contact time and pH at the absorption site, and cell membrane transport mechanisms.

4. Drugs are distributed throughout the body to the cells by way of the cardiovascular system. Distribution depends on drug flow to the tissues, the drug's ability to leave the vascular system and enter cells, the drug's lipid affinity (lipophilic) or water affinity (hydrophilic), and the drug's ability to bind with protein (usually albumin) in the blood.

5. Drug particles that are not bound to protein (ie, are "free") are active and exert an effect. An increase in the number of free drug particles (from low protein levels) will increase the drug's effect, even though the dose of the drug is unchanged.

6. Metabolism changes the drug from its pharmacologically active form to a more water-soluble form so it can be more easily excreted. Most metabolism occurs in the liver. The percentage of drug metabolized each time the drug is circulated to the liver varies from drug to drug. When drugs are highly metabolized during the first circulation to the liver (first pass), little or no active drug is sent to the general circulation.

7. Steady state usually occurs in five half-lives of the drug and may not correlate with the therapeutic effect of the drug.

8. Most drugs are metabolized by at least one CYP isoenzyme Drugs that are metabolized by a specific isoenzyme are called substrates of that isoenzyme.

9. A drug that is a CYP inducer increases the amount or activity of the isoenzyme. More active isoenzyme means that metabolism of the substrates occurs more rapidly and circulating drug levels will be decreased. A drug that is a CYP inhibitor decreases the activity of the isoenzyme; this decreases the metabolism of the isoenzyme's substrates. Less metabolism of a drug will increase its blood level and pharmacologic action.

10. Elimination or excretion of drugs occurs in the kidneys (primarily), liver, gastrointestinal (GI) tract, lungs, sweat and salivary glands, skin, and breast milk. Pathology of these systems (e.g., renal failure) will decrease excretion of the drug. Decreased excretion increases circulating blood levels of the drug even though the dose is unchanged.

KEY TERMS

Matching

Match the following key terms with their definitions.

1. _____ pharmacotherapeutics
2. _____ dose–response curve
3. _____ potency
4. _____ absorption
5. _____ bioavailability
6. _____ distribution
7. _____ active transport
8. _____ first-pass effect
9. _____ passive diffusion
10. _____ facilitated diffusion
11. _____ filtration
12. _____ metabolism
13. _____ pinocytosis

a. Moves gas and liquid molecules from an area of higher concentration to an area of lower concentration to become equally distributed across the cell membrane

b. Fraction of the administered dose that reaches the systemic circulation and produces effects

c. Carrier system that transports substances across the cell membrane without energy expenditure

d. Reason why the drug is prescribed

e. Changing of a drug to a more ionized or water-soluble and less lipid-soluble form

f. Drug's ability as an agonist to stimulate a receptor

g. Drugs entering the body by the enteral route first go through the portal circulation to the liver before reaching the general circulation

h. Passage of a drug through the pores of a semipermeable membrane

i. Delivery of the drug into any and all body compartments it can penetrate

j. Relationship between the dose of a drug administered and the response it produces

k. Movement of a drug from its site of administration to the bloodstream

l. Energy source is required to move molecules across the cell membrane against a concentration gradient

m. Cell membrane engulfs a substance on its outer surface, forms a membrane-covered vesicle, and carries it inside the cell

Match the following key terms with their definitions.

1. _____ steady state
2. _____ volume of distribution
3. _____ plasma protein binding
4. _____ competitive binding
5. _____ blood–brain barrier
6. _____ placental barrier
7. _____ metabolite
8. _____ inducer
9. _____ inhibitor
10. _____ enterohepatic cycling
11. _____ excretion
12. _____ clearance
13. _____ half-life

a. Removal of a drug (or its metabolites) from the body

b. Drugs circulate in the plasma bound to plasma proteins

c. When the administration rate of a drug equals the rate of drug elimination

d. Decreases the isoenzyme and, consequently, decreases the metabolism of isoenzyme's substrates

e. Dose of a drug is distributed into all of the body compartments and tissues that it is physically able to penetrate

f. Reabsorption of a drug or its metabolites from bile in the small intestines

g. Rate of disappearance of the drug molecules from the circulation

h. Time needed for the plasma concentration of a drug to be reduced by 50%

i. End product of a chemical change of one drug into another

j. If two drugs are given and each drug has a high affinity for albumin, they will compete for the available binding sites

k. Thick membranes of the placenta do not create an absolute barrier to the passage of drugs from mother to fetus

l. Increases the amount of the isoenzyme, thus increasing its activity

m. Selective mechanism that opposes the passage of most ions and large molecular compounds from the blood to the brain tissue

CORE DRUG KNOWLEDGE: JUST THE FACTS

Multiple choice

Circle or fill in the option that best answers the question or completes the statement.

1. Which of the following routes of administration provides the greatest control over the actual dose of the drug delivered to the patient?

   a. enteral

   b. sublingual

   c. parenteral

   d. rectal

2. _____ administration is the most common parenteral route.

   a. intravenous

   b. subcutaneous

   c. intramuscular

   d. intradermal

3. Which of the following is most likely to be affected by ischemia?

   a. absorption

   b. distribution

   c. metabolism

   d. excretion

4. Which of the following statements regarding the blood–brain barrier is correct?

   a. All drugs pass freely from the vasculature into the brain.

   b. Drugs must be lipid soluble or have a transport system to be effective in the brain.

   c. Most antimicrobial agents cross the blood–brain barrier without difficulty.

   d. Steroids and sedative-hypnotic agents have difficulty diffusing through the blood–brain barrier.

5. Which of the following organs of the body is the primary site for metabolism?

   a. lungs

   b. kidneys

   c. liver

   d. skin

6. For a drug to be excreted by the kidneys, the drug must be

   a. lipid soluble.

   b. water soluble.

   c. metabolized from adipose stores.

   d. able to diffuse through the blood–brain barrier.

7. The ability of a drug to dissolve and form a solution is called

   a. solubility.

   b. efficacy.

   c. potency.

   d. affinity.

8. The attraction of certain molecules to specific sites is called

   a. solubility.

   b. efficacy.

   c. potency.

   d. affinity.

9. Biotransformation is also known as

   a. absorption.

   b. distribution.

   c. metabolism.

   d. excretion.

Essay

1. In addition to the kidneys, what other routes of excretion are available?

2. Describe the difference between active reabsorption and passive reabsorption.

CORE PATIENT VARIABLES: PATIENTS, PLEASE

Multiple choice

Circle the option that best answers the question or completes the statement.

1. Which of the following patients would most likely receive a drug by the rectal route?

   a. Mrs. Langly, age 63, with a history of diverticulitis

   b. Robin Short, age 9, with nausea and vomiting

   c. Mr. Taunt, age 36, with peptic ulcer disease

   d. Charlie Galt, age 11, with irritable bowel syndrome

2. Susan Wiles takes metoclopramide (Reglan), a drug that stimulates the upper GI system. Which of the following pharmacokinetics would be affected?

   a. absorption

   b. distribution

   c. metabolism

   d. excretion

3. Mrs. King has both liver and kidney disease. She takes several enteral medications. You would expect the duration of action of these medications to

   a. increase.

   b. decrease.

   c. be absent.

   d. stay the same.

4. Melissa Reyes, age 4, has been diagnosed with juvenile rheumatoid arthritis. Her age and body composition may affect which of the following?

   a. absorption

   b. distribution

   c. metabolism

   d. excretion

5. Mr. Palmer takes Drug A, which is highly protein bound. Today, he began to take Drug B, which is 90% protein bound. What is most likely to occur?

   a. Drug A becomes less pharmacologically active.

   b. Drug B becomes less pharmacologically active.

   c. Drug A becomes more pharmacologically active.

   d. Drug B becomes more pharmacologically active.

NURSING MANAGEMENT: EVERY GOOD NURSE SHOULD . . .

Multiple choice

Circle the option that best answers the question or completes the statement.

1. Before initiating a patient on oral drug therapy, the nurse should assess for

   a. dysphagia.

   b. circulatory impairment.

   c. skin integrity.

   d. visual acuity.

2. Mr. Johnson has chronic renal failure. He is receiving medication that is renally excreted. The nurse should expect that he will need

   a. a larger dose than normal to achieve the desired effect.

   b. a smaller dose than normal to achieve the desired effect.

   c. more frequent dosing than normal to achieve the desired effect.

   d. no changes in the normal dose to achieve the desired effect.

3. Ms. Harris has liver disease and receives medication that is metabolized in the liver. A toxic effect from this drug is thrombocytopenia. Based on this information, a nursing diagnosis appropriate for Ms. Harris is

   a. ineffective individual coping related to liver disease.

   b. risk for injury related to potentially high drug serum levels.

   c. anxiety related to adverse effects of medication.

   d. risk for altered skin integrity related to poor liver function.

4. Ilga Sorenson's blood work shows a low serum albumin level. She is receiving medication that is normally 95% protein bound. The nurse should monitor Ms. Sorenson for signs of

   a. hyperalbuminemia.

   b. drug toxicity.

   c. hypokalemia.

   d. CNS depression.

5. Gordon Stemmers has been taking a drug (Drug A) that is highly metabolized by the cytochrome P-450 system. He has been on this medication for 6 months. At this time, he is hospitalized and started on a second medication (Drug B) that is an inducer of cytochrome P-450. The nurse should monitor Mr. Stemmers for

   a. increased therapeutic effects of Drug A.

   b. increased adverse effects of Drug B.

   c. decreased therapeutic effects of Drug A.

   d. decreased therapeutic effects of Drug B.

CASE STUDY

Miss Foster is 70 years old. She has peripheral vascular disease and a history of surgical removal of part of her stomach and small intestine. She has been started on medication to treat her peripheral vascular disease.

1. What aspects of pharmacokinetics may be altered because of her pathologies?

2. What effect will her pathologies have on the dosage of drugs she receives?

3. What factors must the nurse monitor to evaluate Miss Foster's reaction to her prescribed medications?

CRITICAL THINKING CHALLENGE

Georgia Rowland is started on a heparin drip solution for a deep venous thrombosis. The half-life of heparin is 1.5 h. The physician writes these orders:

Heparin drip solution 1,000 units per minute.
Check clotting time (aPTT) every 4 hours until patient's clotting time is two times the normal.
Titrate the heparin drip by increasing it 500 units per hour until aPTT is two times the normal.

Four hours after the heparin infusion is started, the aPTT is one and one-half times the normal. The nurse increases the infusion rate by 500 units per hour. Eight hours after the heparin infusion is started, the aPTT is two and one-half times the normal.

Use the principles of pharmacokinetics to determine what contributed to the excessively high aPTT 8 hours after beginning the infusion.

CHAPTER 5

Pharmacodynamics

TOP TEN THINGS TO KNOW ABOUT PHARMACODYNAMICS

1. Pharmacodynamics are the effects of the drug on the body.
2. Pharmacodynamic processes include uptake, movement, binding, and interactions of pharmacologically active molecules with their site(s) of action.
3. There are three main characteristics of drugs: (1) Drugs do not create a response in the body; they modify the body's response. (2) Drugs exert multiple effects on the body rather than a single effect. (3) Drug action occurs due to an interaction of the drug with a molecule or structure in the body.
4. Most drugs produce their effects from drug-receptor interactions (agonist/antagonist effects), drug-enzyme interactions, or nonspecific drug interactions.
5. Receptors are areas on a cell wall that, when activated by a particular chemical, will cause the cell to respond in a certain, preprogrammed way. Drugs are designed to fit certain receptors. If the drug activates the response when it is on the receptor, it is said to be an *agonist* or *stimulant* of the receptor. If the drug blocks another chemical from activating the receptor, the drug is called an *antagonist* or *blocker* of the receptor.
6. The potency of a drug refers to how many particles of a drug (measured in milligrams or grams) are needed to produce a desired effect. Efficacy is the innate ability of the drug to produce a desired effect. Two drugs may have the same efficacy but different potencies. Usually the potency of a drug is less important than the efficacy (i.e., it doesn't matter if it requires a 10-mg pill or a 20-mg pill as long as it is effective in achieving the therapeutic effect).
7. A loading dose is one that is larger than the standard dose. It is given at the beginning of drug therapy to quickly raise the blood level of the drug into therapeutic range. It is used when the desired therapeutic response is required more quickly than can be achieved with the standard dose.
8. A maintenance dose is the dose that continues to keep the drug in the desired therapeutic range. It is used after a loading dose. For many drugs, patients receive the maintenance dose at both the start of therapy and throughout therapy.
9. The therapeutic index relates to the drug's margin of safety (ratio of effective dose to lethal dose). The closer the therapeutic index is to 1 the more dangerous the drug is and the more closely the patient must be monitored.
10. Tolerance to a drug's effect means that a larger dose is needed to bring about the same response.

KEY TERMS

True/false

Mark true or false for each of the following statements. If the statement is false, replace the underlined words with the correct words to make a correct statement.

1. _____ <u>Pharmacodynamics</u> is the effect of what the drug actually does to the body.

2. _____ An <u>enzyme</u> is a specialized area on the cell wall or within the cellular cytoplasm.

3. _____ An <u>antagonist</u> is a drug that has the ability to initiate the desired therapeutic effect by binding to a receptor.

4. _____ An <u>agonist</u> is a drug that has affinity for a receptor, but does not achieve a response.

5. _____ <u>Mixed agonists</u> compete with agonist molecules for the same receptor.

6. _____ <u>Noncompetitive antagonists</u> irreversibly bind to a number of receptors, thus decreasing the availability for other molecules to bind and create an action.

7. _____ A <u>competitive agonist</u> has both <u>agonist</u> and antagonist effects at the receptor site.

8. _____ The tendency of a drug to attach to a specific receptor site is called <u>efficacy.</u>

9. _____ The power of a drug to produce a therapeutic response is known as <u>affinity.</u>

10. _____ The term <u>potency</u> means the drug's ability to initiate a biologic activity at its maximum therapeutic ability.

11. _____ An increased rate or dose of a drug to achieve faster steady state is called a <u>maintenance dose.</u>

12. _____ The amount of drug needed to sustain a therapeutic effect is called the <u>loading dose.</u>

13. _____ When a fixed dose of a drug no longer produces a therapeutic effect, <u>tolerance</u> has developed.

CORE DRUG KNOWLEDGE: JUST THE FACTS

Multiple choice

Circle the option that best answers the question or completes the statement.

1. The theory/theories that explain the ability of a drug to exert an effect at a particular receptor or subtype is called
   a. nonspecific drug interaction.
   b. drug–enzyme interaction.
   c. drug–receptor interaction.
   d. all of the above.

2. Which of the following is NOT a common characteristic of drugs?
   a. Drugs do not create responses.
   b. Drugs exert multiple rather than single effects on the body.
   c. Drug action results from a physiochemical interaction between the drug and a molecule or structure in the body.
   d. Drugs developed in the last 5 years have the ability to target a subtype receptor to create a single response.

3. Which phase of drug action includes the absorption, distribution, metabolism and excretion of a drug?
   a. pharmaceutical phase
   b. pharmacokinetic phase
   c. pharmacodynamic phase
   d. all of the above

Essay

Define therapeutic index.

CORE PATIENT VARIABLES: PATIENTS, PLEASE

Multiple choice

Circle the option that best answers the question or completes the statement.

1. Holly S., age 24, has an opiate dependence. She has received nalbuphine (Nubain), an opioid agonist-antagonist, from her doctor. Which of the following may occur when Holly takes this drug?
   a. She may experience increased euphoric effects.
   b. She may experience withdrawal symptoms.
   c. She will not develop tolerance to this drug.
   d. She will have increased sedative effects.

2. Mr. L. has renal and liver dysfunction. Which of the following interactions by the nurse is most appropriate for Mr. L.?
   a. Monitor frequently and carefully for signs of adverse effects or toxicity
   b. Refuse to administer any medications that are metabolized solely by the liver
   c. Decrease the dose of medication by one third should signs of toxicity occur
   d. Decrease the dose, but increase the frequency of drug administration

NURSING MANAGEMENT: EVERY GOOD NURSE SHOULD . . .

Multiple choice

Circle the option that best answers the question or completes the statement.

1. Your patient is asking you about over-the-counter analgesics (pain relievers). She says, "The commercials say this one is more potent. Is the most potent drug the best drug?" You should respond:
   a. Yes, you always want to take the drug that is most potent.
   b. Yes, a more potent drug has a more rapid effect.
   c. No, a more potent drug is dangerous.
   d. No, you want to take a drug that is more effective, not necessarily more potent.

2. Your patient has liver disease and is receiving a drug that is highly metabolized by the liver. To achieve the usual pharmacodynamic response of the drug, you would expect the drug's dose to be
   a. greater than a "standard" dose.
   b. smaller than a "standard" dose.
   c. the same as a "standard" dose.
   d. the same as a "standard" dose, but given more frequently.

3. Your patient has been on a narcotic analgesic for chronic pain from cancer. The dose he has been receiving is no longer bringing about the same pain relief as it once did. The patient asks you why the medicine doesn't work anymore. In your patient teaching, you should explain to him about
   a. tolerance.
   b. potency.
   c. receptor agonists.
   d. efficacy.

4. If your patient is exhibiting tolerance to a drug's desired effects, you, as the nurse, should
   a. increase the dose per written order or protocol.
   b. decrease the dose per written order or protocol.
   c. give the same dose more frequently.
   d. give the same dose less frequently.

CASE STUDY

Ann Faraday has atrial fibrillation and an increased ventricular rate (150 to 160 beats per minute). She is to be started on digoxin (a drug that slows the heart rate). Digoxin has a very long half-life of about 30 to 40 hours. The onset of action is 30 to 120 minutes if given orally and 5 to 30 minutes if given by IV. Ann's orders are as follows:

Digoxin 0.375 mg IV now
Digoxin 0.188 mg IV 4 hours from now and repeat again in another 4 hours
Digoxin 0.25 mg PO every day, starting tomorrow morning

1. Explain why IV doses were chosen to be given today but oral doses tomorrow.

2. Explain why the combined IV dose today (all three doses) is larger (more milligrams) than the oral dose ordered for tomorrow.

CRITICAL THINKING CHALLENGE

Digoxin is a drug with a narrow therapeutic index.
What are the risks to Ann Faraday while she is
receiving the loading dose of digoxin? What actions of
the nurse are important now?

CHAPTER 6

Adverse Effects and Drug Interactions

TOP TEN THINGS TO KNOW ABOUT ADVERSE EFFECTS AND DRUG INTERACTIONS

1. An adverse effect of drug therapy is any nontherapeutic response to the drug therapy; its consequences may be minor or significant.
2. A drug interaction is the action of one drug on a second drug or other element creating increased or decreased therapeutic effect of either or both drugs, a new effect, or an increase in the incidence of an adverse effect.
3. Allergic reactions are altered physiologic reactions to a drug because a prior exposure to the drug stimulated the immune system to develop antibodies. Anaphylaxis is the most serious allergic reaction.
4. Drugs accumulate in the body whenever the dosage exceeds the amount the body can eliminate through metabolism and excretion.
5. Drug accumulation that causes damage to a tissue or organ is called drug toxicity.
6. Common drug toxicities are neurotoxicity, hepatotoxicity, immunotoxicity, cardiotoxicity, nephrotoxicity, and ototoxicity.
7. Drug interactions may be due to gastrointestinal (GI) absorption, enzyme induction, renal excretion, radiopharmaceutical use, and pharmacodynamic effects.
8. Pharmacodynamic interactions of drugs may produce additive effects (similar to $1 + 1 = 2$), synergistic effects (similar to $1 + 1 = 3$), potentiation effects (similar to $0 + 1 = 2$), and antagonistic effects (similar to $1 + 1 = 0$).
9. The core patient variables may predispose a patient to adverse effects and drug interactions.
10. Collecting a thorough drug history prior to the start of new drug therapy will help minimize the occurrence of adverse effects and drug interactions.

KEY TERMS

Anagrams

Using the following definitions, unscramble each of the following sets of letters to form a word. Write your response in the spaces provided.

1. When one drug and a second drug or element (e.g., food) have an effect on each other

   A C T E I N N R T O I

   ☐☐☐☐☐☐☐☐☐☐☐

2. An effect other than the desired effect

   E S E V D A R

   ☐☐☐☐☐☐☐

3. An effect that is uncomfortable or undesirable, but not significant

   D E I S

   ☐☐☐☐

4. An effect to an organ or system that is serious or potentially life threatening

   X T O C I I Y T

   ☐☐☐☐☐☐☐☐

5. The most serious type of allergic reaction

   H N A A P A X Y L S I

   ☐☐☐☐☐☐☐☐☐☐☐

6. An unusual, abnormal, or peculiar response to a drug

   Y C D I S I C A O T R I N

   ☐☐☐☐☐☐☐☐☐☐☐☐☐

7. The process of binding with the object drug

   L A N H C T E I O

   ☐☐☐☐☐☐☐☐☐

8. An interacting effect in which 1 + 1 = 2

   D D I V I T A E

   ☐☐☐☐☐☐☐☐☐

9. An interacting effect in which 1 + 1 = 3

   G E I T S N I C R Y S

   ☐☐☐☐☐☐☐☐☐☐☐

10. An interacting effect in which 1 + 1 = 0

    S I I G N A A N C T O T

    ☐☐☐☐☐☐☐☐☐☐☐☐

11. The effect if only one of the two interacting drug is increased

    N O A N P E T O I T I T

    ☐☐☐☐☐☐☐☐☐☐☐☐

12. A compound used in both diagnosis and treatment

    M A T L A D P R A O I R A H U E C I C

    ☐☐☐☐☐
    ☐☐☐☐☐☐☐☐☐☐☐☐

13. Injury to the nervous system related to drug therapy

    T N O E X U I R C O I T Y

    ☐☐☐☐☐☐☐☐☐☐☐☐☐

14. Injury to the immune system related to drug therapy

    M T I O X M I C U I N T O Y

    ☐☐☐☐☐☐☐☐☐☐☐☐☐☐

15. Injury to the liver related to drug therapy

    E H T O P X A I C T O T I Y

    ☐☐☐☐☐☐☐☐☐☐☐☐☐☐

16. Injury to the kidneys related to drug therapy

    C R T Y E O P O N X H I I T

    ☐☐☐☐☐☐☐☐☐☐☐☐☐☐

17. Injury to the 8th cranial nerve related to drug therapy

    T C O I O I T X T Y O

    ☐☐☐☐☐☐☐☐☐☐☐

18. Injury to the heart related to drug therapy

    R T C Y I T D C O I A O I X

    ☐☐☐☐☐☐☐☐☐☐☐☐☐☐

CORE DRUG KNOWLEDGE: JUST THE FACTS

1. Drug A and Drug B, given in combination, increase the incidence of thrombocytopenia. This is an example of _____.

2. List the common signs and symptoms of an allergic reaction.

3. List the most common classes of drugs that may cause an allergic reaction.

4. Identify the classic symptoms of anaphylaxis.

5. Identify potential signs and symptoms of neurotoxicity.

6. Identify potential signs and symptoms of hepatotoxicity.

7. Identify potential signs and symptoms of ototoxicity.

8. List five potential interactions involving GI absorption.

9. Write an example of a beneficial additive drug–drug interaction.

10. What is the difference between potentiation and synergism?

11. You have just hung an IV piggyback of phenytoin (Dilantin) using the primary line of D5W. Ten minutes later, you return and note that the tubing has a cloudy precipitant. What do you suspect has occurred?

CORE PATIENT VARIABLES: PATIENTS, PLEASE

Multiple choice

Circle the option that best answers the question or completes the statement.

1. Mrs. Kite is allergic to several antibiotic agents. She has been diagnosed with acute bilateral pneumonia and prescribed an antimicrobial agent that she has never taken before. Which of the following interactions would you do?

    a. Place an emesis basin next to the bed in easy reach of Mrs. Kite.

    b. Obtain an order for calamine lotion in case of rash.

    c. Monitor Mrs. Kite's vital signs every 4 hours.

    d. Have epinephrine available for quick access.

2. Jeremy Jones, age 45, is given chloral hydrate for his insomnia. Two hours later, as you are doing your routine rounds, you find Mr. Jones sitting in bed, anxious and hypervigilant. This is an example of a(an)

    a. adverse effect.

    b. allergic reaction.

    c. idiosyncratic response.

    d. drug toxicity.

3. Mr. Kenny was admitted to your unit with a diagnosis of acute cellulitis of the right foot 4 days ago. He is receiving IV penicillin G but has had only a mild improvement of his symptoms. After reviewing Mr Kenny's health status, you note that he has a seizure disorder and is taking phenobarbital (Luminal) TID. You would expect his antimicrobial dosage may need to be

    a. increased.

    b. decreased.

    c. discontinued.

    d. left alone.

4. Mrs. Smith is taking verapamil (Calan) and cimetidine (Tagamet). She should be monitored for

    a. idiosyncratic drug interactions.

    b. efficacy of therapy.

    c. toxicity.

    d. antagonistic effects.

5. Audrey Thompson is receiving penicillin VK potassium and probenecid (Benemid) for a tooth abscess. Why would the dentist give these two drugs in combination?

    a. Probenecid and penicillin VK, in combination, have a synergistic effect.

    b. Probenecid interacts with the kidneys and prevents renal excretion of penicillin VK, thus prolonging its duration.

    c. Probenecid and penicillin VK have a drug–drug interaction that binds them together, resulting in an antagonistic effect.

    d. Penicillin VK is destroyed in the acidic environment of the stomach. Probenecid inhibits its destruction.

6. Which of the following drugs does smoking cigarettes NOT diminish?

    a. benzodiazepines

    b. antibiotics

    c. narcotic analgesics

    d. anticoagulants

7. Mr. Quincy Harris is an alcoholic. What process of pharmacokinetics may be affected by his disease?

    a. absorption

    b. distribution

    c. metabolism

    d. excretion

8. Mary Dodge, age 86, takes nitroglycerin (NTG) for her chest pain. Because Mary has arthritis, she places the NTG in a larger pill container for easier access. Mary has noticed that she does not have a burning sensation under her tongue when she takes the NTG and it is less effective. This is an example of a (an)

    a. health status interaction.

    b. life span and gender interaction.

    c. environment interaction.

    d. cultural interaction.

NURSING MANAGEMENT: EVERY GOOD NURSE SHOULD . . .

Multiple choice

Circle the option that best answers the question or completes the statement.

1. When a patient is receiving drug therapy that has the known adverse effect of causing nephrotoxicity, the nurse should monitor the patient's
   a. ALT and AST levels.
   b. intake and output levels.
   c. balance when standing.
   d. cognitive level.

2. Mr. Roberts has liver disease. He is receiving a drug that is metabolized by the liver. The nurse needs to *most* carefully monitor this patient for signs of
   a. therapeutic effects.
   b. allergic effects.
   c. adverse effects.
   d. idiosyncratic effects.

3. Mrs. George has hypertension and receives both a diuretic and a beta blocker drug as drug therapy for this condition. They are both prescribed to be taken twice a day. The nurse knows that these two drugs
   a. should never be given at the same time.
   b. should only be given 1 hour apart.
   c. may be given at the same time.
   d. may have antagonistic effects.

4. A patient, before being discharged from a hospital on a new drug therapy, should receive education about
   a. possible adverse effects of the drug therapy.
   b. how to cope with possible adverse effects.
   c. foods that may interact with the drug therapy.
   d. all of the above.

5. In assessing the patient's core patient variables, you learn that the patient is 75 years old and is receiving drug therapy for asthma. The nurse recognizes that this patient is likely to have an altered response to drug therapy and should closely monitor the patient for
   a. increased adverse effects.
   b. decreased therapeutic effects.
   c. decreased pharmacodynamics.
   d. increased allergic response.

CASE STUDY

Amy Lohman has rheumatoid arthritis and hypertension. She is receiving aspirin and furosemide, a loop diuretic, as drug therapies for these conditions. Describe the patient education you, the nurse, would provide to minimize the serious adverse effects from these therapies. (Hint: Need help? See Chapters 25 and 31.)

CRITICAL THINKING CHALLENGE

Amy remains on aspirin and furosemide for 6 months, at which time she returns to the clinic for follow-up. She complains that the aspirin is upsetting her stomach. She states her stomach feels too acidic and burns.

1. What aspects of core patient variables should the nurse assess at this time?

2. What strategies might the nurse suggest to minimize the adverse effect of aspirin?

UNIT III

Core Patient Variables

CHAPTER 7

Life Span: Children

TOP TEN THINGS TO KNOW ABOUT
LIFE SPAN: CHILDREN

1. Children are different from adults in many ways, and safe, appropriate drug therapy must reflect these differences.
2. A child's age, growth, and maturation affect the core drug knowledge of drug therapy.
3. Pediatric drug dosages must be accurate to reduce risk of adverse effects and prevent overdosage.
4. Two nurses should always check drug dosage calculations to prevent overdosage from math errors.
5. The child's stage of growth and development must be considered when assessing core patient variables and the interaction of core drug knowledge and core patient variables.
6. Choice of appropriate route and/or site of drug administration will vary by the child's age and size, and the drug therapy.
7. Special techniques may be needed when administering drug therapy to minimize traumatic effects to the child (e.g., use of EMLA cream to numb an area before an injection, use of Popsicle or ice chips to numb taste buds before unpleasant oral drugs, not mixing drug therapy into infant formula).
8. The parent is an important source of information about the child, source of comfort for the child, and partner in the care of the child requiring drug therapy.
9. Education about drug therapy should be provided to the patient, at a developmentally appropriate level, and to the family.
10. Health education aimed at promoting health and preventing illness and injury will prevent the need for many types of drug therapy, thus reducing the risk of adverse effects from drug therapy.

KEY TERMS

Matching

Match the following key terms with their definitions.

1. _____ body surface area

2. _____ play therapy

3. _____ kernicterus

4. _____ pediatric patient

5. _____ nomogram

a. Measuring device such as a chart or graph

b. Under age 16 and under 50 kg

c. External surface of the body expressed in square meters

d. Effective technique to prepare a child for drug therapy

e. Life-threatening condition resulting from an accumulation of bilirubin

CORE DRUG KNOWLEDGE: JUST THE FACTS

1. In the pediatric patient, what physiologic differences affect core drug knowledge?

2. In pharmacotherapeutics for a pediatric patient, what is the major difference between a child and an adult?

3. What is the standard formula for calculating body surface area (BSA)?

4. For the absorption of drugs, at what age will a child's pH equal an adult's pH of the stomach?

5. How is distribution of drugs different in children compared to adults?

6. List initial education for parents of children receiving drug therapy.

Matching

Match the following developmental levels with strategies for drug administration.

1. _____ have parent in room during administration

2. _____ allow to choose which medication to take first

3. _____ use ventrogluteal site for intramuscular (IM) injections

4. _____ place liquid medication in buccal fold of mouth

5. _____ remember privacy and patient control when administering medication

a. Infant

b. Toddler

c. Preschool

d. School age

e. Adolescent

CORE PATIENT VARIABLES: PATIENTS, PLEASE

Multiple choice

Circle the option that best answers the question or completes the statement.

1. Melissa Counts, age 14 months, is to receive penicillin V. Melissa weighs 11.9 kg. The order reads administer 50 mg/kg in 4 divided doses. Using the body weight method, how much penicillin V will you give Melissa in one dose?

   a. 595 mg

   b. 150 mg

   c. 100 mg

   d. 1 g

2. Mrs. Lewis has three children: 2 boys ages 5 and 8, and a daughter age 9 months. She is going to treat all her children for a heat rash with hydrocortisone cream. What instructions would you give?

   a. Apply the same amount of hydrocortisone for all the children.

   b. Use less of the hydrocortisone for the boys.

   c. Use less of the hydrocortisone for her daughter.

   d. Do not use cream for any of the children.

3. Use of water-soluble drugs in children may result in an increased risk for

   a. toxicity.

   b. rapid elimination of drugs.

   c. subtherapeutic levels of drugs.

   d. enhanced pharmacodynamics.

4. Michael Ray, age 6, is hospitalized for seizures. He has been prescribed phenobarbital (Luminal). In comparison to an adult, you would expect the frequency of drug administration to be

   a. increased.

   b. decreased.

   c. no difference.

5. Emily Ann White, age 4, is hospitalized with appendicitis. Which of the following should be done to reduce Emily's anxiety about drug therapy?

   a. Use parents to restrain child in order to give an injection.

   b. Explain the pharmacodynamics of each drug and the rationale for therapy.

   c. Tell Emily she will be a "good girl" if she allows you to administer her medications.

   d. Demonstrate drug therapy using a rag doll.

NURSING MANAGEMENT: EVERY GOOD NURSE SHOULD . . .

Multiple choice

Circle the option that best answers the question or completes the statement.

1. You are preparing to give vitamin K to a newborn infant. It is given intramuscularly. You should

   a. use the ventrogluteal site.

   b. select a needle longer than 5/8 inch.

   c. use a fine-gauge needle.

   d. avoid aspirating before injecting.

2. You are going to administer multivitamin drops to an infant. You should

   a. use a calibrated measuring cup to measure the dose.

   b. mix the measured dose into infant's formula.

   c. explain the rationale for the drug to gain cooperation.

   d. gently squeeze the mouth open and place the drops in the buccal pouch.

3. Brenda, an active 2-year-old girl, is receiving an intravenous (IV) infusion of heparin, an anticoagulant. To minimize adverse effects from the drug therapy, the nurse should

   a. run the IV solution by way of gravity.

   b. activate the lock feature on the pump's infusion rate.

   c. place enough volume in the microdrip calibrated chamber to last 4 hours.

   d. check the IV infusion site once a shift.

4. Which of the following statements made by the nurse would most likely gain cooperation from the preschooler during drug administration?

   a. "Would you like to take the liquid medicine or the pill first?"

   b. "Take your medicine pills or I will have to give you a shot."

   c. "Do you want to take your medicine for me?"

   d. "Only bad children don't want to take their medicine."

5. When administering drug therapy to an adolescent, the nurse should

   a. direct all questions to the parents.

   b. provide stickers and prizes for taking drug therapy.

   c. offer explanations and teaching directly to the patient.

   d. maintain tight control over all aspects of drug administration.

CASE STUDY

Jordan is 11 years old and is to be discharged from the hospital on oral theophylline, a bronchodilator, for his asthma. Theophylline is similar to caffeine in chemical structure. Cigarette and marijuana smoking will decrease the effectiveness of theophylline.

1. To maximize therapeutic effect of the theophylline therapy, the nurse should assess what aspect of Jordan's core patient variables?

2. To minimize adverse effects of the theophylline therapy, the nurse should assess what aspect of Jordan's core patient variables?

CRITICAL THINKING CHALLENGE

Marshall is a newborn infant who was born by cesarean section. The mother receives morphine for pain after the cesarean section and is breast-feeding Marshall. What are the major risks to Marshall and why?

CHAPTER 8

Life Span: Pregnant or Breast-Feeding Women

TOP TEN THINGS TO KNOW ABOUT LIFE SPAN: PREGNANT OR BREAST-FEEDING WOMEN

1. Drug therapy may be indicated for pregnant or breast-feeding women to manage preexisting conditions or those that are newly developed.
2. The normal physiologic changes that occur during pregnancy may alter absorption, distribution, and elimination of drug therapy.
3. Drug therapy may produce therapeutic effects in the pregnant woman but adverse effects, including teratogenic effects, in the fetus or infant.
4. Potential fetal risks must be compared to maternal benefits when drug therapy is required.
5. The minimum therapeutic dose should be used for as short a time period as possible to minimize adverse effects in the fetus. If possible, drug therapy should be delayed until after the first trimester, especially if the drug has teratogenic effects.
6. FDA pregnancy categories for safety of use of drugs in pregnancy include five divisions—A through D and X. Categories A and B most likely carry no or little risk to the fetus, C and D most likely carry some risk to the fetus, and X is contraindicated in pregnancy.
7. Health status of the woman may indicate the need for drug therapy due to chronic conditions (e.g., epilepsy, diabetes) or conditions that develop secondary to pregnancy (e.g., hyperemesis gravidarum, preeclampsia and eclampsia, and thrombus formation).
8. Adverse effects of drug therapy may be misinterpreted as discomforts commonly associated with pregnancy.
9. Many drugs also cross into breast milk, although the dosage that reaches the infant is very small. Nursing mothers need to be educated about possible risks to the infant.
10. Nonpharmacologic alternatives to drug therapy should be used if possible.

KEY TERMS

Fill in the blanks

Read each statement carefully and, using the chapter's key terms, write your answer in the space provided.

1. Hypertension, edema and proteinuria are classic signs of _____.

2. The first trimester is the critical period of _____.

3. _____ is another term for pernicious vomiting of pregnancy.

4. Severe growth retardation, mental retardation, and microencephaly are signs of _____.

5. The secretion of breast milk is called _____.

6. Preeclampsia may lead to _____, characterized by cerebral edema and convulsions.

7. _____ is caused by secretion of placental hormones.

8. A _____ effect causes physical defects in the developing fetus.

9. Craniofacial abnormalities, limb defects, and growth deficiency are signs of _____.

CORE DRUG KNOWLEDGE: JUST THE FACTS

Multiple choice

Circle the option that best answers the question or completes the statement.

1. Which of the following pharmacokinetics is UNAFFECTED by pregnancy?
   a. absorption
   b. distribution
   c. metabolism
   d. excretion

2. During pregnancy, the pharmacodynamics of a drug must be carefully considered due to changes in the
   a. integumentary system.
   b. cardiovascular system.
   c. renal system.
   d. gastrointestinal (GI) system.

3. Distribution of drugs is altered during pregnancy due to
   a. hemodynamic changes.
   b. increased hormone secretion.
   c. decreased renal function.
   d. increased attachment to plasma proteins.

4. Which of the following types of drugs most readily enter fetal circulation?
   a. highly protein-bound drugs
   b. ionized drugs
   c. lipophilic drugs
   d. large molecular drugs

5. What percentage of a drug taken by the mother passes into the fetus during breast-feeding?
   a. 5%
   b. 10%
   c. 2%
   d. 20%

Matching

Match the following pregnancy categories with the correct statement.

1. _____ Category A
2. _____ Category B
3. _____ Category C
4. _____ Category D
5. _____ Category X

a. Used in life-threatening situations.
b. Drugs are given if benefit justifies the risk to the fetus.
c. Human studies fail to demonstrate a risk to the fetus.
d. Fetal risk outweighs potential benefit.
e. Animal studies do not indicate a risk, but no human studies confirm lack of risk to fetus.

CORE DRUG KNOWLEDGE: PATIENTS, PLEASE

Multiple choice

Circle the option that best answers the question or completes the statement.

1. Which of the following patients is most likely to develop teratogenic effects of drug therapy?
   a. Mona S., with first-trimester intrauterine pregnancy
   b. Donna T., with second-trimester intrauterine pregnancy
   c. Mary Y., with third-trimester intrauterine pregnancy
   d. They all have equal potential for teratogenic effects.

2. Mary Reilly has preeclampsia. Which of the following classes of drugs would you expect to be prescribed?
   a. alpha-adrenergic blocking agent
   b. angiotensin-converting enzyme inhibitor
   c. benzodiazepine
   d. direct vasodilator

3. Barbara Bauman comes to the clinic with suspected pregnancy. She is concerned because she has multiple preexisting health problems and takes Lasix (furosemide), Tenormin (atenolol), insulin, and Dilantin (phenytoin). Her urine test is positive. Which of her current medications should be changed immediately?
   a. Lasix (furosemide)
   b. Tenormin (atenolol)
   c. insulin
   d. Dilantin (phenytoin)

4. Gina Miglin has recurrent headaches. She states she has tried nonpharmacologic interventions but is unable to obtain relief. Which of the following analgesics would be best during Gina's pregnancy?
   a. acetaminophen
   b. aspirin
   c. ibuprofen
   d. codeine

NURSING MANAGEMENT: EVERY GOOD NURSE SHOULD . . .

Multiple choice

Circle the option that best answers the question or completes the statement.

1. Your patient is still in the first trimester and has developed gestational diabetes. The physician has ordered her to be started on NPH insulin daily. The nurse should
   a. contact the physician and request that oral hypoglycemics be ordered instead of NPH insulin.
   b. verify that blood glucose levels remain at levels above normal (> 120) while on insulin.
   c. teach the patient that she will need to take insulin even after delivery.
   d. teach the patient that the insulin dose may need to be changed throughout the pregnancy.

2. Your pregnant patient has developed hyperemesis gravidarum. She is now in week 12 of the pregnancy. Antiemetic therapy of meclizine (a piperazine) has been prescribed. She expresses concern to you about taking a drug while pregnant. In your patient education, you should include
   a. the risks of taking medicine while in the second trimester.
   b. that piperazines have not been found to be teratogenic.
   c. the importance of taking this drug as frequently as possible.
   d. the benefits of hyperemesis gravidarum.

3. Your patient is 22 weeks pregnant and has developed a cardiac arrhythmia. Drug therapy has been prescribed. Prior to administering the first dose of the prescribed drug, the nurse should
   a. verify the FDA pregnancy category of the drug.
   b. determine if the patient is allergic to the prescribed drug.
   c. verify if the dose is appropriate for the patient's age, weight, and health status.
   d. do all of the above.

4. Your patient is in the second trimester of pregnancy and has developed some swelling of the ankles, feet, and hands. To minimize adverse effects, the nurse should first
   a. consult with the physician about ordering a mild diuretic.
   b. recommend a diet high in sodium.
   c. suggest the patient consume large amounts of coffee with caffeine for diuresis.
   d. instruct the patient to rest with her feet elevated several times a day.

5. You are working in a postpartum care unit. Your patient is a 17-year-old new mother who is an admitted abuser of heroin and cocaine. She tells you she is considering breast-feeding, because it would be cheaper than bottle feeding. However, she is not sure that she wants to breast-feed. In your teaching with this patient, it is most important that you include information on
   a. the value to the infant from commercial formulas.
   b. heroin and cocaine being contraindicated with breast-feeding due to the effects on the infant.
   c. the importance of postpartum rest for the mother.
   d. positions for effective breast-feeding.

CASE STUDY

In the middle of January, Anita Rodrigez is 26 weeks' pregnant and presents to the emergency room having difficulty breathing. She is having bronchial constriction from bronchitis that developed after a bad cold. The physician orders aminophylline, a bronchodilator, administered by IV drip infusion. Aminophylline is a pregnancy Category C drug.

1. What assessments should be made while Anita receives IV aminophylline?

2. When should the aminophylline be discontinued?

CRITICAL THINKING CHALLENGE

After delivery of a full-term, healthy baby, Anita develops continuing problems with bronchitis and is started on ipratropium (Atrovent) inhaler. This is a pregnancy Category B drug and is an anticholinergic bronchodilator. Anita is breast-feeding.

1. Should you be concerned that Anita is breast-feeding while on this drug therapy?

2. Are there other core patient variables that should be assessed with this patient?

CHAPTER 9

Life Span: Older Adults

TOP TEN THINGS TO KNOW ABOUT LIFE SPAN: OLDER ADULTS

1. Older adults share common age-related changes and risk factors that alter drug administration, dosage, and expected response to drug therapy.
2. Aging alters all of the pharmacokinetic processes, placing older adults at higher risk for adverse drug effects.
3. It is likely that disease processes alter the older adult's absorption patterns more than changes related to aging.
4. Decreased body mass, reduced levels of plasma albumin, and a less effective blood–brain barrier alter the older adult's distribution of drugs.
5. Hepatic metabolism is slowed and renal efficiency is decreased due to aging changes. Serum creatinine levels will remain normal even though kidney function is impaired.
6. Pharmacodynamics of drug therapy may be decreased in the older adult due to changes in the receptor systems.
7. Many of the signs and symptoms of health problems in older adults are due to the normal age-related decline in organ or system function. These symptoms of health problems often mimic the adverse effects of drug therapy.
8. Polypharmacy in older adults increases the risk for drug interactions and adverse effects.
9. Lifestyle of the older adult may affect the pharmacokinetics of drug therapy. Likewise, the adverse effects of drug therapy may affect the quality of life for the older adult.
10. To increase adherence, simplify the therapeutic regimen, give memory aids (if necessary), give written instructions, determine financial access to drug therapies, assess cultural barriers, and titrate the dose upward slowly to minimize adverse effects.

KEY TERMS

True/false

Mark true or false for each of the following statements. If the statement is false, replace the underlined words with the correct words to make a correct statement.

1. _____ The margin between desired therapeutic effects and adverse consequences of drug therapy is called the <u>therapeutic index.</u>

2. _____ <u>Nonadherence</u> is the inability to follow a recommended drug therapy regimen.

3. _____ A patient who responds with hyperactivity to a drug that normally causes sedation has an adverse effect known as <u>idiosyncratic</u> excitement.

4. _____ A geriatric patient is also known as an <u>older adult.</u>

5. _____ The practice of one patient taking several drugs simultaneously is called <u>drug abuse.</u>

6. _____ An <u>older adult</u> is any patient over the age of 65 with a debilitating medical problem.

PHYSIOLOGY AND PATHOPHYSIOLOGY: THE BODY HUMAN

Essay

1. Summarize the normal physiologic changes with age that affect absorption in an elderly patient receiving drug therapy.

2. Summarize the normal physiologic changes with age that affect distribution in an elderly patient receiving drug therapy.

3. Summarize the normal physiologic changes with age that affect metabolism in an elderly patient receiving drug therapy.

4. Summarize the normal physiologic changes with age that affect excretion in an elderly patient receiving drug therapy.

CORE DRUG KNOWLEDGE: JUST THE FACTS

Multiple choice

Circle the option that best answers the question or completes the statement.

1. Because of age-related changes of the body, absorption of drugs in the elderly
   a. delays the onset of action.
   b. enhances the intensity of the peak response.
   c. is minimal compared with a younger adult.
   d. increases the risk for toxicity.

2. In the elderly patient, the dosage of fat-soluble drugs may need to be _____ in order to avoid toxicity.
   a. increased
   b. decreased
   c. neither of the above

3. Which of the following may occur as a result of physiologic changes in the elderly patient's metabolism?
   a. increased half-life
   b. decreased half-life
   c. decreased potential for adverse effects
   d. decreased potential for drug–drug interactions

4. Because of the reduction of creatinine production in the elderly patient, the creatinine clearance test may be normal. This is an indication of
   a. normal renal function.
   b. impaired renal function.
   c. more information concerning renal status is needed to make an assessment.
   d. impaired metabolism.

5. Which of the following is the least likely effect of drug therapy in the elderly?
   a. subtherapeutic drug regimens
   b. overdose or toxicity
   c. increased drug–drug interactions
   d. increased incidence of adverse effects

CORE PATIENT VARIABLES: PATIENTS, PLEASE

Multiple choice

Circle the option that best answers the question or completes the statement.

1. Sara Smith, age 87, has been admitted to your unit with deep vein thrombosis of the left leg. Mrs. Smith is receiving a heparin drip at the standard rate according to the standing protocol of the unit. Because of Mrs. Smith's age, how may her aPTT be affected?

   a. It will not be affected.

   b. It may be 2 to 2½ times the control.

   c. It may be more than 2 to 2½ times the control.

   d. It may be less than the control.

2. Jim Wright has taken ibuprofen for his arthritis for the past 5 years. As Jim advances with age, you would expect the onset of action to be

   a. delayed.

   b. shortened.

   c. the same, despite his age.

3. Mary Gerard, age 89, is taking chloral hydrate, a hypnotic, for her insomnia. Mary has an increased risk for which of the following adverse effects?

   a. sedation

   b. rash

   c. nausea

   d. paradoxical excitement

4. Which of the following questions should be included in an assessment of an elderly patient before initiating drug therapy in an outpatient setting?

   a. "Do you have stairs at your home?"

   b. "Do you have difficulty opening the medication bottle?"

   c. "Do you have difficulty swallowing or chewing?"

   d. All of the above

Essay

Identify strategies that may decrease nonadherence to drug therapy in the elderly.

NURSING MANAGEMENT: EVERY GOOD NURSE SHOULD . . .

Multiple choice

Circle the option that best answers the question or completes the statement.

1. Frank Goodwin is 75 years old. He tells you that he needs to have his food cut finely because he has trouble chewing and swallowing large pieces. The nurse recognizes that this fact has implications for drug therapy in which of the following ways?

   a. Drugs will not be absorbed as easily.

   b. The oral route cannot be used.

   c. Drugs will not be eliminated as easily.

   d. Oral drugs may need to be crushed or in liquid form.

2. Ethel Thomas is an 80-year-old widow who lives alone. To assess potential problems with adherence to a prescribed drug regimen, the nurse should determine

   a. whether Mrs. Thomas visits with friends during the week.

   b. the way Mrs. Thomas usually obtains her prescription and refills.

   c. the amount of fluid Mrs. Thomas drinks in a day.

   d. whether Mrs. Thomas has renal or hepatic disease.

3. Irma Humphreys is 68 years old and is receiving gentamycin for a severe infection. Gentamycin has the adverse effect of causing renal toxicity. The nurse would expect that the ordered dose of gentamycin for Ms. Humphreys to be

   a. larger than the average adult dose.

   b. smaller than the average adult dose.

   c. the same as the average adult dose.

   d. larger than the average adult dose but given less frequently.

4. Ralph Greenbaum is 70 years old and has been started on phenytoin, an anticonvulsant, for a new onset of seizures. When he returns to the clinic for his 3-week checkup after starting the drug, his daughter confides that she thinks her father is getting old. He falls asleep during the daytime frequently now and seems to have difficulty following conversations. The best response for the nurse is

   a. "Yes, it's a shame to get older, isn't it?"

   b. "You need to expect these changes with aging."

   c. "These are signs that he is not getting enough drug therapy."

   d. "These are signs of adverse effects."

5. Gertrude Hanson is 84 years old and had surgery to repair a broken hip. She has been ordered morphine, a narcotic, for pain relief. The order states that she may have 4 to 10 mg every 4 hours as needed. If giving the first dose of pain medication to Ms. Hanson, the nurse should select

   a. 4 mg.

   b. 6 mg.

   c. 8 mg.

   d. 10 mg.

CASE STUDY

Antonio Vibaldi, 68 years old, is admitted to your unit with uncontrolled hypertension. He also has a history of chronic obstructive pulmonary disease (COPD) and congestive heart failure. He was recently in the hospital for exacerbation of his COPD. In your assessment, you ask him about his drug therapies and if he takes them as prescribed. He replies that he is always taking some pill or other. He admits that he might forget sometimes to take some of his doses because there are so many. You write down what he says he takes and compare it to his discharge orders for drug therapy, written at the end of his last hospitalization.

Mr. Vibaldi's List	Discharge Orders for Drug Therapy
"fluid pill" 2 × day	furosemide (Lasix) 40 mg BID
"pressure pill" 2 or 3 × day	captopril (Capoten) 100 mg TID
"heart pill" every day	nicardipine (Cardene) 30 mg BID
potassium 2 × day	potassium (K-Dur 10) one tablet BID
"breathing pill" 2 × day	theophylline (Theo-Dur) 100 mg q 12 hours

1. Determine what times Mr. Vibaldi should be taking drug therapy at home.

2. What can you do to help Mr. Vibaldi remember to take his drug therapy when it is due?

CRITICAL THINKING CHALLENGE

What other issues should you explore with Mr. Vibaldi to determine whether nonadherence with the prescribed drug therapy is contributing to frequent hospitalizations?

CHAPTER 10

Lifestyle: Substance Abuse

TOP TEN THINGS TO KNOW ABOUT SUBSTANCE ABUSE

1. Substance abuse is a problem occurring throughout the life span, and in all socioeconomic, ethnic, and cultural groups.
2. Three components must be present for drug addiction to have occurred: psychological dependence, physical dependence, and tolerance. Physical dependence and tolerance may occur independently without psychological dependence (behavioral changes and cravings). When this happens, addiction has not occurred.
3. Genetic disposition, developmental and environmental influences, personality traits, mood disorders, availability of drugs, cultural attitudes, and socioeconomic factors may all contribute to substance abuse in an individual.
4. Most abused drugs affect the central nervous system (CNS) as stimulants, depressants, or hallucinogens.
5. Alcohol is the most widely abused CNS depressant. Nicotine is the most widely abused CNS stimulant.
6. Prescription drugs may be abused either for their own effects or the combined effect that is similar to that from an illegal drug, to increase the duration or "high" of an illegal drug, or to prevent withdrawal from an illegal drug.
7. Cocaine, a CNS stimulant, increases neurotransmitter (dopamine, norepinephrine, and serotonin) activity, leading to ease of addiction; prolonged, intense craving during withdrawal; and high rates of relapse.
8. Abused substances have significant adverse effects on developing fetuses, infants, and children. Effects from substance abuse may be misinterpreted as signs of aging in the older adult.
9. Substance abuse may create health problems requiring drug therapy, may require drug therapy to prevent or treat withdrawal, or may interact with drug therapy for another physiologic problem.
10. Nurses need to assess patients for substance abuse, act to prevent life-threatening or debilitating effects from a substance or its withdrawal, administer drugs to treat withdrawal or its symptoms, and provide education about the substance, addiction, drug therapy, and rehabilitation.

KEY TERMS

Crossword puzzle

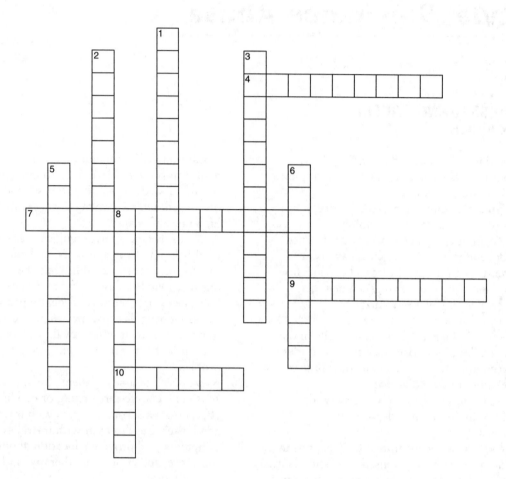

Across

4. Type of abuse involving self-administration of drug substance for nonmedical purposes
7. Type of dependence that results from the influence of drugs on brain chemistry
9. State of having a physical or psychological need for a drug
10. Type of dependence when actual changes in body cells cause the body to "need" a drug for homeostasis

Down

1. Another term for hallucinogens
2. Another term for opioids
3. Another term for CNS stimulants
5. A syndrome caused by sudden cessation of drug ingestion
6. The body develops a natural resistance to a drug's physical or euphoric effects
8. Another term for addiction

PHYSIOLOGY AND PATHOPHYSIOLOGY: THE BODY HUMAN

Matching

Identify the correct physiologic effects during intoxication in the right-hand column with the correct drug in the left-hand column.

1. _____ inhalants
2. _____ amphetamines
3. _____ opiates
4. _____ alcohol

a. Ataxia, nystagmus, slurred speech
b. Motor agitation, pupillary dilation, tachycardia
c. Pinpoint pupils, euphoria, apathy
d. Distorted perceptions, light-headedness, euphoria

Matching

Identify the correct physiologic effects during withdrawal in the right-hand column with the correct drug in the left-hand column.

1. _____ inhalants
2. _____ amphetamines
3. _____ opiates
4. _____ alcohol

a. Myalgia, piloerection, yawning
b. Fatigue, nightmares, depression, increased appetite
c. None, appreciably
d. Nausea, vomiting, tremors, seizures

CORE DRUG KNOWLEDGE: JUST THE FACTS

True/false

Mark true or false for each of the following statements.

1. _____ Psychological dependence occurs because the patient has a preexisting mental health disorder.

2. _____ Chronic stress is an environmental factor that may influence a person's substance abuse.

3. _____ There is a clearly identified addictive personality.

4. _____ Drug abuse occurs most frequently in lower socioeconomic groups.

5. _____ Individuals with a personality disorder may use drugs initially to become socially acceptable.

6. _____ The three main categories of abusable drugs are CNS stimulants, CNS depressants, and hallucinogens.

7. _____ Designer drugs are difficult to develop but are very popular due to their safety profile.

8. _____ Common adverse effects to anabolic-androgenic steroids include sex hormone imbalances, permanent sterility, and hepatic cancer.

9. _____ Alcoholism may induce hypertension.

10. _____ Cocaine has a very long half-life and can sustain a "high" for 12 hours.

CORE PATIENT VARIABLES: PATIENTS, PLEASE

Multiple choice

Circle the option that best answers the question or completes the statement.

1. In the alcoholic patient, liver damage may attributed to the
   a. mechanism by which alcohol is metabolized.
   b. increased absorption of alcohol.
   c. interference of nerve impulses.
   d. utilization of the P450 enzyme system.

2. Mr. Leer is admitted to the hospital for acute anemia. He has been diagnosed with esophageal varices. Knowing this information, for which of the following would you monitor?
   a. symptoms of opiate withdrawal
   b. symptoms of alcohol withdrawal
   c. symptoms of cocaine withdrawal
   d. symptoms of hallucinogen withdrawal

3. In the patient who abuses cocaine, which of the following vital signs would you expect to see?
   a. BP 100/90; P 88; R 22
   b. BP 122/88; P 60; R 16
   c. BP 150/100; P 100; R 22
   d. BP 140/90; P 82; R 12

4. In the patient who abuses heroin, which of the following would you expect to see?

   a. frequent bronchitis

   b. abscess formation

   c. pruritus

   d. renal failure

5. You notice that your patient has very labile moods—one minute he is quiet and the next he is yelling loudly. Which of the following is most likely the substance that he has used?

   a. heroin

   b. cocaine

   c. glue

   d. LSD

6. Leslie Town, age 16, comes to the school nurse with a complaint of decreased mental and physical abilities. With your knowledge of substance abuse, which of the following drugs may be responsible for these symptoms?

   a. PCP

   b. cannabis

   c. inhalants

   d. CNS stimulants

7. Jenna Raymond, age 32, has just delivered a baby with microencephaly and craniofacial abnormalities. What drug of abuse may be responsible?

   a. alcohol

   b. heroin

   c. cocaine

   d. marijuana

8. Alissa Wande is concerned about her baby who was delivered yesterday and confides to you that she had been unable to stop her use of heroin during pregnancy. You would expect to find which of the following behaviors in Alissa's baby?

   a. microencephaly

   b. cleft palate

   c. tremor, respiratory distress, or hyperirritability

   d. weak cry, lethargy, decreased muscle tone

NURSING MANAGEMENT: EVERY GOOD NURSE SHOULD . . .

Multiple choice

Circle the option that best answers the question or completes the statement.

1. When the nurse is performing a complete drug history and health assessment, the patient should be questioned about use of which of the following substances?

   a. cigarettes

   b. alcohol

   c. street or recreational drugs

   d. all of the above

2. Your patient is a recovered alcoholic and has been started on disulfiram (Antabuse). Which of the following should be included in the teaching about this drug?

   a. Take this drug whenever you have a desire to drink.

   b. This drug has no adverse effects at all.

   c. If you drink any alcohol while you are on this drug, you will feel ill.

   d. Moderate drinking is allowed while on this drug.

3. Seventeen-year-old Jena is brought to a busy emergency room by some friends. Jena is screaming, covering her ears and eyes with her hands, and appears to be having hallucinations. Her friends say Jena used some LSD at a party. An initial nursing action for Jena should include

   a. placing her on a stretcher in the middle of the emergency room to observe her.

   b. administering phenothiazines if ordered.

   c. staying with her and speaking calmly and soothingly.

   d. referring her to an inpatient psychiatric facility.

4. As a middle-school nurse, you are called to a classroom to help Lee, a 12-year-old boy who is short of breath after sniffing White-Out correction fluid. An item of priority that you should bring with you from the health suite is

   a. a syringe of epinephrine.

   b. portable oxygen.

   c. an emesis basin.

   d. a defibrillator.

CASE STUDY

Jordan Taylor is a 35-year-old successful lawyer admitted to your unit on a Monday morning after surgery, with general anesthesia, to repair a torn rotator cuff. He received the narcotic morphine in the recovery room for complaints of pain. It is now 2 hours after his surgery and 1 hour after his morphine injection. He is somewhat more difficult to arouse than most patients after surgery. His history states that he drinks "socially on weekends." When asked to clarify this, his wife states that he usually has one or two drinks before dinner, a bottle of wine with dinner, one or two drinks after dinner, and then usually another drink or two later in the evening on Friday, Saturday, and Sunday nights. What factors might be contributing to the difficulty in arousing this patient after surgery?

CRITICAL THINKING CHALLENGE

On Tuesday, Jordan Taylor is somewhat irritable and anxious. You note a very fine tremor in his hands when he offers you his arm to take his pulse. His pulse is 90 beats per minute.

1. What assessment might you make from this data? What actions should you take?

2. Assessment of a patient's physical condition may be influenced by bias or stereotypical thinking of the health care provider. What factors may lead a nurse or other health care providers to overlook alcohol abuse and possible withdrawal in Jordan Taylor?

CHAPTER 11

Lifestye, Diet, and Habits: Nutritional Considerations

TOP TEN THINGS TO KNOW ABOUT LIFESTYLE, DIET, AND HABITS: NUTRITIONAL CONSIDERATIONS

1. The use of dietary supplements, herbs, and other botanicals, to promote wellness is considered a complimentary therapy.
2. A well-balanced diet may prevent chronic illness, indirectly decreasing the need for drug therapy.
3. Nutritional deficiencies may occur due to chronic illness, or as an adverse effect from drug therapy.
4. Nutritional supplements may be prescribed by the physician or may be taken independently by the patient without the physician's knowledge.
5. Some foods, beverages, and dietary supplements can affect the pharmacokinetics of a drug.
6. Some foods, beverages, and dietary supplements can alter the effectiveness of some drugs or produce an adverse effect.
7. Adverse drug–nutrient interactions are most likely to occur with medications taken for chronic conditions, if several medications are taken, or if nutritional status is poor or deteriorating.
8. The nurse should encourage the patient to inform all health care providers about all dietary supplements (including herbs) used.
9. The nurse should teach the patient and family about any potential interactions of their drug therapy with herbal preparations.
10. The nurse should always ask if the patient uses dietary supplements because patients may not realize the importance of mentioning this use.

KEY TERMS

Essay

1. Differentiate between the terms *alternative therapy* and *complementary therapy*.

2. Define *herbal* and *botanical* preparations.

3. Identify the major mineral cations.

4. Define *phytomedicines*.

5. Identify the most important trace elements.

6. Define the word *vitamin*.

CORE DRUG KNOWLEDGE: JUST THE FACTS

Multiple choice

Circle the option that best answers the question or completes the statement.

1. Which of the following should encompass approximately 50% to 60% of a healthy diet per day?
   a. protein
   b. fats
   c. carbohydrates
   d. dietary fiber

2. Which of the following major mineral cations plays a role in the transmission of nerve impulses; contraction of cardiac, skeletal, and smooth muscle; acid–base balance; and the maintenance of normal renal function?
   a. calcium
   b. magnesium
   c. potassium
   d. sodium

3. Which of the following types of vitamins requires frequent consumption to maintain adequate body levels?
   a. water-soluble vitamins
   b. lipid-soluble vitamins
   c. both of the above

4. Which of the following trace elements is essential to form red blood cells?
   a. chromium
   b. copper
   c. iron
   d. selenium

CORE PATIENT VARIABLES: PATIENTS, PLEASE

Multiple choice

Circle the option that best answers the question or completes the statement.

1. Your patient has taken an overdose of a vitamin/mineral supplement. You assess central nervous system changes, hypotension, and an abnormal electrocardiogram. Which of the following minerals is most likely to cause these symptoms?
   a. calcium
   b. magnesium
   c. potassium
   d. sodium

2. Your patient has hypertension and is prescribed furosemide (Lasix) 40 mg QD. In this patient, it is important to monitor
   a. trace elements
   b. protein.
   c. dietary fiber.
   d. major mineral cations.

3. Your patient is admitted to the medical-surgical unit for management of a deep vein thrombosis (DVT). During your admission assessment, you find that the patient is homeless and consumes alcohol on a daily basis. In order for therapy to be successful, which of the following nutritional states should be further evaluated?
   a. vitamin consumption
   b. use of dietary fiber
   c. protein intake
   d. carbohydrate intake

NURSING MANAGEMENT: EVERY GOOD NURSE SHOULD...

Multiple choice

Circle the option that best answers the question or completes the statement.

1. Which of the following should be included in a drug history?
   a. Do you use any vitamin or nutritional supplements?
   b. Do you use any herbal supplements?
   c. Who recommended that you use this supplement?
   d. all of the above
   e. none of the above

2. Bob James is 94 years old. He has a history of hypertension, cardiac arrhythmias, hyperlipidemia, and an enlarged prostate. He takes five different prescription drugs for these problems. The nurse should assess Mr. James for

   a. nutritional deficiencies.

   b. typical daily diet.

   c. the time of day prescribed medications are taken.

   d. all of the above.

   e. none of the above.

3. Doris Wright has chronic obstructive pulmonary disease (COPD) and takes prednisone as an immune suppressant as part of her drug therapy. At her clinic visit for follow-up, she tells you, the nurse, that because the weather is getting colder, she is going to start taking echinacea to keep her from getting pneumonia. Your best response is

   a. "That's a good idea. You should also take vitamin C."

   b. "Echinacea will be beneficial to your COPD and will make you feel better."

   c. "Echinacea may counteract the immunosuppressant effect of the prednisone, and you might actually have more respiratory problems."

   d. "Be sure you buy your echinacea from a reputable source."

CASE STUDY

Jerome Morrison is malnourished due to a history of alcohol abuse. He is hospitalized with a deep vein thrombosis in his left leg. He is prescribed intravenous heparin as treatment for his thrombosis. Heparin is an anticoagulant and is highly protein bound. After 24 hours on heparin, his coagulation time is much longer (i.e., he bleeds longer) than would be expected from the heparin infusion.

1. What might be contributing to his altered coagulation time?

2. How would you confirm your assessment?

CRITICAL THINKING CHALLENGE

Jerome Morrison is discharged to home on warfarin, an oral anticoagulant, which is also highly protein bound. His coagulation times at discharge are lengthened appropriately to be therapeutic from the warfarin. When he returns to the clinic for follow-up in 4 weeks, he tells you that he has been trying to improve his health by cutting down on his drinking and using herbs. He tells you that he has been drinking chamomile tea several times a day as a substitute for some of the alcohol that he drank, also because it soothes his stomach pain from a gastric ulcer that flared up from alcohol use. He also tells you that he is taking garlic tablets to bring down his cholesterol levels. His lab results show that his coagulation time is excessively elevated.

What might be contributing to his altered lab values?

CHAPTER 12

Environment: Influences on Drug Therapy

TOP TEN THINGS TO KNOW ABOUT ENVIRONMENT: INFLUENCES ON DRUG THERAPY

1. The environment in which drug therapy occurs may vary. It may be the acute care hospital, acute rehabilitation unit, transitional care unit, outpatient center, long-term care facility, or the patient's home.

2. Each type of environment has limitations as to which drugs may be given, or which route of drug administration may be used. These limitations are related to the need for close monitoring of the patient, specialized equipment, life-saving equipment and drugs, and specialized personnel.

3. Environmental conditions, such as pollutants, heat, light, moisture, and temperature, can alter a drug's pharmacokinetics or a drug's pharmacodynamics.

4. Environmental factors may make the patient more susceptible to adverse effects from drug therapy (such as sunlight and photosensitivity).

5. Environmental factors of the home may place the patient at increased risk of injury if a drug adverse effect does occur (such as falls from dizziness when there are no stair railings).

6. The patient's occupation, part of their personal environment, may place them at added risks for some adverse effects from drug therapy.

7. The patient's environment may have contributed to their disease process, causing their need for drug therapy.

8. The nurse should assess the environment in which drug therapy will occur for potential influences on pharmacotherapy.

9. The nurse can create an environment that will maximize the therapeutic effect and minimize the adverse effects of some drug therapies.

10. Providing patient and family education about the potential interactions of drug therapy and the patient environment is an important nursing action.

KEY TERMS

Matching

Match the following key terms with their definitions.

1. _____ carcinogens

2. _____ environment

3. _____ industrial chemicals

4. _____ pollutants

5. _____ hepatic drug metabolizing enzymes

a. Physical setting in which a drug is given

b. A contaminated or noxious substance

c. Agent that may induce cancer in the human body

d. Used to biotransform drugs

e. Compounds that may influence pharmacologic properties of drugs

CORE DRUG KNOWLEDGE: JUST THE FACTS

1. Identify the major environmental settings in which drugs are administered.

2. In addition to the setting, what other concepts are important to the safe administration of medications?

3. Identify possible environmental influences on drug stability.

4. List environmental chemicals that may induce hepatic drug-metabolizing enzymes in susceptible patients.

5. What two environmental factors are most frequently associated with the development of cancer?

CORE PATIENT VARIABLES: PATIENTS, PLEASE

Multiple choice

Circle the option that best answers the question or completes the statement.

1. Mr. B. is a heavy cigarette smoker who has bronchitis and takes a bronchodilator. Because cigarette smoke is an active inducer of hepatic enzymes, Mr. B. should be monitored for

   a. exacerbation of symptoms.

   b. drug toxicity.

   c. both of the above.

   d. neither of the above.

2. Mrs. L. was involved in an auto accident and sustained a fractured collarbone. She has been prescribed a narcotic analgesic for pain. What environmental teaching should Mrs. L. receive?

   a. Change positions slowly to avoid orthostatic hypotension.

   b. Limit alcohol consumption to two drinks per day.

   c. Avoid hazardous tasks until the effects of the drug are assessed.

   d. Keep the drug in a light-resistant bottle.

3. Mrs. K. had total knee replacement surgery today. At 10 PM, the nurse administers a sedative-hypnotic agent to help Mrs. K. fall asleep. When doing rounds at 1 AM, you find Mrs. K. still awake. Which of the following would be appropriate at this time?

   a. Use this time to teach the patient leg-strengthening exercises.

   b. Close the patient's door to decrease external stimuli.

   c. Contact the physician for additional orders.

   d. Offer the patient a snack.

4. Mr. V. is being discharged from the hospital later today. What is the primary role of the nurse regarding drug therapy at this time?

   a. consultation with a pharmacy

   b. patient advocacy with the billing department

   c. patient education

   d. referral

NURSING MANAGEMENT: EVERY GOOD NURSE SHOULD . . .

Multiple choice

Circle the option that best answers the question or completes the statement.

1. It is May and your patient is being sent home with a prescription for tetracycline, an antibiotic that is known to cause photosensitivity reactions. In your assessment of the patient's learning needs related to environmental concerns, you should ask the patient

    a. if they can refrigerate the drug at home.

    b. where they normally store medications.

    c. how many people live in the house.

    d. how much time they spend outdoors.

2. Your patient has been started on a vasodilator for hypertension. The patient tells you he can't wait to get home and take a long soak in the hot tub. The best response to this patient is

    a. "Soaking in hot tubs will be helpful with this drug therapy. Do it every day."

    b. "Excessive heat from hot tubs will cause additional vasodilation and may cause problems for you. Please avoid using them now."

    c. "Hot tubs will not have any effect on this drug therapy. Use them if you wish."

    d. "I'm envious. Can I make a home visit and use the hot tub with you?"

3. Your patient works in the insulation industry and handles polychlorinated biphenyls as part of his job activities. When doing patient education about his prescribed drug therapy (a drug that is highly metabolized in the liver), you would want to emphasize

    a. that he should contact the physician if he has any of the adverse effects that you describe.

    b. that he cannot go to work while he is on this drug therapy.

    c. that adverse effects are less likely to occur in him than in other patients.

    d. none of the above are appropriate to emphasize.

CASE STUDY

Janice Jordan, 20 years old, is 42 weeks' pregnant with her first child, and the obstetrician wishes to start her on oxytocin to induce her labor. The obstetrician has a nurse that works with her in the office, and he can stay with Janice.

Would the obstetrician start the oxytocin infusion in her office?

CRITICAL THINKING CHALLENGE

You are a nurse working on a general medical surgical unit. The admitting department calls and tells you that your unit will be receiving Janice Jordan as a patient because the labor and delivery suite is currently full, and there are no beds on the postpartum floor. The admitting department says Janice can be transferred to the delivery room at the time of delivery, but will return to your floor after giving birth.

What would you do in this situation?

CHAPTER 13

Culture: Considerations in Drug Therapy

TOP TEN THINGS TO KNOW ABOUT CULTURE: CONSIDERATIONS IN DRUG THERAPY

1. The five major cultures in the United States are white American, black American, Asian/Pacific Islander American, Hispanic American, and Native American Indian.

2. Although members of a culture will share certain beliefs and practices, individual variation will still occur. Each patient needs to be considered an individual.

3. Many cultural groups in the United States have beliefs that reflect both their original ethnic culture and the dominant culture of the United States.

4. White Americans (e.g., European Americans) have a linear sense of time, are future oriented, are predominantly Christian, share bioscientific views of disease and health management, and rely primarily on traditional Western medical practices.

5. Black Americans (e.g., African Americans) have a circular view of time, are present oriented, are more relaxed about time than European Americans, tend to be spiritual, are predominantly Christian, may use folk medicine, and, in general, respond to some drugs differently than white Americans.

6. Asian/Pacific Islander Americans (e.g., Chinese Americans) have a concept of time related to the natural cycles of birth, life, and death; believe time is to be integrated into life; may or may not value punctuality; may or may not belong to a formal religion; believe that the body and spirit must be maintained through harmony with nature and yin and yang; have health care practices that include traditional Chinese medicine and Western medicine; and may be affected differently than white Americans by herbal medicines and Western drugs.

7. Hispanic Americans (e.g., Mexican Americans) are more present than future oriented. They may or may not value punctuality, may believe that life is ruled by chance or luck or may be deeply religious, are primarily Catholic, believe that disease occurs when there is an imbalance between opposing life forces (hot, cold, wet, dry), and may metabolize some drugs differently from other cultural groups.

8. Native American Indians (e.g., Navaho Indians) are present oriented; attach little value to planning for the future; view time as nonimportant; are spiritual but do not practice formalized religions; believe good health depends on maintaining a balance among the elements of the body, mind (or spirit), and environment; and use herbal remedies to treat disease. Younger Native American Indians are more accepting of Western medical practices than older Native American Indians. Responses to drug therapy may vary by tribe, but this has not been studied adequately.

9. The nurse should consider the patient's cultural background, religious preferences, personal practices, and ethnic background when providing nursing management in drug therapy.

10. Patient education related to drug therapy needs to consider cultural variations to be effective.

KEY TERMS

Anagrams

Use the following anagrams to define the key terms in the chapter:

1. Specific physical, biological, and psychosocial variations in ethnic and racial groups

   O I B L R A T L U C U L O Y G C O E

   □□□□□□□□□□□□ □□□□□□

2. Assumption that all members of a particular ethnic or cultural group will have the same response

   G S Y R P E E T I T O N

   □□□□□□□□□□□□

3. Shared customs and traditions of a group

   T E U C U L R   □□□□□□□

4. The inability to accept the culture of others

   N E S T E T C R H O M I N

   □□□□□□□□□□□□□

5. Group that shares common cultural heritage linked by race, nationality, and/or language

   I I Y C T T N H E

   □□□□□□□□□

6. Awareness of one's own values and beliefs without letting it have undue influence on those of other backgrounds

   T L C L U U A R E C N E T E M P C O

   □□□□□□□□ □□□□□□□□

7. Inability to recognize differences between groups or individuals within a group

   T L U C R U L A D N I L N S B S E

   □□□□□□□□ □□□□□□□□□

CORE DRUG KNOWLEDGE: JUST THE FACTS

Multiple choice

Circle the option that best answers the question or completes the statement.

1. Despite cultural differences, the goal of the nurse is to
   a. provide appropriate nursing care.
   b. "normalize" patient behaviors.
   c. integrate all cultural customs into drug therapy.
   d. be aware of each culture's acceptable practices.

2. A nurse with cultural competence
   a. is able to provide care for an individual from a particular culture.
   b. understands the difference between cultural beliefs that coincide with Western medicine and those that do not.
   c. accepts and respects cultural and ethnic differences.
   d. is able to assist patients of different cultures to attain acculturation.

3. Biocultural ecology
   a. integrates commonalities among different cultures to the care of a patient.
   b. examines physical, biologic, and psychological variations in ethnic or racial groups.
   c. predicts common behavior patterns of a particular culture or ethnic group.
   d. categorizes cultures according to geographic locality.

4. Which of the following is NOT an identified worldview health belief?
   a. biomedical
   b. magico-religious
   c. holistic
   d. isolated

5. The philosophy of yin and yang is prevalent in which of the following groups?
   a. Chinese Americans
   b. African Americans
   c. European Americans
   d. Native Americans

6. In planning drug therapy for a Chinese-American patient, which of the following drugs does NOT need consideration for a lower dose of medication?

    a. amitriptyline (Elavil), a tricyclic antidepressant

    b. diazepam (Valium), a benzodiazepine

    c. penicillin (Pen V K), an antibiotic

    d. propranolol (Inderal), a beta-adrenergic antagonist

Essay

List the 12 domains of Purnell's Model for Cultural Competence.

CORE DRUG KNOWLEDGE: PATIENTS, PLEASE

Multiple Choice

Circle the option that best answers the question or completes the statement.

1. Which of the following influences may be associated with a white American patient?

    a. They tend to place little emphasis of the importance of obtaining medications.

    b. Primarily, they have a magico-religious view of disease and health management.

    c. They are usually future oriented and have a strong work ethic.

    d. They tend to be late for appointments or meetings.

2. Which of the following influences may be associated with an African-American patient?

    a. They have a linear view of time.

    b. Most families have a nuclear family with the father being the head of the family.

    c. They are very religious and are accepting of medical treatment unless it is viewed contrary to their religious beliefs.

    d. The drug response and adverse effects profile of drug therapy is the same as white Americans.

3. Which of the following influences may be associated with a Chinese-American patient?

    a. Time is of little value and can be mastered for their benefit.

    b. Harmony with nature is essential for spiritual and physical well-being.

    c. They rarely use herbal medications.

    d. They metabolize drugs the same as other cultures.

4. Which of the following influences may be associated with a Hispanic-American patient?

    a. They tend to seek medical attention rather than use self-care practices.

    b. They believe an imbalance of hot, cold, wet, and dry may induce disease.

    c. The families tend to be matriarchal.

    d. They metabolize drugs the same as other cultures.

5. Which of the following influences may be associated with a Native American patient?

    a. They believe good health depends on maintaining a balance among the elements of the body, mind or spirit, and environment.

    b. The families tend to be patriarchal.

    c. They tend to be very punctual for appointments.

    d. Frequency of disease is the same for all tribal groups.

6. To be an effective culturally competent nurse, it is important to

    a. develop cultural blindness when giving patient care.

    b. integrate all cultural practices into patient care.

    c. remember that cultural patterns are helpful, but a wide range of responses is possible within each group.

    d. assist the patient to acculturation.

NURSING MANAGEMENT: EVERY GOOD NURSE SHOULD . . .

Multiple choice

Circle the option that best answers the question or completes the statement.

1. Why is it important to assess the patient's cultural background before beginning drug therapy?

    a. Patients may respond to drug therapy differently depending on their cultural and racial background.

    b. Patients' attitudes about the value of drug therapy may contribute to their adherence to the drug therapy regimen.

    c. Patients may use folk or herbal remedies based on their cultural background that may interact with the prescribed drug therapy.

    d. all of the above

2. You have worked with Carlos Miguel, a Mexican American, for several days. You have come to learn that he is generally present time oriented. He has been hospitalized for osteomyelitis, a severe infection of the bone. He has received antibiotic therapy intravenously and is to be discharged on oral antibiotics for 6 more weeks. In your teaching about the drug, you most likely want to emphasize that

a. failure to take all of the prescription will cause him to be hospitalized again.

b. evenly spaced daily doses will help to keep the drug levels up to treat the infection.

c. skipping doses may eventually cause permanent damage to the bone.

d. all of the above.

3. Mr. Lee, an elderly Chinese American, was hospitalized for a heart attack. He tells you he did not come to the hospital sooner because he thought he only had indigestion. He had treated himself for the "indigestion" with ginseng. To minimize adverse effects from currently prescribed drug therapy, the most effective response of the nurse would be to

a. tease Mr. Lee about his use of herbs.

b. tell Mr. Lee that he is foolish to use herbs.

c. emphasize that Western medicine is much safer than using herbs.

d. ask Mr. Lee to describe other herbs that he uses regularly.

4. Robert Blackfeather is a Native American Indian, Albert Clark is a white American, and Thomas Chan is an Asian/ Pacific Islander American. They are all to be started on isoniazid for tuberculosis. The nurse would expect that the ordered interval between doses might be longer for which of these patients?

a. Albert Clark

b. Robert Blackfeather

c. Thomas Chan

d. The interval would be the same for all three.

CASE STUDY

Susan Sam is a Chinese American. Joshua Marshall is an African American. Both patients are started on the same sulfonamide antibiotic for a urinary tract infection. At a 3-week follow-up appointment, Susan is found to be anemic, but Joshua has normal hemoglobin levels.

What factors might be contributing to this different response to the identical drug therapy?

CRITICAL THINKING CHALLENGE

What other core patient variables might have placed Susan at increased risk for developing anemia?

UNIT IV

Peripheral Nervous System Drugs

CHAPTER 14

Drugs Affecting Adrenergic Function

TOP TEN THINGS TO KNOW ABOUT DRUGS AFFECTING ADRENERGIC FUNCTION

1. Adrenergic receptors are divided into alpha-1, alpha-2, beta-1, and beta-2. Drugs that stimulate the receptors are called agonists; those that block are antagonists or blockers. Most drugs stimulate or block more than one receptor at a time, although some drugs are relatively selective in their stimulation or blockade.

2. Stimulation of alpha-1 receptors causes vasoconstriction, increased peripheral resistance, increased blood pressure, pupil dilation (mydriasis), and increased closure of the internal sphincter of the bladder. Blocking causes the opposite effects.

3. Stimulation of alpha-2 receptors decreases release of norepinephrine, reducing sympathetic outflow from the brain, and produces vasodilation. Blocking causes the opposite effects.

4. Stimulation of beta-1 receptors causes tachycardia, increased myocardial contractility, increased rate of conduction, and the release of renin. Blocking causes the opposite effects.

5. Stimulation of beta-2 receptors causes bronchodilation, vasodilation, slightly decreased peripheral resistance, increased muscle and liver glycolysis, increased release of glucagon, and relaxation of uterine smooth muscle. Blocking causes the opposite effects.

6. Epinephrine stimulates all alpha and beta receptors (nonselective adrenergic agonist). It has many uses, primarily to treat cardiopulmonary arrest, ventricular fibrillation, anaphylactic shock, and asthma. Adverse effects are related to stimulation of all receptors. CNS and cardiac adverse effects are most common and may be most serious.

7. Phenylephrine is an alpha-1 stimulant and a potent vasoconstrictor used to treat vascular failure, hypotension, and related shock. It is also used as a nasal decongestant and to cause pupil dilation (mydriasis). Avoid IV extravasation.

8. Prazosin, an alpha-1 blocker, is used to treat hypertension. The first dose may cause syncope.

9. Isoproterenol is a nonselective beta-2 stimulant used to treat emergency conditions (various types of shock, hypoperfusion, congestive heart failure) and chronic respiratory conditions (asthma, bronchitis, emphysema). Adverse effects are primarily related to cardiac stimulation.

10. Propranolol is a nonspecific beta blocker used primarily for cardiovascular disorders. Adverse effects are due to cardiac and respiratory effects. It should be discontinued slowly to prevent rebound tachycardia leading to angina, and possibly myocardial infarction.

KEY TERMS

Fill in the blanks

Read each statement carefully and, using the chapter's key terms, write your answer in the space provided.

1. The _____ is comprised of the brain and spinal cord.

2. The _____ consists of all neurons that are found outside the brain and spinal cord.

3. The _____ has been identified as an involuntary system responsible for the control of smooth muscle (e.g., bronchi, blood vessels, and gastrointestinal [GI] tract), cardiac muscle, and exocrine glands (e.g., gastric, sweat, and salivary glands).

4. Adrenergic _____ are drugs that mimic the action of the sympathetic nervous system.

5. Drugs that block the receptor's ability to respond to a stimulus are known as _____.

6. Norepinephrine and epinephrine are the major _____ in the sympathetic nervous system.

7. _____ initially involves the synthesis of neurotransmitters in the nerve terminal with subsequent storage of the neurotransmitter awaiting an action potential that allows the neurotransmitter to be released.

8. Agents that stimulate multiple adrenergic subtype receptors are called _____.

9. A _____ targets a specific subtype receptor.

10. The autonomic nervous system is divided into the _____ and the _____.

11. Another term for the sympathetic nervous system is the _____.

PHYSIOLOGY AND PATHOPHYSIOLOGY: THE BODY HUMAN

Matching

Match the following body response with the correct adrenoceptor.

1. _____ tachycardia

2. _____ vasoconstriction

3. _____ relaxed uterine smooth muscle

4. _____ mydriasis

5. _____ inhibition of norepinephrine

6. _____ increased myocardial contractility

7. _____ increased blood pressure

8. _____ increased peripheral resistance

9. _____ bronchodilation

10. _____ increased glucagon release

a. Alpha-1
b. Alpha-2
c. Beta-1
d. Beta-2

CORE DRUG KNOWLEDGE: JUST THE FACTS

Multiple choice

Circle the option that best answers the question or completes the statement.

1. Phenylephrine works by stimulating which of the following receptors?
   a. alpha-1
   b. alpha-2
   c. beta-1
   d. beta-2
   e. all of the above

2. Which of the following is NOT a contraindication or precaution to phenylephrine therapy?
   a. hypertension
   b. pregnancy
   c. hypothyroidism
   d. narrow-angle glaucoma

3. Epinephrine works by stimulating which of the following receptors?
   a. alpha-1
   b. alpha-2
   c. beta-1
   d. beta-2
   e. all of the above

4. Which body systems are most affected by epinephrine therapy?
   a. renal and respiratory
   b. respiratory and cardiovascular
   c. cardiovascular and integumentary
   d. CNS and respiratory

5. Which of the following drugs is classified as a nonselective beta agonist?

    a. phenylephrine

    b. albuterol

    c. dobutamine

    d. isoproterenol

6. Isoproterenol should not be used for patients with which of the following disorders?

    a. asthma

    b. digitalis toxicity

    c. cardiopulmonary failure

    d. glaucoma

7. Prazosin (Minipress), an alpha antagonist, is used in the treatment of

    a. COPD.

    b. hypertension.

    c. hypotension.

    d. urinary frequency.

8. Which of the following drugs is similar to prazosin?

    a. doxazosin (Cardura)

    b. yohimbine

    c. propranolol (Inderal)

    d. isoproterenol (Isuprel)

9. Which of the following disorders CANNOT be managed by beta-adrenergic antagonists such as propranolol?

    a. tachycardias

    b. essential tremor

    c. bradycardia

    d. migraine headaches

10. Which of the following adverse effects is not associated with propranolol therapy?

    a. hallucination and psychosis

    b. hypoglycemia

    c. hyperthyroidism

    d. weight loss

CORE DRUG KNOWLEDGE: PATIENTS, PLEASE

Multiple choice

Circle the option that best answers the question or completes the statement.

1. Jennifer Taylor has chronic allergies and takes phenylephrine on a daily basis. What potential adverse effects may Jennifer experience?

    a. hypotension

    b. hypoglycemia

    c. hyperglycemia

    d. hypertension

2. Mary Gelrud, age 78, is a patient in the coronary intensive care unit with a diagnosis of cardiogenic shock. What is the goal of epinephrine therapy for Mary?

    a. control arrhythmias

    b. reduce intraocular pressure

    c. treat hypotension

    d. increase circulating glucose

3. Carey Pitts, age 17, has a severe allergy to bees. She has just been stung and needs to self-administer epinephrine. Which of the following routes of administration would be best for Carey in this situation?

    a. inhalation

    b. sublingual

    c. intramuscular

    d. subcutaneous

4. Carey, in the above situation, calls you after she has self-administered epinephrine. She states that she feels like she "will jump out of my skin" and that she can feel her knees shaking. What is the best response to Carey?

    a. "These are expected effects from the dose of epinephrine."

    b. "You should drive to your doctor's office right away."

    c. "You need to call 911 immediately and come to the hospital."

    d. "Take another dose of medication to stop the symptoms."

5. Allen Saylor takes albuterol for his asthma. Craig Little takes isoproterenol for the same condition. Which of these two patients has a higher risk for cardiovascular adverse effects?

    a. Allen

    b. Craig

    c. They have the same risk.

    d. Neither has a risk.

6. Isoproterenol is being given to Monica Lewis, age 76, for cardiogenic shock. The anticipated cardiovascular response of isoproterenol is

    a. increased myocardial contractility and decreased heart rate.

    b. decreased myocardial contractility and increased heart rate.

    c. decreased myocardial contractility and decreased heart rate.

    d. increased myocardial contractility and increased heart rate.

7. Calista Reynolds, age 55, has been prescribed prazosin for her hypertension. What instructions should you give her so she may safely self-administer the first dose?

    a. "It is important for you to void before taking your medication so your bladder will be empty."

    b. "Take your dose with a small amount of food at bedtime, then lie down."

    c. "Take three deep breaths then cough forcefully before you take the medication."

    d. "After you have taken the medication, do not eat for 2 hours."

8. Which of the following patient instructions is inappropriate for the patient on prazosin therapy?

    a. "It is OK to drink beer, but you should stay away from the hard stuff."

    b. "You should have your blood pressure and pulse checked periodically."

    c. "It would be best not to drive or do anything that requires alertness until you see how the medication affects you."

    d. "You should change positions slowly to avoid getting dizzy."

9. Jennifer Alston takes propranolol for her migraine headache. In the past, she has been noncompliant because she prefers narcotic analgesics. Which of the following physical findings would indicate that Jennifer may be noncompliant with her propranolol?

    a. BP 132/88

    b. respirations 20

    c. temperature 98.2

    d. pulse 110

10. Allison Leach has asthma and uses an albuterol inhaler as needed. She has just been diagnosed with migraine headaches. Why would propranolol be an inappropriate drug for Allison's migraine prophylaxis?

    a. It is not inappropriate—she may use it without problems.

    b. It may increase her blood pressure, which may result in increased headaches.

    c. It may induce bronchospasm, which may result in an asthma attack.

    d. It may induce cerebral hypotension and hypoperfusion, thus increasing the intensity of her headache.

NURSING MANAGEMENT: EVERY GOOD NURSE SHOULD . . .

Multiple choice

Circle the option that best answers the question or completes the statement.

1. Thelma Broughton is receiving IV phenylephrine, an alpha-1 agonist, to treat drug-induced hypotension. The drug is infusing into a vein in the antecubital space of the left arm. The IV infusion infiltrates, and the drug extravasates into the tissues. The first action of the nurse should be to

    a. check the blood pressure.

    b. turn off the IV infusion.

    c. lower the left arm below heart level.

    d. place a tourniquet around the left forearm.

2. To treat Thelma Broughton's extravasation, the nurse should use

    a. epinephrine SC.

    b. epinephrine IV.

    c. phentolamine SC.

    d. phentolamine IV.

3. Don Winkler is brought to the emergency room after a severe allergic response to a new prescribed drug therapy. He is having difficulty breathing and is in anaphylactic shock. He receives epinephrine, a mixed adrenergic stimulator, IV. The nurse should monitor him for

 a. hypotension.

 b. electrocardiogram (ECG) changes.

 c. decreased urinary output.

 d. fever.

4. William Jeffries is to be started on isoproterenol, a nonselective beta agonist, for asthma. Before starting drug therapy, the nurse should assess him to determine the presence of

 a. orthopnea.

 b. hypervolemia.

 c. hypothyroidism.

 d. tachycardia.

5. Jessie Faulkner is to start on prazosin, an alpha-1 blocker for treatment of his blood pressure. Patient education regarding this drug therapy should include which of the following?

 a. It is important to come to a standing position quickly after lying flat.

 b. Alcohol may be consumed without concerns.

 c. Avoid driving for about 4 hours after the first dose.

 d. Take the first dose in the morning after a hot shower.

6. Gordon Sheeler is receiving propranolol, a beta blocker, for his angina. However, he has developed depression while on the drug and wishes to stop taking the propranolol. Education for this patient should include that

 a. the depression will stop after he adjusts to taking the propranolol.

 b. the drug should not be abruptly stopped.

 c. depression is not related to beta blocker use.

 d. the dose needs to be increased if he is depressed.

CASE STUDY

Judy Brenner is 14 years old and uses an inhaler of isoproterenol, a beta agonist, when she has severe asthmatic episodes. She complains to you that sometimes the inhaler is effective and other times it is not. What questions might you ask Judy to help determine the cause of her complaints?

CRITICAL THINKING CHALLENGE

As a nursing student, you are preparing to send your patient to the operating room for an inguinal hernia repair. He is expected to be in the operating room and recovery room a total of 2 1/2 hours. He is NPO now, but he should be able to receive oral fluids after he has fully awakened from anesthesia. The patient takes propranolol, a beta blocker, for hypertension. His blood pressure is currently 126/80. He is due a dose of propranolol now but cannot have it because he is NPO. His last dose was last night. Your instructor asks you if you think the patient will suffer adverse effects from skipping this dose.

1. What should you respond?

2. Can you safely withhold this dose?

CHAPTER 15

Drugs Affecting Cholinergic Function

TOP TEN THINGS TO KNOW ABOUT DRUGS AFFECTING CHOLINERGIC FUNCTION

1. The autonomic nervous system (ANS) is made up of the sympathetic and parasympathetic systems.
2. The parasympathetic neurotransmitter is acetylcholine; the receptors are muscarinic or nicotinic.
3. Muscarinic receptors are particularly concentrated in the heart, smooth muscle, and exocrine glands. Nicotinic receptors are found in the central nervous system (CNS), the neuromuscular junction, autonomic ganglia, and the adrenal medulla.
4. Cholinergic stimulants are also known as cholinergic agonists or, simply, cholinergics; cholinergic blockers are known as cholinergic antagonists or anticholinergics.
5. Excess cholinergic effects from cholinergic agonist drugs cause decreased intraocular pressure, mitosis (constriction of pupil), sweating, increased salivation, increased bronchial secretions, bronchial constriction, increased gastrointestinal (GI) tone, diarrhea, decreased blood pressure, bradycardia, and contraction of bladder detrusor muscle.
6. Excess anticholinergic effects from anticholinergic drugs cause increased intraocular pressure, mydriasis (pupils dilate), photophobia, decreased sweating, dry mouth, decreased bronchial secretions, respiratory depression, decreased GI motility, constipation, decreased then increased blood pressure, tachycardia and possibly palpitations, urinary retention, vasodilation, and drowsiness, confusion, and agitation.

7. Pilocarpine is a direct-acting cholinergic used topically to treat simple and acute glaucoma, pre- and postoperative elevated intraocular pressure, and drug-induced mydriasis.
8. Nicotine stimulates the CNS. Its use as a drug is limited to preparations to assist in smoking cessation. Adverse effects are related to its effects on the cardiovascular and central nervous systems.
9. Neostigmine is an indirect-acting cholinergic drug that acts by reversibly inhibiting postsynaptic cholinesterase. Because acetylcholine is not broken down as quickly, it has more opportunity to stimulate cholinergic receptors and create an effect. It is used in the treatment of myasthenia gravis to minimize muscle fatigue. Cholinergic crisis is the most serious adverse effect.
10. Atropine is an anticholinergic drug. It is the antidote for cholinergic poisoning. It is used preoperatively to dry secretions, in acute cardiac emergencies, topically (homatropine) to treat ophthalmic disorders, and to treat motion sickness and diarrhea. Adverse effects are related to loss of acetylcholine stimulation on receptors. The most serious adverse effect is anticholinergic overdose (or poisoning).

KEY TERMS

Matching

Match the following key terms with their definitions.

1. _____ autonomic nervous system

2. _____ cholinergic agonist

3. _____ cholinergic antagonist

4. _____ cholinergic crisis

5. _____ miosis

6. _____ muscarinic receptors

7. _____ nicotinic receptors

8. _____ parasympathetic nervous system

9. _____ sympathetic nervous system

a. Cholinergic receptor with subtypes M_1 through M_5

b. Division of the ANS with acetylcholine as the terminal neurotransmitter

c. Drugs that block the action of acetylcholine

d. Division of the ANS with norepinephrine as the terminal neurotransmitter

e. Caused by cholinergic toxicity and results in medullary paralysis

f. Drugs that mimic the action of acetylcholine

g. Cholinergic receptors found in the CNS, neuromuscular junction, autonomic ganglia, and adrenal medulla

h. Involuntary system controlling smooth muscle, cardiac muscle, and exocrine glands

i. Constriction of the pupil in the eye

PHYSIOLOGY AND PATHOPHYSIOLOGY: THE BODY HUMAN

True/false

Mark true or false for each of the following statements. If the statement is false, replace the underlined word with the word that will make the statement correct.

1. _____ Cholinergic stimulation of the eyes results in <u>dilation</u> of the pupil.

2. _____ The heart beat <u>increases</u> when stimulated by the cholinergic system.

3. _____ Digestion <u>increases</u> with cholinergic stimulation.

4. _____ Cardiovascular effects of cholinergic stimulation include <u>hypertension</u>.

5. _____ In the respiratory system, cholinergic drugs may <u>decrease</u> bronchial secretions.

6. _____ Blocking cholinergic stimulation may induce urinary <u>frequency</u>.

7. _____ <u>Constipation</u> is a potential effect of blocking cholinergic stimulation.

8. _____ To dilate the bronchioles, drugs that <u>mimic</u> the cholinergic nervous system may be used.

9. _____ Nicotinic receptors respond to acetylcholine and have a <u>low</u> affinity for nicotine.

10. _____ <u>Muscarinic</u> receptors are concentrated in the heart, smooth muscle, and exocrine glands.

CORE DRUG KNOWLEDGE: JUST THE FACTS

Multiple choice

Circle the option that best answers the question or completes the statement.

1. Which of the following is NOT a contraindication to the use of pilocarpine?
   a. glaucoma
   b. hypersensitivity
   c. acute iritis
   d. uncontrolled asthma

2. Pilocarpine should be instilled
   a. directly over the pupil.
   b. in the inner canthus of the eye.
   c. at the lateral edge of the eye.
   d. in the conjunctival sac.

3. Nicotine replacement is used primarily
   a. in patients with hypoactive states.
   b. for smoking-cessation programs.
   c. for patients with adrenal insufficiency.
   d. in alcohol recovery programs.

4. Which of the following adverse effects may be induced by nicotine replacement therapy?
   a. constipation
   b. hyperactivity
   c. sedation
   d. headache

5. Some indirect-acting cholinergic agonists are also known as
   a. cholinesterase inhibitors.
   b. cholinesterase agonists.
   c. anticholinergics.
   d. cholinergic blockers.

6. Myasthenia gravis, a neuromuscular disorder, may be treated with
   a. pilocarpine.
   b. neostigmine.
   c. atropine.
   d. nicotine.

7. The antidote for neostigmine overdose is
   a. pilocarpine.
   b. atropine.
   c. nicotine.
   d. oxygen.

8. Pralidoxime (PAM) is used in the treatment of
   a. myasthenia gravis.
   b. urinary hesitancy.
   c. overexposure to irreversible anticholinesterase drugs.
   d. acetaminophen overdose.

9. In the preoperative patient, atropine is used to
   a. diminish bronchial secretions.
   b. prevent dysentery.
   c. treat of muscarinic excess.
   d. decrease cardiac stimulation.

10. Mrs. Kay receives atropine for peptic ulcer disease. Which of the following instructions is MOST important for Mrs. Kay?
    a. "Be sure to monitor your blood sugar."
    b. "Assess how your vision changes before attempting to drive your car."
    c. "Decrease the amount of fluids you normally drink to avoid constipation."
    d. "Let us know if you are having difficulty with urinary frequency."

Essay

1. Identify the principal actions of atropine.

2. List the potential symptoms of a cholinergic crisis.

CORE PATIENT VARIABLES: PATIENTS, PLEASE

Multiple choice

Circle the option that best answers the question or completes the statement.

1. In the patient with _____, pilocarpine should be used with caution.
   a. cancer
   b. AIDS
   c. cardiovascular disease
   d. depression

2. Which of the following patients who smoke would benefit most from nicotine replacement therapy?
   a. John Culver, a 46-year-old male with cardiac arrhythmias
   b. Julie Bright, a 35-year-old female with chronic bronchitis
   c. Astrid Love, a 50-year-old female with angina
   d. Jeremy Tilden, a 67-year-old male with an acute myocardial infarction

3. Which of the following strategies may be ineffective for patients using nicotine replacement therapy?
   a. Encourage participation in stop-smoking programs.
   b. When cravings occur, have just one cigarette to abate the symptoms.
   c. Advise the patient to adhere to the recommended dosage and frequency to minimize craving.
   d. Encourage the patient to avoid exposure to others who smoke.

4. Marley Janes has myasthenia gravis and is in crisis. To differentiate between a myasthenic crisis and a cholinergic crisis, she is given edrophonium (Tensilon). What effect from edrophonium would indicate Marley is in cholinergic crisis?
   a. increase in muscle weakness
   b. decrease in muscle weakness
   c. sedation
   d. cough

5. Which of the following may predispose a patient to psychogenic effects of neostigmine?
   a. pregnancy status
   b. gender
   c. culture
   d. age

6. Gabriel Torres, age 68, has symptomatic bradycardia and is being transported to the hospital by paramedics. On the way to the hospital, Mr. Torres' heart rate drops to 38. As the mobile intensive care nurse on the radio, what drug would you order?

   a. neostigmine

   b. pralidoxime

   c. atropine

   d. digoxin

7. Mac Vitale, age 60, takes an anticholinergic agent for his pronounced motion sickness. Due to his therapy, as well and his age and gender, what adverse effect would you anticipate?

   a. constipation

   b. urinary retention

   c. blurred vision

   d. dry mouth

8. Mr. Lane takes a medication that contains atropine for his peptic ulcer disease. He tells you that he frequently feels his heart beating very quickly. Which of the following may interact with atropine to induce this symptom?

   a. over-the-counter (OTC) or herbal medications

   b. ice cream

   c. fat-soluble vitamins

   d. green, leafy vegetables

Essay

List important ongoing assessments to make for the patient receiving neostigmine for myasthenia gravis.

NURSING MANAGEMENT: EVERY GOOD NURSE SHOULD . . .

Multiple choice

Circle the option that best answers the question or completes the statement.

1. James O'Connor is 70 years old and is receiving pilocarpine eyedrops for his simple glaucoma. The nurse should instruct Mr. O'Connor to

   a. avoid or be very cautious with night driving.

   b. drink additional fluids.

   c. place the drop directly over the eyeball.

   d. suck on hard candy to relieve a dry mouth.

2. Sam Harris wants to stop smoking, and nicotine patches have been prescribed. Mr. Harris tells you that he thinks he should not use the first few patches with the higher nicotine dosage but should start with the lowest dose possible so he can stop smoking sooner. Appropriate patient education for Mr. Harris would be to

   a. start with the lowest dosage of nicotine and use the higher doses last.

   b. start with the highest dosage of nicotine and then decrease the dose.

   c. place the patch on the skin when there is an urge to smoke.

   d. smoke while using the nicotine patch.

3. Barbara Fisher has been newly diagnosed with myasthenia gravis and is to be started on neostigmine 45 mg every 8 hours. You have looked up the time of onset and duration of action of neostigmine and learned that onset is 45 to 75 minutes with duration being 2 to 4 hours. She wants to take the drug at 7 AM, 3 PM, and 11 PM. What would be the best times for her to perform her daily activities that are most tiring?

   a. 6 AM, 2 PM, and 10 PM

   b. 7 AM, 3 PM, and 11 PM

   c. Between 8:30 AM and noon, and between 4:30 PM and 8 PM

   d. Between 1 PM and 3 PM, and between 9 PM and 11 PM

4. Jane is one year old and is rushed to the emergency room by her grandmother. The grandmother reports that Jane was found playing with the grandmother's pilocarpine drops and appeared to have swallowed some of the pilocarpine. Jane is sweating, drooling, flushed, and she has vomited. The nurse suspects that Jane is demonstrating

   a. nicotinic poisoning.

   b. cholinergic poisoning.

   c. anticholinergic overdose.

   d. parasympathetic blockage.

5. To treat Jane, in the scenario above, the nurse would expect to administer

   a. pilocarpine.

   b. atropine.

   c. ipecac.

   d. neostigmine.

CASE STUDY

Jack Fitzsimmons comes to the clinic. He tells you he would like medication to help prevent motion sickness because he is going on a fishing trip. You know that scopolamine transdermal patch, an anticholinergic drug, is often prescribed to prevent motion sickness. What other information should be assessed before requesting that the nurse practitioner or doctor write an order for scopolamine?

CRITICAL THINKING CHALLENGE

Mr. Fitzsimmons is found to be a suitable candidate and is given a prescription for scopolamine patches. He returns to the clinic 2 days later complaining of blurred vision. His pupils are dilated. He tells you he removed the scopolamine patch this morning. Shortly after that, he began to have blurred vision and photosensitivity. What could have caused Mr. Fitzsimmons' eye problems?

UNIT V

Central Nervous System Drugs

CHAPTER 16

Drugs Producing Anesthesia and Neuromuscular Blocking

TOP TEN THINGS TO KNOW ABOUT DRUGS PRODUCING ANESTHESIA AND NEUROMUSCULAR BLOCKING

1. Isoflurane is an inhaled anesthetic. As part of balanced anesthesia, it is used to induce and maintain anesthesia. It can also be used for sedation and analgesia.

2. Respiratory depression occurs with isoflurane, like all inhaled anesthetics, and the patient requires mechanical ventilation. Prolonged hypotension during induction of anesthesia may occur. Postoperative respiratory depression and cardiovascular problems are possible, and are more likely if the patient has ongoing chronic respiratory or cardiac problems preoperatively, or is significantly obese.

3. Postoperatively, the nurse minimizes adverse effects to isoflurane by monitoring blood pressure, pulse, and temperature; supporting respiratory function; preventing aspiration; keeping the patient warm; and assessing for return of normal bowel sounds and urinary output.

4. Propofol is a nonbarbiturate hypnotic used as a parenteral anesthetic as part of balanced general anesthesia. When propofol is used to induce anesthesia, loss of consciousness occurs rapidly after IV administration although the effects are short lived. Thus, it is administered as a continuous infusion.

5. Lidocaine is a local anesthetic with multiple uses, creating anesthesia in a confined area without loss of consciousness. It works by diminishing the permeability of the nerve membrane to sodium; this reversibly blocks nerve conduction.

6. Neuromuscular blockade occurs at acetylcholine receptors in the neural muscular joint (NMJ) where the neurotransmitter acetylcholine reacts with the muscle cell membrane causing depolarization and subsequent muscle relaxation.

7. Nondepolarizing drugs prevent the muscle from contracting (muscle stays relaxed). Depolarizing drugs cause depolarization (muscle contraction) but then prevent the muscle from being stimulated again (contraction followed by flaccid paralysis).

8. Tubocurarine, a nondepolarizing neuromuscular blocker, is used as an adjunct to general anesthesia to facilitate endotracheal intubation and with mechanically ventilated patients to conserve energy and prevent "fighting" the respirator. Neuromuscular blockade can be reversed with anticholinesterases (neostigmine, pyridostigmine, and edrophonium).

9. Tubocurarine does not depress the central nervous system (CNS). Although the patient cannot speak, move, or breathe unassisted, hearing, thought processes, and sensation are not affected. General anesthetics should be administered before administering tubocurarine for surgical intubation. The nurse should provide reassurance to ventilated patients on tubocurarine.

10. Succinylcholine is a depolarizing neuromuscular blocker used in endotracheal intubation and short procedures such as endoscopy or electroconvulsant therapy (ECT). It is not used as an adjunct to anesthesia. A small amount of a nondepolarizing neuromuscular blocker is used before succinylcholine to prevent or decrease muscle fasciculations.

KEY TERMS

True/false

Mark true or false for each of the following statements. If the statement is false, replace the underlined word with the word that will make the statement correct.

1. _____ The use of sedating drugs to help uncover unconscious material during psychoanalysis is called neuroleptanesthesia.

2. _____ Depolarizing drugs prevent neural communication by depolarizing the muscle.

3. _____ General anesthesia is the condition that results when sensory transmission from a local area of the body to the CNS is blocked.

4. _____ The inability to move or function is called anesthesia.

5. _____ The site of communication between a nerve and a muscle is called the end-plate.

6. _____ Paralysis is a loss of feeling or sensation.

7. _____ Narcoanalysis is also known as conscious sedation.

8. _____ Nondepolarizing drugs cause muscle depolarization and prevent repolarization.

9. _____ Local anesthesia is a combination of drugs to produce a lighter stage of anesthesia.

10. _____ Dissociative anesthesia is a loss of perception of certain stimuli while that of others remains intact.

11. _____ Balanced anesthesia is characterized by a state of unconsciousness, analgesia, and amnesia.

PHYSIOLOGY AND PATHOPHYSIOLOGY: THE BODY HUMAN

Essay

Match the following stages of anesthesia with their descriptions.

1. _____ Unless rapid intervention and support occur, coma and death follow.

2. _____ The patient remains conscious.

3. _____ Contains four planes or levels.

4. _____ Systolic pressure rises, and the patient may experience excitation.

a. Stage I
b. Stage II
c. Stage III
d. Stage IV

CORE DRUG KNOWLEDGE: JUST THE FACTS

Multiple choice

Circle the option that best answers the question or completes the statement.

1. Surgical anesthesia is _____ anesthesia.
   a. stage I
   b. stage II
   c. stage III
   d. stage IV

2. The onset of action of isoflurane (Forane) is
   a. 30 to 60 minutes.
   b. 2 to 3 minutes.
   c. 20 to 30 seconds.
   d. 7 to 10 minutes.

3. Isoflurane (Forane) is contraindicated for use in patients with:
   a. hyperthyroidism.
   b. head trauma.
   c. orthopedic injuries.
   d. glaucoma.

4. Which of the following drugs is similar to isoflurane (Forane)?
   a. ketamine (Ketalar)
   b. droperidol (Inapsine)
   c. halothane (Fluothane)
   d. fentanyl (Sublimaze)

5. Ketamine (Ketalar) is contraindicated for adult patients with a history of psychiatric disorders because it may induce
   a. nausea and vomiting.
   b. anaphylaxis.
   c. emergence reaction.
   d. syncope.

6. An unusual potential adverse effect associated with long-term or high-dose propofol (Diprivan) therapy is
   a. headache.
   b. bright green urine.
   c. decreased albumin levels.
   d. amnesia.

7. To minimize potential bacterial growth, propofol (Diprivan) should be discarded after _____ hours.
   a. 6
   b. 2
   c. 24
   d. 12

8. Local anesthetics such as lidocaine (Xylocaine) are NOT useful in the management of
   a. laceration repair.
   b. regional blocks.
   c. ophthalmic anesthesia.
   d. general anesthesia.

9. What is the anticipated onset of action of tubocurarine (Tubarine) when given intravenously?
   a. 90 minutes
   b. 20 to 30 minutes
   c. 2 minutes
   d. 60 minutes

10. Tubocurarine (Tubarine) is an acetylcholine antagonist. This results in
    a. flaccid paralysis.
    b. CNS anesthesia.
    c. spastic paralysis.
    d. muscle fasciculations.

11. Which of the following drugs is NOT used to reverse the action of tubocurarine (Tubarine)?
    a. edrophonium (Tensilon)
    b. neostigmine (Prostigmin)
    c. pyridostigmine (Mestinon)
    d. succinylcholine (Anectine)

12. During tubocurarine (Tubarine) therapy, relaxation of arterial muscles may result in
    a. hypertension.
    b. hypotension.
    c. pasty white complexion.
    d. bronchospasm.

13. Succinylcholine (Anectine) is used during _____ because of its rapid and complete neuromuscular blockade.
    a. electroconvulsive therapy
    b. long and protracted surgeries
    c. anaphylaxis
    d. mechanical ventilation

14. What is the major difference between tubocurarine (Tubarine) and succinylcholine (Anectine) mechanism of action?
    a. Tubocurarine produces paralysis by excitation of muscles, and succinylcholine produces paralysis by relaxation of muscles.
    b. Tubocurarine produces paralysis by relaxation of muscles, and succinylcholine produces paralysis by excitation of muscles.
    c. Tubocurarine has a slower onset and shorter duration than succinylcholine.
    d. Succinylcholine has a slower onset and longer duration than tubocurarine.

Essay

Identify important differences between the local anesthetic agents groups: esters and amides.

CORE PATIENT VARIABLES: PATIENTS, PLEASE

Multiple choice

Circle the option that best answers the question or completes the statement.

1. Which of the following patients has an increased risk for adverse effects from isoflurane (Forane)?
   a. Manual Flores, age 70, with COPD
   b. Donna Hickson, age 66, with hypothyroidism
   c. Sean Morell, age 16, with anorexia
   d. Virginia Palmer, age 80, with Parkinson's disease

2. Keeghan Davis, age 32, had isoflurane (Forane) anesthetic during her surgery. She is now in the recovery room. With your knowledge of isoflurane, which of the following questions would you ask Ms. Davis?
   a. "Would you like me to remove the blanket and just cover you with the sheet?"
   b. "Would you like some pain medication?"
   c. "Would you like a light snack?"
   d. all of the above

3. Your patient has just returned to your unit after having surgery. Which of the following should be documented?

   a. vital signs

   b. bowel sounds

   c. urine output

   d. all of the above

4. Henry Lanum was involved in a severe motor vehicle accident and sustained a closed head injury. To keep Mr. Lanum in a protective coma, the nurse administers propofol (Diprivan). Which of the following lab tests should be done before and during administration of propofol?

   a. triglycerides

   b. hemoglobin

   c. urinalysis

   d. arterial blood gas

5. Which of the following nursing interventions is important during the administration of propofol (Diprivan)?

   a. due to paralysis, turn the patient frequently

   b. due to potential diarrhea, place the patient on plastic sheets

   c. to enhance propofol's effects, keep environmental stimuli to a minimum

   d. to enhance propofol's effects, keep the patient on a ventilator

6. Melissa Fait came to the Emergency Department with a full-thickness laceration. The doctor anesthetized the area with lidocaine (Xylocaine) before suturing. Melissa asks, "When will that wear off?" Which of the following is correct?

   a. 10 minutes

   b. 4 hours

   c. 1 to 3 hours

   d. 12 hours

7. Megan Jones has just received viscous lidocaine to treat an ulceration in her throat. Which of the following nursing interventions should you do?

   a. withhold food and fluids for 1 hour

   b. take her blood pressure every 15 minutes

   c. give an antacid to decrease stomach acids

   d. place an icebag over her neck

8. Allysa James has a history of COPD. Why would tubocurarine (Tubarine) be a poor choice for her surgery?

   a. Patients with COPD may have decreased efficacy with tubocurarine.

   b. Tubocurarine releases histamine, which may exacerbate COPD.

   c. Tubocurarine induces electrolyte disturbances, which may induce bronchospasm.

   d. Drugs used in the treatment of COPD inactivate tubocurarine.

9. Monica Packard, age 65, was involved in a motor vehicle accident and has head trauma. Review of her health status reveals chronic renal failure. She was intubated and became very agitated. Mrs. Packard was given tubocurarine (Tubarine) for paralysis to decrease potential increased intracranial pressure from her agitation. Which of the following nursing implications is important with this patient?

   a. Monitor paralysis every 5 minutes because she may not have adequate response to tubocurarine.

   b. Monitor intake and output because of her renal status.

   c. Monitor Mrs. Packard's respiratory status carefully after extubation because tubocurarine may have prolonged effects in this patient.

   d. Pad the side rails because Mrs. Packard has increased risk for seizures.

10. Kimberly Myers is on mechanical ventilation and tubocurarine (Tubarine) therapy. Her family has come to visit. Which of the following statements by the nurse is most appropriate?

    a. "Stroke her arm. She will be able to feel your touch although she cannot move."

    b, "Talk to her. She may be afraid because she cannot move, but she can still hear what is going on around her."

    c. "She can hear what you are saying but will not understand because the drug has made her unconscious."

    d. "She cannot feel your touch below the neck, but you can touch her head and she will feel it."

11. Your patient is scheduled for surgery and will be induced with tubocurarine (Tubarine). After reviewing your patient's health status, you note a history of COPD and renal insufficiency. Which of the following interventions would be most appropriate?

    a. Call the surgical suite and cancel the surgery.

    b. Contact the anesthesiologist and advise him/her of the patient's history.

    c. Write a note on a sticky pad and place it on the progress notes in the chart.

    d. Call the patient's family and advise them of the risks of anesthetic agents for this patient.

12. James Grey, age 66, has a history of cardiac arrhythmias. Why would succinylcholine (Anectine) be a poor choice for Mr. Grey's surgery? Succinylcholine

    a. produces profound CNS obtundation and Mr. Grey could not tell the staff he was experiencing chest pain.

    b. slows the conduction of the heart and may induce CHF.

    c. releases potassium from intense muscle contraction, which may induce cardiac arrhythmias.

    d. requires pseudocholinesterase for degradation, which is enhanced by cardiac insufficiency.

13. Benny Welsh has been on metoclopramide for nausea and vomiting. Mr. Welsh is now diagnosed with a bowel obstruction and is being readied for surgery. How may the use of metoclopramide (Reglan) affect the action of succinylcholine (Anectine)?

    a. The duration of action may be shorter.

    b. The duration of action may be longer.

    c. The onset may be quicker.

    d. The onset may be delayed.

NURSING MANAGEMENT: EVERY GOOD NURSE SHOULD . . .

Multiple choice

Circle the option that best answers the question or completes the statement.

1. You are the nurse responsible for admitting patients into the operating room holding area and performing the final checks and preparation for surgery. You anticipate that a patient will receive isoflurane, an inhaled anesthetic. To help maximize the therapeutic effect of the isoflurane, you would

    a. involve the patient in an active conversation about politics or sports to distract him.

    b. place the patient in a busy hallway so he can be easily observed.

    c. tell the patient as little as possible about the events that will occur during induction of anesthesia in order not to frighten him.

    d. keep the holding room as quiet as possible with subdued lighting to promote relaxation.

2. You are the nurse working in the recovery room of an outpatient surgical center. Your patient has received general anesthesia with isoflurane, an inhaled anesthetic. Before discharging him from the recovery room and allowing him to go home, you should verify

    a. that his vital signs are stable and have returned to baseline.

    b. that he has voided.

    c. that he has someone to drive him home.

    d. all of the above.

3. James Brooks is intubated and receiving mechanical ventilation. He is receiving tubocurarine, a nondepolarizing NMJ blocker. Which of the following should be included in his nursing care?

    a. Turn and reposition every 1 to 2 hours.

    b. Keep skin clean and dry.

    c. Explain all activity and care that will be performed.

    d. all of the above

    e. none of the above

4. Brenda Wilton received succinylcholine before receiving ECT. The day after the treatment she complains to you, the nurse, that her muscles hurt all over. The most appropriate nursing action would be to

   a. administer another dose of succinylcholine.

   b. contact the anesthesiologist immediately.

   c. explain that these feelings may be expected.

   d. complete an incident sheet.

CASE STUDY

Dennis Kornevitz is to receive lidocaine as a local anesthetic while a chest tube is to be inserted. You are to prepare the lidocaine for use during the procedure.

1. Through what route would you expect the lidocaine to be administered?

2. Do you need any other information to prepare the medication?

CRITICAL THINKING CHALLENGE

Dennis Kornevitz requires several doses of lidocaine before he tells the physician that adequate anesthesia has occurred. As the physician prepares to proceed with inserting the chest tube, Mr. Kornevitz begins to act confused and disoriented. You check his vital signs, and his pulse is 55 and irregular, his blood pressure is 86/50.
What could account for these findings?

CHAPTER 17

Drugs That Are Sedatives, Hypnotics, and Anxiolytics

TOP TEN THINGS TO KNOW ABOUT DRUGS THAT ARE SEDATIVES, HYPNOTICS, AND ANXIOLYTICS

1. Drugs that produce sedation create a soothing, calming effect. They will cause drowsiness, which will lead to sleep. Drugs that are hypnotics will initially produce sleep but will also induce a loss of consciousness and pain sensation. The same drug may do either function, depending on dose, route, and duration of administration. These drugs depress the central nervous system (CNS).

2. Drugs that reduce anxiety are called anxiolytics. Depending on the dose and route, these drugs can also promote a calming effect, lead to drowsiness, and sleep. Some of them can be used in creating conscious sedation and as adjuncts for anesthesia. These drugs depress the CNS.

3. The barbiturates (prototype phenobarbital) induce a state of generalized CNS depression. They are used primarily for hypnotic effects. Phenobarbital is also used to treat seizures. Barbiturates are seldom used to treat insomnia due to their narrow therapeutic index, with potential for overdose and death.

4. Phenobarbital and other barbiturates cause adverse effects that are from CNS depression. Respiratory depression is the most serious. The larger the dose, the more respiratory depression that occurs. Paradoxical excitement may occur—especially in children or older adults.

5. Phenobarbital has a long half-life and induces the metabolism of many other drugs. Always check for drug interactions.

6. The benzodiazepines (prototype lorazepam) potentiate the effect of GABA, an inhibitory CNS neurotransmitter. This results in CNS depression.

7. Benzodiazepines, like lorazepam, are used to treat anxiety disorders, insomnia, seizures, muscle spasms and tension, and acute alcohol withdrawal symptoms. IV doses of certain benzodiazepines (midazolam) are used in conscious sedation and preanesthesia. Selection of the benzodiazepine for a particular use is related to the half-life of the drug (some have short half-lives; some have long half-lives).

8. Lorazepam, and other benzodiazepines, produce adverse effects from CNS depression; sedation and ataxia are most common. Anticholinergic effects are also likely. Paradoxical excitatory reactions are possible.

9. The risk for fatal overdose is small with benzodiazepines, compared to barbiturates, due to their wide therapeutic index.

10. Caution patients to avoid taking other CNS depressants when taking either a barbiturate or a benzodiazepine due to additive CNS depression that may occur. Caution patients not to drive or do potentially hazardous activities until the effects of the barbiturate or benzodiazepine on them are known.

KEY TERMS

Definitions

Define the following:

1. anxiety
2. neurotransmitters
3. synapse

Essay

List the most common pathologic anxiety disorders.

PHYSIOLOGY AND PATHOPHYSIOLOGY: THE BODY HUMAN

Essay

1. What is the function of the thalamus?

2. What is the function of the limbic system?

3. Explain the motor and sensory functions of the reticular activating system (RAS).

4. Identify the major neurotransmitters believed to be involved in mental illnesses.

5. What is the importance of stage 3 and 4 sleep?

CORE DRUG KNOWLEDGE: JUST THE FACTS

Multiple choice

Circle the option that best answers the question or completes the statement.

1. Which of the following types of barbiturates is used in the management of seizure disorders?
   a. ultrashort-acting
   b. short-acting
   c. intermediate-acting
   d. long-acting

2. Death from phenobarbitol (Luminol) overdose is usually caused by
   a. respiratory depression.
   b. seizure activity.
   c. cardiac arrhythmias.
   d. blood dyscrasias.

3. Which of the following contraindicates the use of phenobarbitol (Luminol) and the other barbiturates?
   a. seizure disorder
   b. migraine headache
   c. severe hepatic dysfunction
   d. cardiac arrhythmias

4. Which of the following symptoms may occur after rapid IV administration of phenobarbitol (Luminol)?
   a. hypertension
   b. seizure activity
   c. hypotension
   d. tachypnea (rapid breathing)

5. Which of the following contraindicates the use of lorazepam (Ativan) and the other benzodiazepines?
   a. anemia
   b. severe renal dysfunction
   c. hypertension
   d. hyperthyroidism

6. The most common adverse effects of benzodiazepines such as lorazepam (Ativan) are
   a. sedation and ataxia.
   b. urinary retention and headache.
   c. sedation and cardiac arrhythmias.
   d. respiratory depression and hypertension.

7. CNS effects of lorazepam (Ativan) may be potentiated when given concurrently with
   a. phenytoin (Dilantin).
   b. flumazenil (Romazicon).
   c. alcohol.
   d. levodopa (Dopar).

8. Benzodiazepines can impair ability to
   a. recall long-term memories.
   b. produce white blood cells.
   c. digest fats and carbohydrates.
   d. remember events following drug administration.

CORE PATIENT VARIABLES: PATIENTS, PLEASE

Multiple choice

Circle the option that best answers the question or completes the statement.

1. Haley, age 6, is receiving phenobarbitol (Luminol) for a seizure disorder. Due to her age, which of the following adverse reactions may occur?

   a. paradoxical excitement

   b. respiratory depression

   c. development of a rash

   d. migraine headaches

2. Kimberly Kay, age 26, is taking phenobarbitol (Luminol) for her seizure disorder. What patient education is extremely important for Mrs. Kay?

   a. "Call the office if you feel any sedation."

   b. "Be sure to use contraceptive measures while taking this drug."

   c. "It is important that you eat at least six times a day with this medication."

   d. "Double the dose in the evening if you forget to take it in the morning."

3. James Glover, age 45, has been taking phenobarbitol (Luminol) for 5 years. Mr. Glover calls the office and states, "I almost fell asleep driving home from work last night. This is the first time I felt so sedated." Which of the following additions to Mr. Glover's lifestyle may have increased his sedation?

   a. over-the-counter (OTC) herbal medications

   b. smoking

   c. increased exercise routine

   d. increased coffee intake

4. Which of the following patients should avoid the use of phenobarbitol (Luminol)?

   a. Hugh, age 50, with hyperthyroidism

   b. Lester, age 45, with hypertension

   c. Pat, age 60, with benign prostatic hypertrophy

   d. Ian, age 55, with morbid obesity

5. Which of the following patients should avoid the use of lorazepam (Ativan)?

   a. Malcolm, with a history of mitral valve prolapse

   b. Christy, with a history of peptic ulcer disease

   c. Tyler, age 45

   d. Myrna, 18 weeks' pregnant

6. Which of the following assessments would potentially decrease the sedative effects of lorazepam? The patient

   a. has COPD.

   b. smokes two packs of cigarettes per day.

   c. is a vegetarian.

   d. is Asian.

7. Mary Steele has been taking lorazepam (Ativan) for her anxiety disorder for the past year. She is now admitted to your unit for appendicitis. What nursing intervention related to her long-term lorazepam use would you do?

   a. Monitor intake and output daily.

   b. Obtain an order for a blood gas.

   c. Obtain an order for a benzodiazepine to avoid withdrawal syndrome.

   d. Tell the patient care technician to take her vital signs every ½ hour.

8. Myron Beach, age 70, has been ordered a benzodiazepine for sleep during his hospitalization. You note that Mr. Beach is Asian. You would expect the dose of benzodiazepine to be

   a. higher than normal.

   b. lower than normal.

   c. the same as for any adult.

NURSING MANAGEMENT: EVERY GOOD NURSE SHOULD . . .

Multiple choice

Circle the option that best answers the question or completes the statement.

1. Patient teaching for phenobarbital therapy should include

   a. "Use contraceptive backup method if taking birth control pills."

   b. "Sedation is a common adverse effect."

   c. "Avoid drinking alcohol."

   d. all of the above.

   e. none of the above.

2. Jonas Taylor is 24 years old and experiencing delirium tremens from alcohol withdrawal. You are to administer lorazepam, a benzodiazepine, IM as treatment. To maximize the therapeutic effect and minimize adverse effects you should

   a. use a 25-gauge and ⅝-inch length needle.

   b. administer into dorsal gluteal or ventrogluteal muscle.

   c. inject using a 45-degree angle.

   d. do all of the above.

3. Gina Jenkins, 33 years old, has been prescribed lorazepam, a benzodiazepine, as an anxiolytic. What teaching should be done regarding this drug therapy?

   a. Avoid activities requiring mental alertness initially.

   b. Avoid drinking alcohol.

   c. Avoid becoming pregnant while on this drug.

   d. all of the above

4. Henry Marzeti is 70 years old and is to receive lorazepam as a sedative tonight before surgery tomorrow morning. The nurse would expect to administer to Mr. Marzeti

   a. an average adult dose.

   b. a dose larger than the average adult dose.

   c. a dose smaller than the average adult dose.

   d. none of this drug, because it is contraindicated in older adults.

5. Julia Farrow, 60 years old, was seen today in the outpatient department. She is to be started on lorazepam to treat anxiety she has had since her husband died suddenly a month ago. She is to take the drug twice a day. She has told you, the nurse, that she has a two-story house, with her bedroom and bathroom upstairs. To minimize adverse effects, teach Mrs. Farrow to

   a. use the handrail when going down the stairs.

   b. take the evening dose at bedtime.

   c. take the larger portion of the day's dose at night.

   d. do all of the above.

   e. do none of the above.

CASE STUDY

John Williamson, 68 years old, has CHF and takes digoxin, hydrochlorothiazide, and captopril daily. He currently has an inguinal hernia and goes to surgery for correction. He receives IV lorazepam before being anesthetized. After surgery, he confides in you, the nurse, that he "must be getting old" because he can't remember anything that happened from before surgery until he was back in his bed.
What would you say to Mr. Williamson?

CRITICAL THINKING CHALLENGE

The morning after surgery, Mr. Williamson is complaining of feeling very weak and lethargic, and nauseous. He also states he sees a yellowish halo around objects.

1. What is your assessment of a possible cause of these complaints?

2. What lab work would confirm your assessment?

CHAPTER 18

Drugs for Treating Mood Disorders

TOP TEN THINGS TO KNOW ABOUT DRUGS FOR TREATING MOOD DISORDERS

1. The two major mood disorders are depression and bipolar disorder (alternating mania and depression). Mood disorders are believed to be due to an alteration in neurotransmitters or the function of neurotransmitter receptors.

2. Antidepressants are divided into tricyclic, selective serotonin reuptake inhibitors (SSRI), monoamine oxidase inhibitors (MAOI), and miscellaneous categories. They bring about long-term changes in norepinephrine (NE) and serotonin (5-HT) receptor symptoms. This may be why the full therapeutic (antidepressant) effect from drug therapy may take several weeks to occur.

3. Tricyclic antidepressants (prototype desipramine) block the reuptake of norepinephrine and serotonin, allowing more effect to occur from these transmitters. Blockage of the neurotransmitters is nonselective. This accounts for many of the adverse effects.

4. The most frequent adverse effects of desipramine are sedation and anticholinergic effects, although tolerance will develop to these adverse effects. Hypotension is possible due to alpha-1 receptor blockade. Cardiotoxicity is also possible.

5. Phenelzine is an MAOI used for depression that does not respond to other antidepressants. Phenelzine acts in peripheral adrenergic nerve endings to increase norepinephrine there, although it prevents the release of norepinephrine in response to normal nerve activity.

6. Common adverse effects of phenelzine and other MAOIs are anticholinergic effects and central nervous system (CNS) depression effects. Severe drug–drug interactions (mixed acting sympathomimetics) or drug–food interactions (tyramine or tryptophan-rich foods) will produce severe hypertensive crisis due to excessive norepinephrine stimulation. These interactions have limited the use of phenelzine.

7. Fluoxetine is an SSRI, meaning it has little effect on other neurotransmitters. This accounts for the few adverse effects. Adverse effects tend to be mild and transient. Anticholinergic effects are not common. Fluoxetine has a long half-life, allowing for once-daily dosing.

8. Lithium is a mood stabilizer (prevents mood swings) used in bipolar affective disorder; its effectiveness is believed to be due to increased norepinephrine uptake and increased serotonin receptor sensitivity.

9. As the body perceives lithium ions to be sodium ions, the two compete for reabsorption in the proximal tubule. Decreased sodium intake will cause the body to reabsorb more lithium.

10. Lithium toxicity is dose related, and there is a narrow therapeutic index. Signs of lithium toxicity include serious CNS effects ranging from coarse hand tremor and vertigo to seizures and coma. Adverse effects can be minimized by monitoring drug blood levels and maintaining consistent sodium intake and blood levels.

KEY TERMS

Anagrams

Use the following anagrams to explain the key terms in the chapter:

1. Drugs use to treat depressive disorders

   S S T N A S E R P E D T I N A

   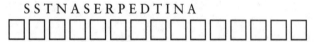

2. Often associated with decreased productivity, work absenteeism, unemployment, alcohol and drug abuse, and risk for suicide

   E N R O P I E S D S

   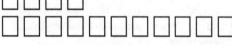

3. Drugs that manage or prevent mood swings in patients with bipolar disorder

   O O M D L S A E S R B I T Z I

   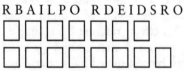

4. A conscious state of mind or predominant emotion

   D O M O   ▢▢▢▢

5. Characterized by recurrent episodes of depression, mania, or mixed states

   R B A I L P O R D E I D S R O

   ▢▢▢▢▢▢
   ▢▢▢▢▢▢

6. Depression may be caused by dysregulation of these

   S N R E E U T R T O I T M R S A N

   ▢▢▢▢▢▢▢▢▢▢▢▢▢▢▢▢▢

PHYSIOLOGY AND PATHOPHYSIOLOGY: THE BODY HUMAN

Essay

1. Identify neurotransmitters thought to influence depression.

2. Identify neurotransmitters thought to influence bipolar disorder.

3. Identify the symptoms that characterize serotonin reuptake inhibitor withdrawal syndrome.

CORE DRUG KNOWLEDGE: JUST THE FACTS

Multiple choice

Circle the option that best answers the question or completes the statement.

1. The most serious effect of tricyclic overdose is
   a. seizures.
   b. hyperpyrexia.
   c. metabolic acidosis.
   d. cardiac arrhythmias.

2. The unlabeled pharmacotherapeutics of desipramine (Norpramin) include
   a. enuresis in children.
   b. chronic pain syndromes.
   c. bipolar disorder.
   d. atypical psychoses.

3. Adverse effects to desipramine (Norpramin) therapy may include
   a. anticholinergic effects.
   b. hypertension.
   c. hypervigilance.
   d. diarrhea.

4. Phenelzine (Nardil), a monamine oxidase inhibitor, is used in the treatment of
   a. enuresis in children.
   b. manic phase of bipolar disease.
   c. schizophrenia.
   d. atypical depression.

5. Interaction with tyramine-rich foods or beverages may result in
   a. shock.
   b. hypertensive crisis.
   c. bleeding episodes.
   d. sedation.

6. Patients taking phenelzine (Nardil) should avoid which of the following foods?
   a. salmon
   b. veal chops
   c. aged cheese
   d. milk

7. Which of the following is NOT a disorder treated with fluoxetine (Prozac)?
   a. depression
   b. bulimia
   c. atypical psychosis
   d. obsessive-compulsive disorder

8. Optimal therapeutic effect of fluoxetine (Prozac) takes
   a. 4 to 9 days.
   b. 3 days.
   c. 1 to 3 weeks.
   d. 4 weeks.

9. Which of the following drugs is similar to fluoxetine (Prozac)?
   a. lithium carbonate (Eskalith)
   b. nefazodone (Serzone)
   c. phenelzine (Nardil)
   d. venlafaxine (Effexor)

10. In the treatment of bipolar affective disorder, _____ is the drug of choice.
   a. lithium carbonate (Eskalith)
   b. nefazodone (Serzone)
   c. phenelzine (Nardil)
   d. venlafaxine (Effexor)

11. Contraindications for lithium (Eskalith) therapy include
   a. COPD.
   b. dehydration.
   c. hypertension.
   d. peptic ulcer disease.

12. Therapeutic effects of lithium (Eskalith) are demonstrated in approximately
   a. 1 to 3 hours.
   b. 20 hours.
   c. 10 to 21 days.
   d. 3 months.

CORE PATIENT VARIABLES: PATIENTS, PLEASE

Multiple choice

Circle the option that best answers the question or completes the statement.

1. Desipramine (Norpramin) is an acceptable antidepressant for which of the following patients?
   a. Valerie, with a history of asthma
   b. Bernice, with a history of cardiac arrhythmias
   c. Ginger, with a history of hypertension
   d. Julie, with a seizure disorder

2. Which of the following patients should receive a reduced initial dose of desipramine (Norpramin)?
   a. Candice, age 45, with cardiovascular disease
   b. Julie, age 27, who is breast-feeding
   c. Lyle, age 67, with hypothyroidism
   d. Dennis, age 50, with asthma

3. Beatrice has been taking desipramine (Norpramin) for 6 months. Which of the following diagnostic tests is most important for Beatrice?
   a. lipid profile
   b. electrocardiogram
   c. MRI
   d. thyroid function tests

4. Henry Talbet has been taking phenelzine (Nardil) for 4 months without a significant change in his depression. Which of the following precautions should be made before changing Mr. Talbet to another antidepressant?
   a. Discontinue phenelzine for 2 weeks before starting a new medication.
   b. Discontinue phenelzine for 24 hours before starting a new medication.
   c. Administer decreasing doses of phenelzine for 2 weeks, then start the new medication.
   d. No special precautions are needed.

5. Gloria Yates is being discharged from the hospital with a prescription for phenelzine (Nardil). Which of the following patient instructions is INCORRECT?
   a. "You must monitor your diet for foods that contain tyramine or tryptophan."
   b. "You should limit your exposure to sunlight."
   c. "Refrain from drinking alcohol."
   d. "This drug tends to make you gain weight—try using an OTC or herbal weight loss medication."

6. Jennifer Albright comes to the clinic and states, "I'm just not going to take Prozac anymore." She refuses to discuss her decision to discontinue the medication. With your knowledge of fluoxetine, which adverse effect may Mrs. Albright be experiencing?

   a. weight gain

   b. sexual dysfunction

   c. blood dyscrasias

   d. headache

7. Alan Moore, age 77, is taking fluoxetine (Prozac) for depression. Mr. Moore has an increased risk for which of the following adverse effects?

   a. nausea

   b. orthostatic hypotension

   c. blood dyscrasias

   d. weight gain

8. Your patient tells you that after 1 week of fluoxetine (Prozac) therapy, she is still depressed. Your response is based on the fact that

   a. the dose should be increased.

   b. it takes 2 weeks of drug therapy before effects are noted.

   c. the dose should be decreased.

   d. the patient is probably being noncompliant.

9. Fred Walker comes to the clinic with complaints of a coarse hand tremor, severe gastrointestinal (GI) upset and blurred vision. You suspect he is experiencing toxic effects of which of the following drugs?

   a. lithium (Eskalith)

   b. fluoxetine (Prozac)

   c. desipramine (Norpramin)

   d. phenelzine (Nardil)

10. Alice Tau, age 44, takes lithium for bipolar affective disorder. Mrs. Tau states she has been "100% compliant" with her medication, but her lithium level is subtherapeutic. Which of the following could be the etiology of her low lithium level?

    a. age

    b. Japanese ancestry

    c. excessive intake of caffeine-containing foods and beverages

    d. history of congestive heart failure (CHF)

NURSING MANAGEMENT: EVERY GOOD NURSE SHOULD . . .

Multiple choice

Circle the option that best answers the question or completes the statement.

1. Ramona DiPaul has been started on phenelzine, a MAOI to treat depression that has not responded to other drug therapy. To minimize adverse effects, you should teach her to avoid eating

   a. cured meats and aged cheeses.

   b. semolina pasta.

   c. apples.

   d. orange juice.

2. Kerry Harding is taking desipramine, a tricyclic antidepressant. She complains of a severe dry mouth after 1 week on the drug. She says her depression isn't better, and she wants to stop taking the desipramine. Your best response to her would be:

   a. "The dry mouth is a sign of an allergic response. You should stop taking the drug now."

   b. "Dry mouth can occur when you take this drug, but it often goes away after you are on the drug awhile. You will need to stay on the drug for a few weeks until the full antidepressant effect occurs."

   c. "Dry mouth can be bothersome from this drug. But the drug should have relieved your depression by now. Contact the doctor."

   d. "A dry mouth is an unusual occurrence from despiramine. Are you sure you are taking the drug as prescribed?"

3. Robert Haynes has been prescribed fluoxetine, an SSRI antidepressant. Teaching for Mr. Haynes should include:

   a. Minimize the intake of caffeine-rich drinks and foods to prevent insomnia.

   b. Increase the intake of carbohydrates to promote the antidepressant effect.

   c. Watch total calorie intake to prevent overeating and weight gain.

   d. All of the above.

   e. None of the above.

4. Susan Atwater is severely depressed. She tells you that life isn't worth living and that she would like to end it all. She has been prescribed desipramine, a tricyclic antidepressant. To maximize therapeutic effects and minimize adverse effects, the nurse should

  a. instruct her to discontinue the drug if she is still depressed after 1 week of therapy.

  b. verify that the prescription is only for a limited number of pills.

  c. discourage her from continuing with psychotherapy now that she is on drug therapy.

  d. do all of the above.

5. To minimize adverse effects from lithium, the nurse should monitor

  a. blood lithium levels.

  b. blood potassium levels.

  c. tyramine intake.

  d. dairy intake.

CASE STUDY

Larry Viceroy is 40 years old and was started on lithium as drug therapy for bipolar-affective disorder about 2 weeks ago. He tells you that he doesn't feel any different than when he first started the drug therapy. He has had one manic episode, although it was not quite as severe as before starting lithium. He also complains of an upset stomach after taking the lithium in the morning.
What patient-related variables should you assess to obtain more information related to his comments?

CRITICAL THINKING CHALLENGE

Larry returns to the clinic for follow-up 3 months later. At this time, he complains of blurred vision and vertigo. You note a hand tremor in his left hand. His blood lithium levels are 2 mEq/L. You ask if he has had any other recent changes, and he tells you that he has cut his salt intake to "practically zero" because he heard that salt wasn't good for his "pressure."

1. What is your assessment of Larry's current condition?

2. What factors contributed to his current blood lithium levels?

3. Explain how these factors contributed to his condition.

CHAPTER 19

Drugs for Treating Thought Disorders

TOP TEN THINGS TO KNOW ABOUT DRUGS FOR TREATING THOUGHT DISORDERS

1. Antipsychotic drugs are used in the treatment of acute and chronic psychotic illnesses, such as schizophrenia. Drug therapy is needed for several weeks before the full therapeutic effect will occur. Antipsychotics are divided into two groups, the typical and the atypical. They may also be grouped by their chemical structure.

2. Typical antipsychotic drugs block dopamine receptors. Additionally, these drugs will also bind to some nondopamine receptors (histamine, alpha-1 adrenergic, and cholinergic). Many of the adverse effects from these drugs are from binding to these other receptor sites.

3. Typical antipsychotic drugs vary in their potency, although all are similarly effective in controlling psychotic symptoms. More potent drugs tend to have more extrapyramidal (EPS) adverse effects; less potent drugs tend to have more anticholinergic adverse effects.

4. Chlorpromazine, a typical phenothiazine antipsychotic, also has significant antiemetic, hypotensive, sedative, and anticholinergic effects. Adverse effects include production of extrapyramidal symptoms (akinesia, dystonia, pseudo-parkinsonism) in the first weeks of therapy and, with long-term use, tardive dyskinesia (abnormal involuntary movements of mouth, tongue, face). Tardive dyskinesia is irreversible. Anticholinergic adverse effects (dry mouth, blurred vision, constipation, urinary retention) and effects from alpha receptor blockade (orthostatic hypotension, tachycardia) are also common. Adverse effects may limit a patient's acceptance of and adherence to drug therapy. Teach the patient how to manage or deal with these adverse effects.

5. Atypical antipsychotic drugs block at dopaminergic receptors, but not as much as the typical antipsychotics. Atypical antipsychotics have significant attraction for serotonin receptors, alpha adrenergic receptors, histamine receptors, and muscarinic receptors and produce a blockade at these sites. Atypical antipsychotics are unlikely to cause the extrapyramidal symptoms that are common with the typical antipsychotics.

6. Clozapine, an atypical antipsychotic drug, is used in the management of severely ill schizophrenic patients. Onset of antipsychotic effects can take several weeks; several months of drug use may be needed to obtain the maximum therapeutic effects.

7. Clozapine may cause agranulocytosis, which is fatal. This adverse effect has been minimized with close monitoring of patients in the "Clozaril National Registry." (Clozaril is the trade name for clozapine.) White blood cell monitoring is required prior to therapy, weekly or biweekly during therapy, and for 4 weeks after the drug is stopped.

8. The most common adverse effects of clozapine are anticholinergic effects. Other adverse effects are weight gain and constipation.

9. Rivastigmine is used in the treatment of mild to moderate dementia from Alzheimer disease. It enhances memory, language and orientation and improves ability to perform activities of daily living. Rivastigmine inhibits acetylcholinesterase, and thus increases the concentration of acetylcholine.

10. The most common adverse effects of rivastigmine are GI (nausea, vomiting, anorexia, weight loss).

KEY TERMS

Fill in the blanks

Read each statement carefully and, using the chapter's key terms, write your answer in the space provided.

1. _____ are effective in the treatment of hallucinations, delusions, and thought disorders, regardless of their etiology.

2. Antipsychotic agents are also known as _____ , because of their ability to induce extrapyramidal side effects.

3. The classic antipsychotic drugs (APs) are also called _____ agents.

4. _____ involve the nerves and muscles controlling movement and coordination.

5. A late complication of neuroleptic therapy characterized by involuntary and often persistent movements of the facial muscles and tongue is called _____ .

6. Catatonia, stupor, fever, unstable blood pressure and myoglobinemia are symptoms of _____ .

7. _____ have less potential to produce undesirable side effects related to antipsychotic drug treatment.

8. Loss of memory and cognitive skills is called _____ .

9. A form of progressive dementia, _____ is one of the most common chronic conditions and causes of dementia in the elderly.

10. _____ is a particular kind of psychosis that is characterized mainly by a clear sensorium but a marked disturbance in thinking.

11. It is unknown whether antagonism of any receptor other than _____ plays any antipsychotic role.

12. _____ is the inability to perceive and interpret reality accurately, think clearly, respond correctly, and function in a socially appropriate manner.

PHYSIOLOGY AND PATHOPHYSIOLOGY: THE BODY HUMAN

Essay

1. Identify the primary functions of the left and right hemispheres of the brain.

2. What are the functions of the frontal lobes of the brain?

3. Identify the other CNS functional systems and their responsibilities.

4. What role do the brain neurotransmitters play in the treatment of psychosis?

CORE DRUG KNOWLEDGE: JUST THE FACTS

Multiple choice

Circle the option that best answers the question or completes the statement.

1. Chlorpromazine (Thorazine) is commonly used in the treatment of
   a. schizophrenia.
   b. bipolar-affective disorder.
   c. major depression.
   d. all of the above.

2. Adverse effects commonly associated with antipsychotic drugs such as chlorpromazine (Thorazine) include
   a. gastrointestinal (GI) bleeding.
   b. profound sedation.
   c. extrapyramidal syndrome.
   d. diarrhea.

3. In men, the antidopaminergic effects of chlorpromazine (Thorazine) may induce
   a. anemia.
   b. headache.
   c. decreased libido.
   d. hyperthyroidism.

4. Concurrent use of chlorpromazine (Thorazine) with other CNS depressants may result in
   a. liver dysfunction.
   b. anemia.
   c. galactorrhea.
   d. excessive sedation.

5. Elderly patients receiving chlorpromazine (Thorazine) have an increased risk for which of the following nursing diagnoses?
   a. Impaired Physical Mobility
   b. Risk for Injury
   c. Noncompliance
   d. Sexual Dysfunction

6. Antipsychotic drugs, such as chlorpromazine (Thorazine), work by
   a. blocking neurotransmitter receptor sites.
   b. increasing the excretion of neurotransmitters.
   c. increasing the metabolism of neurotransmitters.
   d. decreasing the metabolism of neurotransmitters.

7. A potentially fatal adverse effect associated with the administration of clozapine (Clozaril) is
   a. neuroleptic malignant syndrome.
   b. agranulocytosis.
   c. hepatotoxicity.
   d. hypothyroidism.

8. Which of the following statements concerning atypical antipsychotic agents such as clozapine (Clozaril) is INCORRECT?
   a. They are efficacious in treating the symptoms of schizophrenia.
   b. They cause fewer EPS adverse effects.
   c. They block both dopamine and serotonin receptors.
   d. They cause no serious adverse effects.

9. Maximal effects from clozapine therapy should be expected in
   a. 2 weeks.
   b. several months.
   c. 24 hours.
   d. 5 days.

10. Noncompliance with antipsychotic drugs such as clozapine (Clozaril) is frequently related to
    a. changes in sexual patterns.
    b. difficulty with adherence to prescribed diet.
    c. frequency of drug-induced headaches.
    d. EPS symptoms.

11. Effectiveness of clozapine (Clozaril) is affected by intake of
    a. salt.
    b. sugar.
    c. caffeine.
    d. fats.

12. After initiating clozapine (Clozaril) therapy, the patient should be monitored for
    a. sedation.
    b. dermatitis.
    c. upper respiratory illness.
    d. hypervigilance.

13. Alzheimer's disease may be treated with
    a. chlorpromazine (Thorazine).
    b. rivastigmine (Exelon).
    c. haloperidol (Haldol).
    d. clozapine (Clozaril).

14. The drugs used in the management of Alzheimer disease
    a. alter the course of the disease.
    b. do not alter the course of the disease.
    c. increase the symptoms of the disease.
    d. all of the above.

15. Rivastigmine (Exelon) works by
    a. stimulating cholinergic activity.
    b. blocking cholinergic activity.
    c. stimulating sympathetic activity.
    d. stimulating dopaminergic activity.

16. Rivastigmine (Exelon) may induce
    a. bronchodilation.
    b. pupil dilation.
    c. increased gastric acidity.
    d. constipation.

CORE PATIENT VARIABLES: PATIENTS, PLEASE

Multiple choice

Circle the option that best answers the question or completes the statement.

1. Debbie Gentry, age 26, is taking chlorpromazine (Thorazine) for schizophrenia. Which of the following would you include in patient teaching for Debbie? Chlorpromazine may cause
   a. irregular menses.
   b. loss of hair.
   c. coarse dry skin.
   d. acne.

2. Thom Chandler comes to the clinic today for a refill of chlorpromazine. He complains about nausea, "flulike" symptoms, rash, and yellow skin. You understand that
   a. these are expected adverse effects due to the anticholinergic and antidopaminergic properties of the drug.
   b. the nausea is an expected adverse effect, but the yellow skin may mean the dose needs to be increased.
   c. these are annoying symptoms, but nothing needs to be done.
   d. these are symptoms of toxicity, and the drug should be stopped immediately.

3. Which of the following patients has the highest risk for adverse effects from chlorpromazine (Thorazine) therapy?
   a. Louise, age 36, with asthma
   b. Malcolm, age 65, with cardiovascular disease
   c. Terry, age 17, with headaches
   d. Stephanie, age 27, with hyperthyroidism

4. Susan Farmer takes chlorpromazine for schizophrenia. She comes to the clinic today and is very excited about a new horticulture class she is taking. What assessment should the nurse make related to Susan's new class?
   a. "Are you taking precautions to keep away from pesticides?"
   b. "Do you use tools that can be used to injure someone else?"
   c. "How much time do you need to spend in the sunlight?"
   d. "Are you able to handle the increased movement OK?"

5. Georgia Mays complains of EPS related to her chlorpromazine (Thorazine) therapy. You anticipate the health care provider may add
   a. a benzodiazepine.
   b. a barbiturate.
   c. an anticholinergic agent.
   d. an antidepressant.

6. Janice K., age 21, was diagnosed with schizophrenia 3 weeks ago and started taking haloperidol (Haldol). Janice is brought to the emergency department with catatonia, stupor, fever, unstable blood pressure, and myoglobinemia. Which of the following do you suspect?
   a. haloperidol overdose
   b. severe EPS
   c. anticholinergic crisis
   d. neuroleptic malignant syndrome

7. Alex T. has been taking chlorpromazine (Thorazine) for 1 year and has difficulty with recurrent EPS. What do you anticipate should be done for Alex?
   a. Monitor for tardive dyskinesia, then stop the drug should it occur.
   b. Increase the dose of chlorpromazine and add an anticholinergic.
   c. Change to an atypical antipsychotic drug such as clozapine.
   d. Decrease the dose of chlorpromazine and add an antidepressant

8. Phyllis K. has been taking clozapine (Clozaril) for 3 months. At this time, Phyllis has the greatest risk for the development of
   a. neuroleptic malignant syndrome.
   b. agranulocytosis.
   c. severe EPS.
   d. migraine headaches.

9. Jeremy R., age 16, has just been diagnosed with schizophrenia. Jeremy also has a seizure disorder. Use of which of the following antiepileptic drugs would contradict the use of clozapine (Clozaril)?
   a. carbamazepine (Tegretol)
   b. phenytoin (Dilantin)
   c. phenobarbitol (Luminol)
   d. valproic acid (Depakene)

10. Kimberly T. has been taking clozapine (Clozaril) for 1 year. She comes to the clinic today and is excited about her parents installing a hot tub in the back yard. What important patient teaching should be done with Kimberly?
    a. "Soaking for too long can damage your skin."
    b. "Be sure that there is no chlorine in the water."
    c. "You should not get in the hot tub."
    d. "Be sure to always have someone with you."

11. Patrick J. takes clozapine (Clozaril) for schizophrenia. Patient teaching for Patrick should include
    a. foods that will help him gain weight.
    b. nonpharmacologic ways to manage constipation.
    c. relaxation techniques for headaches.
    d. ways to incorporate caffeine into his diet.

12. Leland G. comes to the clinic for a refill of clozapine (Clozaril). He complains of lethargy, weakness, fever, and sore throat. You should
    a. tell the patient to rest and take lots of fluids.
    b. culture his throat.
    c. arrange for a CBC to be drawn.
    d. arrange for LFTs to be drawn.

13. Leo H. has Alzheimer's disease. He is started on rivastigmine (Exelon). Patient teaching for Leo should include
    a. cessation of smoking.
    b. low-fat foods to avoid weight gain.
    c. methods to manage constipation.
    d. need to avoid caffeine products.

14. Carey P. takes rivastigmine (Exelon) for Alzheimer disease. Carey's caregiver should monitor her
    a. breath sounds.
    b. heart rate.
    c. weight.
    d. all of the above.

15. To assess the efficacy of rivastigmine (Exelon) therapy, the nurse should assess for
    a. occurrence of adverse effects.
    b. increased cognition.
    c. weight gain.
    d. control of bladder and bowel.

16. Before administration of rivastigmine (Exelon) to an elderly patient, which of the following diagnostic tests should be done?
    a. chest x-ray
    b. arterial blood gas
    c. bone density
    d. electrocardiogram

NURSING MANAGEMENT: EVERY GOOD NURSE SHOULD . . .

Multiple choice

Circle the option that best answers the question or completes the statement.

1. Rita Gonsalves is being treated with chlorpromazine, a phenothiazine antipsychotic. She complains that her mouth is dry all of the time. The nurse should recommend
   a. rinsing the mouth with hydrogen peroxide.
   b. sucking on hard candies.
   c. increasing dietary intake of sodium.
   d. discontinuation of the chlorpromazine.

2. Vic Torres is 39 years old. He works as a brick mason. He is currently being treated with chlorpromazine, an antipsychotic. Education about his drug therapy should include
   a. the importance of wearing sunscreen and/or protective clothing while working outside.
   b. the importance of needing daily exposure to sunlight.
   c. that he should not be working while on drug therapy.
   d. that his urine may turn blue while on drug therapy.

3. Harry Liebman has been on a daily maintenance dose of chlorpromazine for 3 weeks. He returns to the clinic complaining of feeling dizzy when he first gets out of bed and stands up. He also complains of being sleepy all the time during the daytime. To minimize these adverse effects, the nurse should recommend that he
   a. increase the dose of chlorpromazine.
   b. stand up quickly.
   c. eat six large meals a day.
   d. take the drug at bedtime.

4. Mary Jones is taking clozapine for schizophrenia. She complains to you that she is having trouble with constipation. To minimize this adverse effect you should recommend
   a. limiting her exercise.
   b. encouraging oral fluid intake.
   c. eating more bland, soft foods.
   d. all of the above
   e. none of the above

5. To maximize the therapeutic effect of rivastigmine given for Alzheimer disease, the nurse should do which of the following prior to starting therapy?

   a. Confirm that there are no current, uncorrected hearing problems.

   b. Take away the patient's glasses to prevent injury.

   c. Confirm that the patient is reliable enough to self dose his medications.

   d. All of the above

CASE STUDY

Marty McGinnis, 62 years old, is schizophrenic and lives in a halfway house. He takes chlorpromazine every night. One day when he is in the clinic for a follow-up visit, he tells you, the nurse, that he got in trouble at the halfway house for eating another man's piece of toast at breakfast. He said he couldn't help himself, he was just so hungry.

1. What teaching should you give to Marty?

2. What referrals to community agencies might you give to Marty?

CRITICAL THINKING CHALLENGE

Marty has to be out of the house between 8:00 AM and 6:00 PM. It is a particularly warm summer. One day Marty is found collapsed on the street and is taken to the local hospital's emergency room. He is diagnosed with heat stroke.

Discuss what factors have contributed to heat stroke in Marty.

CHAPTER 20

Drugs For Treating Seizure Disorders

TOP TEN THINGS TO KNOW ABOUT DRUGS FOR TREATING SEIZURE DISORDERS

1. Most antiepileptic drugs (AED) control seizures by altering sodium channels on the neuronal cell membrane (thereby limiting the spread of seizure activity) or by enhancing the activity or concentration of the brain's inhibitory neurotransmitter gamma-aminobutyric acid (GABA), restoring a balance between excitatory and inhibitory neurotransmitters.

2. The choice of AED depends on the type of seizures and on patient-related variables such as age and health status. Monotherapy is the desired goal, although combination therapy may be necessary.

3. AEDs are all central nervous system (CNS) depressants, and CNS depressant adverse effects are common. Other CNS depressants, such as alcohol, will cause additive CNS depression and should be avoided.

4. Sudden withdrawal of AEDs may precipitate seizures or status epilepticus. IV diazepam, a benzodiazepine, is the drug of first choice for status epilepticus. Other benzodiazepines, phenytoin, or phenobarbital may also be used (usually as adjuncts).

5. Nursing management for AEDs include: have patients take prescribed drug at regular intervals, monitor blood drug levels to determine therapeutic or toxic levels, instruct in the importance of wearing Medic-Alert bracelet stating they have epilepsy, encourage good oral hygiene (with phenytoin), teach to avoid sudden cessation of AED, teach safety precautions relevant to CNS depression, and teach to avoid simultaneous use of other CNS depressants.

6. Phenytoin, a hydantoin AED, is the drug of choice for most seizures, except absence seizures. It controls seizures by promoting sodium efflux from the neurons to stabilize the cell membrane, but causes little or no sedative effects. Half-life increases as dose increases. Numerous drug interactions may occur, usually altering metabolism of either drug. Drug absorption will be decreased if given within 2 hours of an antacid or if given via NGI or GT along with tube feedings.

7. The most common adverse effects of phenytoin are related to CNS depression. A fairly common adverse effect is gingival hyperplasia, which may be disfiguring. If phenytoin is given too rapidly IV, cardiovascular collapse, hypotension, and significant CNS depression may occur. A known syndrome of fetal teratogenic effects occurs when phenytoin is used in pregnancy.

8. Clonazepam is a benzodiazepine that is used to treat seizures. Like other benzodiazepines, it suppresses the spread of seizure activity but does not abolish the abnormal focal discharge. Phenobarbital, a generalized CNS depressant and sedative/hypnotic, can also be used to treat seizures. Newer AEDs that cause less CNS depression have generally replaced phenobarbital in AED therapy.

9. Ethosuximide, a succinimide, is used in managing and controlling absence seizures. It elevates seizure threshold and reduces synaptic nerve response to low-frequency repetitive stimulation. Carbamazepine, a miscellaneous AED, treats psychomotor and grand mal seizures. Because of potential fatal adverse effects (agranulocytosis and aplastic anemia), its use is generally restricted to patients who have not responded satisfactorily to other AEDs.

10. Newer AEDs are considered adjunct anticonvulsants and are usually used in combination with other AEDs. They work in various ways. They include gabapentin, lamotrigine, tiagabine, valproic acid, topiramate, felbamate, levetiracetam, zonisamide, and vigabatrin (Canada). Two of them have potential fatal adverse effects: felbamate (aplastic anemia and acute hepatic failure, mostly in adults) and valproic acid (acute hepatic failure, mostly in children 2 years or younger).

KEY TERMS

Fill in the blanks

Read each statement carefully and, using the chapter's key terms, write your answer in the space provided.

1. A systematic, widely accepted categorization of seizure activity is known as _____.

2. When a seizure is in process, this is referred to as the _____ phase.

3. A _____ is caused by disturbances of nerve cells in more diffuse areas and both hemispheres of the brain.

4. The _____ phase of a seizure is when abnormal movements cease.

5. An _____ seizure is also known as a petit-mal seizure.

6. A _____ is paroxysmal involuntary alterations of behavior, movement, or sensation, triggered by an abnormal electric discharge in the brain.

7. A _____ is subdivided into simple, complex, and secondarily generalized seizures.

8. A grand-mal seizure is also called _____.

9. A chronic condition characterized by recurrent, unprovoked seizures is labeled _____.

10. _____ is the main inhibitory neurotransmitter in the mammalian central nervous system.

11. A process known as _____ transforms a presumably normal neural network into one that is abnormally hyperexcitable.

12. A patient who experiences seizure after seizure is said to have _____.

13. _____ is an amino acid that helps carry electrical impulses from one neuron to another.

PHYSIOLOGY AND PATHOPHYSIOLOGY: THE BODY HUMAN

Essay

1. Neuronal cell membrane stability is affected by:

2. Uncontrolled electrical impulses and excessive neuronal firing are prevented by:

3. Seizures result from:

CORE DRUG KNOWLEDGE: JUST THE FACTS

Multiple choice

Circle the option that best answers the question or completes the statement.

1. Which of the following statements concerning phenytoin (Dilantin) is INCORRECT?
   a. widely used AED for tonic-clonic seizure activity
   b. most effective AED for absence seizures
   c. used as prophylaxis for postsurgical neuro patients
   d. may also be used in the treatment of trigeminal neuralgia

2. The therapeutic margin (index) for phenytoin (Dilantin) is
   a. 10 to 20 μg/mL.
   b. 2 to 10 μg/mL.
   c. 40 to 100 μg/mL.
   d. 4 to 12 μg/mL.

3. Phenytoin (Dilantin) inhibits seizure activity by promoting
   a. calcium influx from the neurons in the motor cortex of the brain.
   b. sodium influx from the neurons in the motor cortex of the brain.
   c. calcium efflux from the neurons in the motor cortex of the brain.
   d. sodium efflux from the neurons in the motor cortex of the brain.

4. Which of the following adverse effects would necessitate cessation of phenytoin (Dilantin) therapy?
   a. acne
   b. urine discoloration
   c. gingival hyperplasia
   d. blistered skin rash

5. Which of the following drugs is not acceptable for the treatment of status epilepticus?
   a. diazepam (Valium)
   b. phenobarbital (Luminal)
   c. ethosuximide (Zarontin)
   d. phenytoin (Dilantin)

6. Which of the following adverse effects is NOT associated with clonazepam (Klonopin)?
   a. sedation
   b. gingival hyperplasia
   c. urinary retention
   d. visual disturbances

7. What drug–drug interaction would you anticipate with clonazepam (Klonopin) and alcohol?
   a. decreased renal clearance
   b. decreased absorption
   c. increased sedation
   d. increased rate of metabolism

8. The drug of choice for the treatment of absence seizures is
   a. valproic acid (Depakene).
   b. ethosuximide (Zarontin).
   c. diazepam (Valium).
   d. carbamazepine (Tegretol).

9. The therapeutic margin (index) for ethosuximide (Zarontin) is
   a. 10 to 20 μg/mL.
   b. 40 to 100 μg/mL.
   c. 2 to 10 μg/mL.
   d. 4 to 12 μg/mL.

10. During ethosuximide (Zarontin) therapy, patients with a history of mental health disturbances may experience
    a. emotional disturbances.
    b. sedation.
    c. headache.
    d. hiccups.

11. Pharmacotherapeutics for carbamazepine (Tegretol) include
    a. bipolar disorder.
    b. absence seizures.
    c. restless leg syndrome.
    d. parkinsonism.

12. The therapeutic margin (index) for carbamazepine (Tegretol) is
    a. 10 to 20 μg/mL.
    b. 40 to 100 μg/mL.
    c. 2 to 10 μg/mL.
    d. 4 to 12 μg/mL.

13. Carbamazepine (Tegretol) is contraindicated for patients with a history of hypersensitivity to
    a. monamine oxidase inhibitors.
    b. lithium.
    c. tricyclic antidepressants.
    d. selected serotonin reuptake inhibitors.

14. A benefit of gabapentin (Neurontin) therapy is
    a. minimal drug–drug interactions.
    b. extensive pharmacotherapeutic profile.
    c. once-a-day dosing.
    d. all of the above.

15. One of the most serious potential adverse effects of phenobarbital (Luminol) therapy is
    a. bone marrow depression.
    b. Stevens-Johnson syndrome.
    c. respiratory depression.
    d. migraine headaches.

16. In the elderly, phenobarbital (Luminol) therapy may induce
    a. excitement and confusion.
    b. lethargy and hypertension.
    c. headache and tachypnea.
    d. suicide ideation.

CORE PATIENT VARIABLES: PATIENTS, PLEASE

Multiple choice

Circle the option that best answers the question or completes the statement.

1. Michael Tate, a competitive marathon runner, has a seizure disorder that began after a motor vehicle accident. Which of the following antiseizure drugs may be inappropriate for use with Michael?
   a. phenobarbital (Luminol)
   b. valproic acid (Depakene)
   c. phenytoin (Dilantin)
   d. ethosuximide (Zarontin)

2. Phenytoin (Dilantin) is a pregnancy Category _____ drug.
   a. A
   b. D
   c. C
   d. X

3. Which of the following cultural groups may have a decreased ability to metabolize phenytoin (Dilantin)?

   a. Native American

   b. Hispanic

   c. Pacific Asian

   d. African American

4. Which of the following patients would NOT be a good candidate for clonazepam (Klonopin) therapy?

   a. Jennifer, with a history of drug abuse

   b. Allison, with a history of cardiac arrhythmias

   c. Mary, with a history of hypertension

   d. Eleanor, with a history of peptic ulcer disease

5. To maximize therapeutic effects of clonazepam (Klonopin), the patient should

   a. keep the medication in the refrigerator.

   b. take the medication with milk or food.

   c. take the medication only once a day.

   d. store the medication in a light-resistant container.

6. Murry Amos, age 18, calls the clinic and tells the advice nurse, "My friends all make fun of me because I have to take clonazepam (Klonopin). I'm not coming for my appointment and I'm just going to stop taking this medication." The best response would be

   a. "It doesn't matter what your friends think, but if you want to stop the medication, just go ahead."

   b. "I understand your problem. I'll cancel your appointment."

   c. "If you stop your medication abruptly, you may experience hallucinations or seizures."

   d. "Sounds like you are upset. Would you like to see the psychiatrist?"

7. Jonathan Harris has been prescribed ethosuximide (Zarontin) for his absence seizure disorder. He tells you he has had hepatitis in the past. Which of the following lab tests should be completed before initiating therapy?

   a. CBC

   b. arterial blood gas

   c. AST, ALT

   d. BUN, creatinine clearance

8. Which of the following laboratory tests should be completed before initiating carbamazepine (Tegretol) therapy?

   a. CBC

   b. AST, ALT

   c. BUN, creatinine clearance

   d. all of the above

9. Cody Williams takes carbamazepine (Tegretol) for seizures and works as a crossing guard at the local school. Cody should be cautioned to

   a. take her medication when she returns home from work.

   b. wear protective clothing and wear sunscreen.

   c. take her medication on an empty stomach.

   d. monitor her blood sugar before she goes to work.

10. Wanda Smith takes carbamazepine (Tegretol). She calls the clinic and complains of a sore throat and easy bruising. You would advise Wanda to

    a. stop taking the drug and make an appointment to be seen next week.

    b. continue taking the drug and make an appointment to be seen next week.

    c. come to the clinic to be seen today.

    d. increase her intake of green leafy vegetables and call if the symptoms continue.

11. Valproic acid should be avoided in patients with a history of

    a. hepatic dysfunction.

    b. COPD.

    c. mental health disorders.

    d. Parkinson's disease.

12. Keeghan Morris, age 22, calls the clinic and states she is having trouble swallowing her topiramate (Topamax) tablets. You would advise her to

    a. crush the tablet and place it in a glass of water.

    b. chew the tablet.

    c. continue to swallow the medication whole and make an appointment to discuss the problem with her health care provider.

    d. break the tablet in half and chew it.

13. Leslie W. was brought to the Emergency Department after having a seizure. Leslie states that she has consistently taken her primidone (Mysoline) twice a day. Which of the following STAT tests would be indicated for Leslie?

    a. Mysoline level

    b. phenobarbital level

    c. liver function tests

    d. renal function tests

NURSING MANAGEMENT: EVERY GOOD NURSE SHOULD . . .

Multiple choice

Circle the option that best answers the question or completes the statement.

1. Your patient is receiving phenytoin for seizures. There are new orders to start the patient on cimetidine for a gastric ulcer. You should

    a. administer both drugs as ordered.

    b. administer cimetidine on one day and phenytoin the next day.

    c. verify if drug interactions exist between the drugs.

    d. obtain an order for an oral antacid to be given with both drugs.

2. Your patient has been stabilized on phenytoin and is to start on theophylline, a drug known to increase the metabolism of phenytoin. The nurse should expect to

    a. monitor blood phenytoin levels for a drop compared to before theophylline therapy.

    b. monitor blood phenytoin levels for an increase compared to before theophylline therapy.

    c. monitor blood theophylline levels; they may remain below therapeutic levels due to phenytoin.

    d. monitor blood theophylline levels; they may become toxic due to phenytoin.

3. Alma Rigger is 22 years old and receives phenytoin for seizures. Her disease is well controlled, and she has not had a seizure for 5 years. During her routine follow-up visit, she tells you she is getting married and would like to have children. She asks if she should stay on the phenytoin if she becomes pregnant. Your best response would be that

    a. phenytoin is safe to use during pregnancy.

    b. she should stop using the phenytoin as soon as she becomes pregnant.

    c. before she attempts to become pregnant, she should consult with her health care provider to see if she could be weaned off the phenytoin.

    d. she may remain on the phenytoin as long as her blood levels remain in the therapeutic range.

4. Olive Martin is receiving nutrition through continuous tube feeding (30 mL/hour). She is to receive phenytoin suspension via her G tube every 8 hours. To maximize therapeutic effects of the phenytoin, the nurse should

    a. mix the phenytoin with 200 mL of tube feeding and administer at 30 mL/hour.

    b. mix the phenytoin with 100 mL of tube feeding and administer as a bolus.

    c. turn the tube feeding off for 1 hour before and 1 hour after administering phenytoin.

    d. turn the tube feeding off for 8 hours, then administer all three daily doses of phenytoin as one bolus.

5. You are to give phenytoin IV to your patient who is experiencing status epilepticus and who did not respond to IV diazepam. To minimize the risk of serious adverse effects to this patient, you should

    a. provide good oral hygiene.

    b. administer the drug slowly.

    c. obtain a blood phenytoin level before administering the drug.

    d. warn the patient that he may be drowsy.

3. Jared is 6 years old and is to be started on ethosuximide for absence seizures. What information should be included in teaching for him and his parents?

    a. Initially, he may have drowsiness, but this should go away after he has been on the drug awhile.

    b. Fever is a common and nonserious adverse effect.

    c. If a dose is missed, it may be made up by doubling the dose the next time.

    d. Avoid eating fried foods, as this may produce a drug–food interaction.

7. April Conroy has been started on carbamazepine for her grand mal seizures, which have not been controlled by several other AEDs. To minimize adverse effects, the nurse should teach April the importance of

   a. returning for lab appointments and follow up.

   b. increasing fluid intake.

   c. driving a car, to maintain independence.

   d. all of the above.

   e. none of the above.

CASE STUDY

Elizabeth is 8 years old and is started on phenytoin suspension 125 mg BID (125 mg/5 mL) for seizures. When she returns for her first visit after drug therapy was initiated, her mother reports that the seizures have not improved. Her blood phenytoin level is 4 (therapeutic levels are usually 10 to 20 µg/mL). Based on these findings, Elizabeth's daily dose of phenytoin is increased. Two weeks later, her mother rushes Elizabeth to the emergency room. Her eyes are moving in unusual patterns (nystagmus), and her speech is slurred. Her blood phenytoin level is now 24.

1. What is your assessment of her condition?

2. What questions should you ask the mother to gain understanding as to what may have contributed to her current condition?

CRITICAL THINKING CHALLENGE

Ted Lewis is receiving phenytoin for seizures. He returns for a checkup. He reports that his seizures are well controlled by the drug therapy. His blood phenytoin level is 8. The physician increases the dose so Ted's blood level will be in normal levels. Ted returns in a week complaining of his eyes bothering him, an awkward gait, and confusion. His blood phenytoin level is now 14.

1. What is your assessment of his current findings?

2. What explanation can be made for this assessment?

CHAPTER 21

Drugs Affecting Muscle Spasm and Spasticity

TOP TEN THINGS TO KNOW ABOUT DRUGS FOR TREATING NEUROMUSCULAR FUNCTION

1. A muscle spasm is a sudden violent involuntary contraction of a muscle or group of muscles.

2. Spasticity is a condition in which certain muscles are continuously contracted. This contraction causes stiffness or tightness of the muscles and may interfere with gait, movement, or speech. Damage to the portion of the brain or spinal cord that controls voluntary movement usually causes spasticity.

3. Centrally acting muscle relaxants do not act on painful muscles; rather, they work by their central nervous system (CNS) depressant activity. Most centrally acting muscle relaxants are not effective in the treatment of spasticity.

4. In addition to their CNS depressant effects, centrally acting muscle relaxants have anticholinergic and antihistaminic effects.

5. Cyclobenzaprine is used in the management of muscle spasms associated with acute musculoskeletal disorders, such as low back strain. It relieves muscle spasms through a central action, possibly at the level of the brain stem, with no direct action on the neuromuscular junction or the muscle involved. It reduces pain and tenderness and improves mobility.

6. The common adverse effects of cyclobenzaprine are related to its CNS depression and anticholinergic activity.

7. Baclofen, a centrally acting spasmolytic, is a derivative of the neurotransmitter gamma aminobutyric acid (GABA). It acts at the spinal end of the upper motor neurons at GABA receptors to cause hyperpolarization; this reduces excessive reflex spasms and spasticity, allowing muscle relaxation.

8. Baclofen is used to relieve spasticity from the spinal motor neurons, such as in multiple sclerosis and traumatic lesions of the spinal cord (paraplegia). Baclofen is not useful in spasticity resulting from disorders of the CNS above the spinal motor neurons, such as Parkinson's disease or cerebrovascular accident (CVA). CNS adverse effects, especially sedation, are the most common.

9. Dantrolene, a peripherally acting spasmolytic, acts directly on the muscle cells by reducing the amount of calcium released from the sarcoplasmic reticulum, resulting in muscle relaxation. It does not interfere with neuromuscular communication or have CNS effects.

10. Dantrolene is used to treat or prevent malignant hyperthermia and to treat upper motor neuron disorders. The most common adverse effect is muscle weakness. Fatal hepatitis is possible, especially in women older than 35 taking estrogens.

KEY TERMS

Matching

Match the following key terms with their definitions.

1. _____ spasm

2. _____ spasticity

3. _____ centrally acting

4. _____ peripherally acting

5. _____ spasmolytic

6. _____ tonic spasm

7. _____ clonic spasm

a. Contractions of the affected muscles take place repeatedly, forcibly, and in quick succession, with equally sudden and frequent relaxations

b. Characterized by an unusually prolonged and strong muscular contraction, with relaxation taking place slowly

c. Condition in which certain muscles are continuously contracted

d. Drugs that work in the CNS to reduce excessive reflex activity and allow muscle relaxation

e. Drugs that relax a muscle by a direct action within the skeletal muscle fiber

f. Drugs that act in the CNS to reduce the perception of pain induced from muscle spasm

g. Sudden violent involuntary contraction of a muscle or a group of muscles

PHYSIOLOGY AND PATHOPHYSIOLOGY: THE BODY HUMAN

Essay

1. What two contractile proteins are integral to muscle contraction?

2. Describe the sliding filament theory.

3. List potential etiologies of muscle spasm.

4. List potential etiologies of muscle spasticity.

5. List symptoms of spasticity.

CORE DRUG KNOWLEDGE: JUST THE FACTS

Multiple choice

Circle the option that best answers the question or completes the statement.

1. Optimal effects of cyclobenzaprine (Flexeril) therapy should occur within
   a. 1 week.
   b. 12 hours.
   c. 1 to 2 days.
   d. 2 hours.

2. Cyclobenzaprine (Flexeril) is INEFFECTIVE in the management of
   a. tonic spasms.
   b. clonic spasms.
   c. strained muscles.
   d. cerebral palsy.

3. Cyclobenzaprine (Flexeril) is structurally similar to
   a. tricyclic antidepressants.
   b. lithium.
   c. phenothiazines.
   d. selective-serotonin reuptake inhibitors.

4. Serious adverse effects of cyclobenzaprine (Flexeril) therapy affect the
   a. gastrointestinal (GI) system.
   b. cardiovascular system.
   c. CNS.
   d. integumentary system.

5. Pharmacotherapeutics for baclofen (Lioresal) includes
   a. Huntington's chorea.
   b. Parkinson disease.
   c. cerebral vascular accidents.
   d. multiple sclerosis.

6. Which of the following symptoms is NOT associated with abrupt withdrawal of baclofen (Lioresal)?
   a. agitation
   b. hyperglycemia
   c. exacerbation of spasticity
   d. seizure

7. Which of the following drugs is similar to baclofen?
   a. midazolam (Versed)
   b. tizanidine (Zanaflex)
   c. succinylcholine (Anectine)
   d. orphenadrine (Norflex)

8. Malignant hyperthermia is treated with which of the following drugs?
   a. baclofen (Lioresal)
   b. dantrolene (Dantrium)
   c. tubocurarine (Tubarine)
   d. succinylcholine (Anectine)

9. Dantrolene works by
   a. interfering with pseudocholinesterase.
   b. reducing the amount of calcium from the sarcoplasmic reticulum.
   c. increasing cellular potassium.
   d. interrupting cerebral recognition of pain stimulus.

10. Which of the following disorders is NOT a precaution to dantrolene therapy?
    a. active liver disease
    b. cardiac disease
    c. pulmonary dysfunction
    d. increased intraocular pressure

CORE PATIENT VARIABLES: PATIENTS, PLEASE

Multiple choice

Circle the option that best answers the question or completes the statement.

1. Which of the following patients has the highest risk for increased anticholinergic and CNS depressant effects of cyclobenzaprine (Flexeril)?
   a. Abby, age 45, with asthma
   b. Ben, age 56, with musculoskeletal back pain
   c. Carey, age 68, with hypothyroidism
   d. David, age 17, with chronic sinus infections

2. Jeremy Jones, age 45, was involved in a motor vehicle accident 1 year ago. He has been taking cyclobenzaprine (Flexeril) and ibuprofen (Motrin) since the accident. Mr. Jones is scheduled for back surgery in the morning. The nurse should review the doctor's orders to ensure that
   a. physical therapy has been ordered.
   b. cyclobenzaprine has been ordered as a continuous or tapered medication.
   c. ibuprofen has been ordered as a continuous or tapered medication.
   d. occupational therapy has been ordered.

3. Kimberly Weeks is being discharged from the hospital with a prescription for cyclobenzaprine (Flexeril). Discharge instructions should include
   a. "Assess your level of sedation before driving a car."
   b. "Take this medication only at bedtime."
   c. "Be sure to eat lots of vegetables."
   d. "Limit your alcohol intake to three glasses of wine a day."

4. Elderly patients on baclofen (Lioresal) therapy have an increased risk for
   a. hallucinations.
   b. hyperglycemia.
   c. urinary frequency.
   d. rash.

5. Alan Jones, age 28, is taking baclofen for muscle spasms in his back. What assessment of lifestyle, diet, and habits should the nurse do?
   a. sugar intake
   b. smoking history
   c. alcohol ingestion
   d. all of the above

6. John Deery takes dantrolene for multiple sclerosis. Which of the following adverse effects may occur?
   a. rash
   b. drooling
   c. aplastic anemia
   d. all of the above

7. Johe Henry, age 40, has been prescribed dantrolene for multiple sclerosis. Mrs. Henry denies other medical problems. She takes combination birth control pills to avoid pregnancy. Mrs. Henry may have an increased risk for _____ during dantrolene therapy.

    a. sedation

    b. aplastic anemia

    c. liver damage

    d. dizziness

8. Patient teaching for dantrolene therapy should include

    a. increase fluids to 3 L per day

    b. omit salt from the diet

    c. for missed doses, double the next dose

    d. avoid ultraviolet light

NURSING MANAGEMENT: EVERY GOOD NURSE SHOULD . . .

Multiple choice

Please circle the option that best answers the question or completes the statement.

1. Mary Kay O'Hare, 75 years old, was in a car accident and strained her back muscles. She is started on cyclobenzaprine to treat the painful spasms she is experiencing in her back. Five days after starting treatment, she calls the clinic and complains of a severely dry mouth. As the nurse in the clinic, your best response to her would be

    a. "This is a sign of a significant drug interaction. Stop taking the cyclobenzaprine."

    b. "This is a common adverse effect from cyclobenzaprine. Try sucking on hard candies to relieve your dry mouth."

    c. "This indicates that you are allergic to cyclobenzaprine. Come into the clinic today to be checked."

    d. "This is the desired effect of the drug , and indicates that cyclobenzaprine is working effectively."

2. Steve Andrews, 30 years old, fell off scaffolding at his construction job and was severely injured. He has been on cyclobenzaprine, 10 mg TID, for the last 4 months to treat severe back spasms. At this time, his back spasms have decreased and he would like to stop taking the cyclobenzaprine. His physician has told him he can stop drug therapy whenever the spasms are no longer painful. In providing the patient education to this patient, the nurse should teach Mr. Andrews to

    a. "Stop the drug completely tomorrow."

    b. "Take only 1 pill today and tomorrow and then stop drug therapy."

    c. "Take 2 pills a day for the next month, then 1 pill a day for a month, and then stop drug therapy."

    d. "Take 2 pills a day for the next 7 days, then 1 pill a day for 7 days, and then stop drug therapy."

3. Darryl Ford was started yesterday on baclofen, a centrally acting spasmolytic, to treat his multiple sclerosis. Which of the following is appropriate to minimize adverse effects from the baclofen?

    a. Assist Mr. Ford in ambulating.

    b. Encourage Mr. Ford to stand up and touch his toes.

    c. Offer Mr. Ford a glass of wine with dinner.

    d. Provide Mr. Ford with large, full meals.

4. Barbara Watson has progressing multiple sclerosis. She is on dantrolene, a peripherally acting spasmolytic. Her husband tells the visiting home health nurse that she is not eating well due to difficulty in swallowing. She has periods of choking. He asks if he should discontinue her drug therapy. The best response of the nurse is

    a. "Continue giving the dantrolene as long as she can swallow the capsules."

    b. "Mix the contents of the capsule with a small amount of fruit juice."

    c. "Administer half of the capsule instead of a whole capsule."

    d. "Stop administering the dantrolene."

CASE STUDY

Frank Carlisle, 38 years old, has amyotrophic lateral sclerosis (ALS) and is receiving baclofen to treat the spasms associated with the disease. He also is a diabetic and takes miglitol, an oral antidiabetic drug. When he returns to the clinic for follow-up in 1 month, he complains of fatigue and weakness. He also states that he has urinary frequency.

1. What questions should be asked to determine the exact cause of his symptoms?

2. What lab work should be done to assess for other complications of therapy? (Hint: See the discussion in Chapter 22 on ALS for more information.)

CRITICAL THINKING CHALLENGE

Frank Carlisle adjusts to baclofen therapy and reports that the sedative effects have diminished greatly. After 6 months of baclofen therapy, however, he becomes depressed. He is treated with amitriptyline (Elavil), an antidepressant that he takes once a day in the morning. After 1 week on the amitriptyline, his wife calls to report that he is very lethargic all day and can barely keep his eyes open.

1. What explanation for these effects can you offer to Mrs. Carlisle?

2. What nursing interventions can you suggest to help minimize these adverse effects?

CHAPTER 22

Drugs for Treating Parkinson Disease and Other Movement Disorders

TOP TEN THINGS TO KNOW ABOUT DRUGS FOR TREATING PARKINSON DISEASE AND OTHER MOVEMENT DISORDERS

1. Movement disorders are chronic, severe, and debilitating.
2. None of the currently available drug therapies are curative for movement disorders.
3. Parkinson disease is a disruption in the balanced antagonism between dopamine and acetylcholine.
4. Drug therapy in Parkinson disease is aimed at increasing the amount of dopamine and/or blocking the effect of acetylcholine.
5. Dopaminergic drugs, such as carbidopa-levodopa, work by increasing dopamine in the brain. Anticholinergic drugs, such as benztropine, work by blocking the effect of acetylcholine.
6. Drug therapy for Parkinson disease loses its effectiveness with long-term use; therefore, therapy is usually withheld until activities of daily living are severely compromised by the disease.

7. Neuroleptic malignant syndrome may occur with abrupt cessation of dopaminergic drugs.
8. Bradykinetic episodes may occur with long-term use of dopaminergic drugs.
9. The goal of riluzole drug therapy for ALS is to delay respiratory compromise and the need for tracheostomy or mechanical ventilation.
10. Women and native Japanese are at a higher risk of developing adverse effects from riluzole due to mechanisms of drug metabolism.

KEY TERMS

Anagrams

Using the following definitions, unscramble each of the following sets of letters to form a word. Write your response in the spaces provided.

1. idiopathic parkinsonism

   L S P R A Y A S I G A N A I T S

   ☐☐☐☐☐☐☐☐☐☐

   ☐☐☐☐☐☐

2. clenching of the teeth associated with forceful lateral or protrusive jaw movements

   X B M S U R I   ☐☐☐☐☐☐☐

3. "on–off effect"

   T K D B R C N A E I Y I P D S O E S E I

   ☐☐☐☐☐☐☐☐☐☐☐☐☐

   ☐☐☐☐☐☐☐☐

4. functionally related nuclei located in each cerebral hemisphere

   A B L S A G N L A I A G

   ☐☐☐☐☐ ☐☐☐☐☐☐☐

5. loss of voluntary movement

   A A N I E K S I   ☐☐☐☐☐☐☐☐

6. jerking, flinging movements of an extremity

   S L A B L S M I U

   ☐☐☐☐☐☐☐☐☐

7. group of darkly pigmented cells in the midbrain

   T B S A I A U S N T G I A N R

   ☐☐☐☐☐☐☐☐☐☐

   ☐☐☐☐☐

8. drugs that promote activation of dopamine receptors

   P E G C D O M R I N I A

   ☐☐☐☐☐☐☐☐☐☐☐☐

9. characterized by an abrupt onset of marked rigidity, akinesia, tremor, and hyperpyrexia

   O C R I U T E P N E L G T I N L A A N M

   D E N M Y O S R

   ☐☐☐☐☐☐☐☐☐

   ☐☐☐☐☐☐☐☐

   ☐☐☐☐☐☐☐

10. primary nuclei located deep within the cerebrum

    P R O U S C T R T U S M A I

    ☐☐☐☐☐☐

    ☐☐☐☐☐☐☐

11. abnormal slowness of movement

    K Y E A I B A S I N D R

    ☐☐☐☐☐☐☐☐☐☐☐☐

12. disorder that ceases with withdrawal of the offending drug

    S M N S I I K N R O A P

    ☐☐☐☐☐☐☐☐☐☐☐☐

PHYSIOLOGY AND PATHOPHYSIOLOGY: THE BODY HUMAN

Essay

1. Identify structures in the extrapyramidal "system."

2. Why does the basal ganglia produce the neurotransmitters dopamine and acetylcholine?

3. Parkinson's disease is called a "naturally occurring disease." What does this mean?

4. List the symptoms that result from the imbalance between dopamine and acetylcholine.

5. What is the difference between parkinsonism and Parkinson disease?

6. What is the usual progression of amyotrophic lateral sclerosis (ALS)?

CORE DRUG KNOWLEDGE: JUST THE FACTS

Multiple choice

Circle the option that best answers the question or completes the statement.

1. Carbidopa-levodopa (Sinemet) works by
   a. blocking the action of acetylcholine.
   b. blocking the action of dopamine.
   c. increasing activation of dopamine receptors in the brain.
   d. increasing activation of acetylcholine receptors in the brain.

2. Carbidopa-levodopa (Sinemet) is preferred over plain levodopa in drug treatment of Parkinson disease because
   a. it is better absorbed from the GI tract.
   b. it induces less CNS adverse effects.
   c. it allows more dopamine to reach the brain.
   d. it can be administered once a day.

3. Which of the following adverse effects is not associated with the use of carbidopa/levodopa (Sinemet)?
   a. thrombocytopenia
   b. suicidal tendencies
   c. ballismus
   d. bruxism

4. Drug interactions with carbidopa/levodopa (Sinemet) include:
   a. most antibiotics
   b. thiazide diuretics
   c. hydantoins
   d. cardiac glycosides

5. Centrally acting anticholinergic drugs are used in the management of Parkinson disease to
   a. inhibit the release of dopamine.
   b. increase the release of dopamine.
   c. inhibit the release of acetylcholine.
   d. increase the release of acetylcholine.

6. Tolcapone (Tasmar) is used in the management of Parkinson disease to
   a. increase the amount of levodopa that reaches the brain.
   b. decrease the amount of levodopa that reaches the brain.
   c. block the conversion of levodopa to dopamine.
   d. increase the rate of conversion of levodopa to dopamine.

7. Dopamine agonists such as pramipexole (Mirapex) and ropinirole (Requip) are used to
   a. block the adverse effects of carbidopa-levodopa.
   b. decrease the amount of carbidopa-levodopa needed to control the symptoms of Parkinson disease.
   c. block the action of acetylcholine in the periphery of the body.
   d. increase the conversion of levodopa to dopamine.

8. A therapeutic indication for riluzole (Rilutek) is
   a. Parkinson disease.
   b. multiple sclerosis.
   c. amyotrophic lateral sclerosis.
   d. Alzheimer disease.

9. When given concurrently with riluzole, inhibitors of CYP1A2, such as caffeine or theophylline may induce
   a. an increased risk for toxicity.
   b. subtherapeutic blood levels of riluzole.
   c. delayed absorption.
   d. increased elimination.

10. Which of the following drugs would be INAPPROPRIATE for use in the management of multiple sclerosis (MS)?
    a. bromocriptine (Parlodel)
    b. Interferon β
    c. glatiramer acetate (Copaxone)
    d. oxybutynin (Ditropan)

CORE PATIENT VARIABLES: PATIENTS, PLEASE

Multiple choice

Circle the option that best answers the question or completes the statement.

1. You are assessing the patient's health status for contraindications for carbidopa-levodopa therapy. Which of the following statements would you report to the provider?
   a. "My ophthalmologist says my glaucoma is getting worse."
   b. "I have recurrent urinary tract infections."
   c. "I've been taking amitriptyline (Elavil) for my depression."
   d. "I haven't had a migraine in 6 months."

2. Mrs. X. is taking carbidopa-levodopa. In your assessment of lifestyle, diet, and habits, which of the following statements by the patient would you need to address?
   a. "I just love avocados! I could just eat them every day."
   b. "I tend to watch my meat intake because it just bothers my stomach."
   c. "I eat bran flakes every morning."
   d. "I drink at least 8 glasses of water a day."

3. Which of the following cultural groups may need dosing adjustments for symptom management of Parkinson disease?

   a. Hispanic

   b. African American

   c. Chinese

   d. Caucasian

4. Mrs. K. has Parkinson disease and has been taking carbidopa-levodopa (Sinemet) for several years. Because of many adverse effects, Mrs. K. wishes to stop the drug. What should you tell Mrs. K.?

   a. "Drink lots of water in the next week to flush the drug out of your system."

   b. "You really need to see the doctor before making that decision."

   c. "Just decrease your dose to only once a day and see how you feel."

   d. "That should be fine—I'll make an appointment for you to see the doctor next month."

5. Your patient is taking carbidopa-levodopa (Sinemet) and ropinirole (Requip) for Parkinson disease. She asks, "Why do I need to take both of these drugs?" How would you respond?

   a. "Taking these drugs together decreases the potential for adverse effects."

   b. "That is just the way this disease is treated."

   c. "Why don't you ask the doctor that question?"

   d. Taking these drugs together stops the progression of the disease."

6. Before initiation of therapy with riluzole, the nurse should assess all of the following laboratory data EXCEPT

   a. renal function.

   b. complete blood count.

   c. arterial blood gases.

   d. hepatic function.

7. Which of the following should be assessed related to the core patient variable, environment, for the patient on riluzole therapy?

   a. ability to climb stairs

   b. ability to refrigerate the drug

   c. ability to cover the cost of the drug

   d. ability to store in a warm environment

8. Mrs. L. is prescribed riluzole (Rilutek) for ALS. Patient teaching should include

   a. "Don't worry about your diet—you need all the calories you can get."

   b. "Limit caffeine and high-fat foods."

   c. "Decrease the amount of green leafy vegetables."

   d. "Be sure to drink at least 10 glasses of water a day."

NURSING MANAGEMENT: EVERY GOOD NURSE SHOULD . . .

Essay

Devise a plan of care to maximize therapeutic effects and minimize adverse effects for the patient taking combination therapy benztropine with carbidopa-levodopa.

CASE STUDY

Mrs. Wade, a 65-year-old Caucasian female in your nurse-run clinic, has just been diagnosed with Parkinson disease. She has not been started on pharmacotherapy. She comes to your clinic for her first visit since the diagnosis has been made.

1. What assessments should you make at this time?

2. Why is Mrs. Wade not started on drug therapy at this time?

Mrs. Wade returns to your clinic 9 months later. Her husband tells you she is now unable to dress herself because the tremors in her hands are so severe. The nurse practitioner starts Mrs. Wade on benztropine (Cogentin) and requests a return visit in 1 month.

3. Upon her return, what assessments would you make?

One year later, Mrs. Wade returns to the clinic. She now has an increase in tremors, her gait is mildly ataxic, and she has muscular rigidity to her face and extremities. She is now started on carbidopa-levodopa (Sinemet).

4. What patient teaching should you do at this time?

Two years later, Mrs. Wade comes to the clinic and expresses concern that this medication is not as effective as before.

5. What patient teaching should be done at this time?

CRITICAL THINKING CHALLENGE

Darryl Hackett has been diagnosed with ALS, and the neurologist has prescribed riluzole. Blood work is drawn before Mr. Hackett leaves the clinic to check his ALT and AST levels. After 1 month of therapy, he returns for a follow-up visit. During this visit, his ALT and AST are elevated to approximately twice normal levels. The neurologist instructs Mr. Hackett to continue on the riluzole and return for more follow-up blood work in 2 months. Mr. Hackett asks you, the nurse, to explain why he needs to have more blood work done.

CHAPTER 23

Drugs That Stimulate the Central Nervous System

TOP TEN THINGS TO KNOW ABOUT DRUGS THAT STIMULATE THE CENTRAL NERVOUS SYSTEM

1. Central nervous system (CNS) stimulants may provoke an increased release of neurotransmitters, a decreased reuptake of neurotransmitters, and/or inhibition of postsynaptic enzymes. The net result of these actions is increased stimulation at the receptor and increased arousal.

2. CNS stimulants are used in the treatment of narcolepsy, attention deficit-hyperactivity disorder (ADHD), obesity, and respiratory depression.

3. Dextroamphetamine is used primarily in the treatment of narcolepsy and ADHD. It is an adjunct in the treatment of obesity.

4. Dextroamphetamine causes the release of norepinephrine, causes the release of dopamine in adrenergic nerve terminals (in high doses), and interferes with the reuptake of dopamine.

5. Adverse effects of dextroamphetamine (similar to all CNS stimulants) are signs of CNS overstimulation. They include restlessness, dizziness, insomnia, agitation, tachycardia, palpitations, and elevated blood pressure.

6. Dextroamphetamine, like all amphetamines, has the potential to be abused. Assess the patient for a history of substance abuse.

7. Sibutramine is used in the treatment of obesity, by increasing weight loss. Sibutramine inhibits the central reuptake of dopamine, norepinephrine, and serotonin. It is thought that the serotonin mechanism enhances satiety, whereas the norepinephrine mechanism raises the metabolic rate.

8. The nurse should assess the patient's diet and suggest appropriate modifications because sibutramine is most effective when combined with a low-calorie diet and behavior changes.

9. Caffeine is a mild, direct stimulant at all levels of the CNS. It stimulates the cardiovascular system and the medullary respiratory center, although it relaxes bronchial smooth muscle.

10. Caffeine is used in the management of neonatal apnea, asthma, drowsiness, and fatigue, and in combination with other drugs to treat headache and migraine. When used for neonatal apnea, the nurse should monitor the patient's vital signs carefully.

KEY TERMS

Fill in the blanks

Read each statement carefully and, using the chapter's key terms, write your answers in the space provided.

1. In the disorder _____ , dextroamphetamine has a paradoxical effect.

2. A brief, sudden loss of motor control is known as _____ .

3. Irresistible bouts of rapid-eye movement sleep during nonsleep cycles are characteristic of _____ , a neurologic condition.

4. _____ is characterized by being unable to speak or move before the onset of sleep.

5. An excessive accumulation of adipose is termed _____ .

6. _____ is a buildup of carbon dioxide in the body.

7. Substances used to stimulate the CNS are called _____ .

8. To suppress the appetite, an _____ drug may be ordered.

9. During the transition period between wakefulness and sleep, the appearance of auditory, visual, or kinesthetic sensations in the absence of stimuli is called _____ .

PHYSIOLOGY AND PATHOPHYSIOLOGY: THE BODY HUMAN

Multiple choice

Circle the option that best answers the question or completes the statement.

1. What part of the brain mediates appetite and satiety?
   a. pituitary
   b. pons and medulla
   c. hypothalamus
   d. reticular activating system

2. What part of the brain controls respiration?
   a. pituitary
   b. pons and medulla
   c. hypothalamus
   d. reticular activating system

3. What part of the brain is associated with sleep and arousal?
   a. pituitary
   b. pons and medulla
   c. hypothalamus
   d. reticular activating system

4. Attention deficit-hyperactivity disorder may be associated with a decrease of _____ in the brain.
   a. acetylcholine
   b. dopamine
   c. carbon dioxide
   d. glucose

CORE DRUG KNOWLEDGE: JUST THE FACTS

Essay

1. List five contraindications for dextroamphetamine (Dexedrine) therapy.

2. Name the most common CNS adverse reactions to dextroamphetamine (Dexedrine).

3. Summarize the potential adverse effects of dextroamphetamine (Dexedrine) in relation to the cardiovascular system.

4. Dextroamphetamine (Dexedrine) may lead to cachexia or hypoproteinemia. Why is this a potential problem for drug therapy?

5. What diet considerations must be considered for the patient taking dextroamphetamine (Dexedrine)?

6. How does sibutramine (Meridia) decrease appetite?

7. What are the most common adverse effects to sibutramine (Meridia) therapy?

8. What signs and symptoms may be present when sibutramine (Meridia) is given concurrently with dextromethorphan (Robitussin) or SSRI medications?

CORE PATIENT VARIABLES: PATIENTS, PLEASE

Multiple choice

Circle the option that best answers the question or completes the statement.

1. Hewey Packard, age 14, has ADHD and has been taking dextroamphetamine (Dexedrine) for the past 6 years. Last week, Hewey attempted suicide and was placed on the adolescent unit of your community mental health hospital. Which of the following antidepressants would be a poor choice for Hewey?

    a. amitriptyline (Elavil)

    b. sertraline (Zoloft)

    c. bupropion HCl (Wellbutrin)

    d. phenelzine (Nardil)

2. Janice Elliott, age 7, has been on dextroamphetamine (Dexedrine) for ADHD for the past 2 years. Because of her age, the nurse should evaluate Janice's _____ each recheck.

    a. blood pressure

    b. height and weight

    c. glucose level

    d. liver function

3. Johnny Rider has been taking dextroamphetamine (Dexedrine) for 3 years. Lately he has noticed that he has been having difficulty concentrating and feels the drug "just isn't working." He assures you he has not altered his drug regimen. Which of the following assessments may be implicated in the loss of efficacy of this drug?

    a. assess for diet changes

    b. assess for frequent headaches

    c. assess for tachycardia or palpitations

    d. assess for height or weight changes

4. Mr. and Mrs. Wayne have agreed to start their daughter, Tiffany, on dextroamphetamine (Dexedrine) for ADHD. Which of the following statements would you include in your family teaching when initiating therapy?

    a. "Expect a 25-lb weight loss in the first 6 months."

    b. "Give Tiffany the drug at bedtime so she does not notice the nausea."

    c. "Tiffany may experience a significant growth spurt after a couple of months."

    d. "This is the number for a support group that works with children to increase their self-esteem."

5. Which of the following patients may have an increased risk for adverse effects during dextroamphetamine (Dexedrine) therapy?

    a. Tony, who also takes tetracycline for acne vulgaris

    b. Amber, who wears a nicotine patch for smoking cessation

    c. Calvin, who also takes cimetidine for peptic ulcers

    d. Melissa, who also takes birth control pills

6. Farah T., age 16, is 60 lb overweight. She comes to the clinic and requests sibutramine (Meridia) for weight loss. Before starting sibutramine therapy, Farah should have

    a. testing to exclude organic causes of obesity.

    b. a fasting blood glucose.

    c. triglyceride level.

    d. CBC.

7. Janice K., age 25, is being started on sibutramine (Meridia) therapy for her morbid obesity. Because of her age and gender, it is important to teach Janice

    a. need for diet and exercise.

    b. appropriate diet.

    c. need for consistent birth control.

    d. need for follow-up examinations.

8. Kevin R. is taking caffeine for chronic fatigue. Ken should be advised to avoid taking his medication with

    a. milk.

    b. orange juice.

    c. water.

    d. grapefruit juice.

NURSING MANAGEMENT: EVERY GOOD NURSE SHOULD . . .

Multiple choice

Circle the option that best answers the question or completes the statement.

1. Before starting dextroamphetamine drug therapy for treatment of narcolepsy, the nurse should assess the patient for

    a. symptomatic cardiovascular disease.

    b. hyperthyroidism.

    c. history of drug abuse.

    d. all of the above.

    e. none of the above.

2. Josh is 8 years old and has been prescribed dextroamphetamine to treat his attention deficit-hyperactivity disorder. Patient and family education about the drug therapy should include instructions to

   a. take the drug in the evening to minimize adverse effects.

   b. avoid drinking caffeinated beverages, such as colas.

   c. chew the sustained-release capsules carefully before swallowing.

   d. take a double dose when a dose is skipped accidentally.

3. Dottie Murphy was started on dextroamphetamaine as an adjunct therapy for weight loss. She calls the advice line at her HMO and speaks with you, the "answer nurse." She tells you that she is restless and having problems sleeping at night. She would like a prescription for a sleeping pill. Your best advice would be that--

   a. she should use an over-the-counter sleep aid.

   b. you will contact the prescriber regarding obtaining a prescription sleep aid.

   c. she appears to need more dextroamphetamine and should increase her dose.

   d. she appears to be having adverse effects from the dextroamphetamine and you will contact the prescriber.

4. Sibutramine has been prescribed for Latoya Rydyll to assist in weight loss. Ms. Rydyll confides to you that she really hopes the drug will be effective in helping her lose weight. To maximize the therapeutic effect of sibutramine, the nurse should emphasize to Ms. Rydyll

   a. that the drug should be taken on a full stomach, 1 hour after eating.

   b. that she should continue her normal dietary pattern.

   c. that she should increase her activity level.

   d. that she should take the drug at bedtime.

5. You are administering caffeine to baby Heather, a newborn with apnea. To minimize adverse effects, you should monitor her for

   a. tachypnea.

   b. fever.

   c. hyperglycemia.

   d. all of the above.

   e. none of the above.

CASE STUDY

Mrs. Clemson has come to the clinic for her 4-week postpartum checkup. She is anxious to lose the extra 15 lb she gained from the pregnancy. She states, "Breast-feeding is helping me to lose weight, but I'm not losing fast enough. I was thinking about trying some weight loss pills. Would a prescription pill help me lose weight faster than the ones I can buy over the counter?"
What should you advise Mrs. Clemson regarding the use of anorexics?

CRITICAL THINKING CHALLENGE

What additional advice might you give Mrs. Clemson regarding weight loss?

UNIT VI

Drugs Used to Control Pain and Inflammation

CHAPTER 24

Drugs That Are Narcotic Analgesics

TOP TEN THINGS TO KNOW ABOUT DRUGS THAT ARE NARCOTIC ANALGESICS

1. Pain can be classified by physiologic origin, duration, or pathologic source. Pain may be caused by injury, trauma, disease, diagnostic procedures, or therapy to treat disease or pathologies.

2. Pain is subjective, and the patient must be assessed with an appropriate tool to determine the extent of the pain being experienced. Pain levels should be reassessed after an analgesic is given.

3. Pain is best controlled when analgesics are given before pain becomes severe and the doses are administered around the clock.

4. Doses of narcotic analgesics should be titrated to obtain maximum efficacy with minimal adverse effects. Tolerance and cross-tolerance should be considered when titrating dosages.

5. Patients and families should be educated with the facts concerning pain, pain management, and what will be done if and when they report pain.

6. Morphine, a narcotic agonist used to treat moderate to severe pain, stimulates at the opiate receptors (especially mu), decreasing the release of substance P in the spinal cord and altering pain perception.

7. The most common adverse effects of morphine are respiratory depression, decreased urinary output or urinary retention, delayed return of peristalsis, and constipation. Respiratory depression is treated with naloxone, a narcotic antagonist.

8. Codeine, a moderate narcotic, is used to treat mild to moderate pain, and as a cough suppressant. Codeine, and synthetic forms of codeine, are often combined with nonsteroidal anti-inflammatories for increased pain control.

9. Adverse effects of codeine include drowsiness, dry mouth, nausea and vomiting, and constipation. Respiratory depression and cardiovascular effects can occur in higher doses. Avoid giving to patients who require a cough reflex.

10. Pentazocine is a mixed agonist/antagonist narcotic, meaning it stimulates at some receptors but blocks at others. It will produce analgesia in patients who have not taken other opioid narcotics, but interrupt pain control in patients also receiving narcotic agonists (such as morphine) and produce withdrawal in patients who abuse narcotics.

KEY TERMS

Matching

Match the following key terms with their definitions.

1. _____ acute pain
2. _____ addiction
3. _____ adjunct analgesics
4. _____ analgesics
5. _____ breakthrough pain
6. _____ chronic pain
7. _____ co-analgesics
8. _____ dependence
9. _____ incidental pain
10. _____ narcotics
11. _____ neuropathic pain
12. _____ nociceptors
13. _____ nonsteroidal anti-inflammatory drugs
14. _____ opioid
15. _____ pain
16. _____ rescue doses
17. _____ somatic pain
18. _____ tolerance
19. _____ visceral pain

a. Drugs used to treat pain

b. Spontaneous, or activity-related pain

c. Another term for adjunct analgesics

d. Characterized by a withdrawal syndrome upon cessation of the drug

e. Compulsive use of a drug for a secondary gain

f. Immediate phase of response to an insult or injury

g. Drugs used to treat pain that work on the perception of pain by the brain

h. Pain that persists well beyond actual tissue injury

i. Transitory flare-ups of pain over baseline

j. Drugs used in the management of pain that have another primary pharmacotherapeutic action

k. Unpleasant sensory and emotional experience

l. Results from injury to the peripheral receptors, afferent fibers, or CNS

m. Afferent nuerons found in the skin, muscle, connective tissue, circulatory system, and abdominal, pelvic, and thoracic viscera

n. Body becomes accustomed to the drug and needs a higher dose to relieve pain

o. Results from stimulation within the deep tissues or organs and surrounding structural tissues

p. Another name for a narcotic drug derived from opium

q. Class of drugs used to treat pain that are not narcotics

r. Dose of medication added to the standing doses for pain management

s. Results from ongoing activation of peripheral nociceptors found in structural tissues, such as bone, muscle, and soft tissue

PHYSIOLOGY AND PATHOPHYSIOLOGY: THE BODY HUMAN

Essay

1. In general, what is the theory that explains how CNS depressants work?

2. What is the difference between myelinated A-delta fibers and unmyelinated C fibers in the perception of pain?

3. In addition to the pain stimulus, what other phenomena influence the perception of pain?

4. Identify specific areas of the brain and their function in the perception of pain.

5. List potential sequelae to unresolved pain.

CORE DRUG KNOWLEDGE: JUST THE FACTS

Multiple choice

Circle the option that best answers the question or completes the statement.

1. Equianalgesic dosages are compared to
   a. meperidine.
   b. codeine.
   c. fentanyl.
   d. morphine.

2. Morphine works by
   a. decreasing A-delta fibers.
   b. increasing C fibers.
   c. inhibiting release of substance P.
   d. inhibiting release of acetylcholine.

3. Morphine administration must be used with extreme caution in which of the following disorders?
   a. head injury
   b. COPD
   c. seizure disorder
   d. all of the above

4. The most hazardous adverse effects to the use of morphine occur to the
   a. CNS.
   b. cardiovascular system.
   c. respiratory system.
   d. gastrointestinal system.

5. In addition to pain relief, codeine is also frequently used as a
   a. decongestant.
   b. laxative.
   c. cough suppressant.
   d. sedative.

6. Codeine is used cautiously in patients with respiratory disorders because
   a. it may cause bronchoconstriction.
   b. it may cause bronchodilation.
   c. it may increase respiratory secretions.
   d. it may lead to accumulation of secretions and a loss of respiratory reserve.

7. In addition to CNS depressants, codeine may have drug–drug interactions with
   a. antibiotics.
   b. antiulcer medications.
   c. bronchodilators.
   d. anticoagulants.

8. Which of the following statements about pentazocine (Talwin) is correct?
   a. It is a narcotic agonist.
   b. It is a narcotic antagonist.
   c. It is both a narcotic agonist and antagonist.
   d. None of the above.

9. Because of its pharmacodynamics, intravenous pentazocine (Talwin)
   a. increases the workload of the heart.
   b. decreases the workload of the heart.
   c. increases the workload of the lungs.
   d. decreases the workload of the lungs.

10. Pentazocine (Talwin) should be given cautiously to patients with
   a. severe seizure disorders.
   b. peptic ulcers.
   c. respiratory disorders.
   d. heart murmurs.

CORE PATIENT VARIABLES: PATIENTS, PLEASE

Multiple choice

Circle the option that best answers the question or completes the statement.

1. Your patient has been given morphine 10 mg IM. She now has an increase in her BP and resting pulse and states she feels very anxious. You suspect
   a. an idiosyncratic reaction.
   b. an additive effect.
   c. a synergistic effect.
   d. an agonist response.

2. Jeremy Benz, age 77, is in postsurgical recovery after fracturing his ankle. He is in severe pain and has morphine sulfate ordered to control his pain. With your knowledge of morphine, you would expect the dosage of morphine to
   a. be equal to the dose for a young adult.
   b. be higher than the dose for a young adult.
   c. be lower than the dose for a young adult.

3. Dolly Peterson, age 55, has a fractured rib. She is being released from the emergency room with a prescription for a narcotic analgesic. Before discharging Mrs. Peterson, you assess her lifestyle, diet, and habits. Which of the following questions should be included in this assessment?
   a. "Are you able to drink 3 liters of water a day?"
   b. "Do you drink alcoholic beverages?"
   c. "Do you take other medications?"
   d. "Do you have stairs at your home?"

4. Fred Whatley is taking Tylenol with codeine #3 to control the pain from a fractured arm. Five days later, Mr. Whatley calls the clinic and asks to speak with the advice nurse. Mr. Whatley states he is unable to have a bowel movement since taking the medication. Which of the following is the most appropriate response?

   a. "This is an expected adverse effect to the use of codeine. Increase your fluid intake and take a bulk laxative such as Metamucil."

   b. "This is an additive effect of codeine. Stop taking the medication."

   c. "This is an expected adverse effect to the use of codeine. Double the dose and it will clear out your bowel."

   d. "You are probably allergic to the codeine. Stop taking the medication."

5. Your patient is being discharged from the Emergency Department with a prescription for Tylenol with codeine. Which of the following areas of assessment needs special attention?

   a. health status and environment

   b. culture and lifestyle, diet and habits

   c. health status, lifestyle, diet and habits, and environment

   d. health status and culture

6. Your patient was admitted for observation after a suicide attempt. Upon discharge, the patient is prescribed a narcotic analgesic for an injury sustained during the suicide attempt. Which of the following narcotics would be CONTRAINDICATED for this patient?

   a. propoxyphene (Darvon)

   b. hydrocodone (Vicodin)

   c. codeine

   d. none of the above

7. Susan Peters, age 22, is a recovering narcotic drug abuser. She has not used drugs in 4 years. Susan lists penicillin, ibuprofen, and naloxone as allergies. Which of the following drugs would be inappropriate for Susan to control the pain from her fractured arm?

   a. hydromorphone (Dilaudid)

   b. codeine

   c. pentazocine (Talwin)

   d. oxycodone (Percodan)

8. During a psychiatric intake interview with your patient, she states, "My mom put me here. She's concerned because of my use of 'T's and Blues.'" With your knowledge of this drug combination, you will carefully assess

   a. the heart and lungs.

   b. the lungs and CNS.

   c. kidney and liver function.

   d. the CNS and skin.

NURSING MANAGEMENT: EVERY GOOD NURSE SHOULD . . .

Decision tree

You are the nurse on an orthopedic unit. Your patient, a 64-year-old woman who fell on the ice this morning and has a hip fracture, is in traction and awaiting surgical repair late today. She requests something for pain. The following orders are written for the patient for pain management:

Ibuprofen 400 mg PO q 4 hours prn for mild pain
Percocet one tablet PO q 4–6 hours for moderate pain
Morphine sulfate 5 to 10 mg IM q 4 hours for severe pain

Complete the decision tree to show the steps you would take to assess and treat this patient's pain. (Hint: Ibuprofen is a nonsteroidal anti-inflammatory [NSAID]. See Chapter 25. Percocet is a trade name for a combination drug containing 5 mg oxycodone and 325 mg acetaminophen.)

CASE STUDY

Gordon Richards is 20 years old. He is hospitalized after surgical removal of a bullet from his leg today. You learn from your nursing assessment that he drinks four beers a day and uses cocaine. You assess him for pain using a visual analogue scale, and he indicates that he is having pain at an 8 level on a 0 (no pain) to 10 (worst pain imaginable) scale. He is lying quietly in bed while you talk with him and assess him. He has not received any analgesics in 6 hours. He has orders for Percocet 1 to 2 tablets PO every 4 to 6 hours, and morphine 8 to 10 mg IM every 3 to 4 hours. He last received one Percocet for pain.

1. Does this patient have pain?

Patient Reports Pain

|
Assess pain-using tool

Pain is mild to moderate

Medicate with ☐ per order

Reassess pain level in 60 minutes

Pain diminished/ adequately controlled

Pain diminished but not adequately controlled

Pain increases

Next time c/o similar pain

☐

Next time c/o pain

☐

Seek order to give

☐
now

Reassess pain level in 60 minutes

If effective

Not effective

☐

☐

Pain is moderate to severe

Medicate with ☐ per order

Reassess pain level in 60 minutes

Pain diminished/ adequately controlled

Pain diminished but not adequately controlled

Pain increases

Next time c/o similar pain

☐

Next time c/o pain

☐

Seek order to give

☐
now

Reassess pain level in 30 minutes

Follow decision tree for ☐

Pain is severe

Medicate with ☐

Reassess pain level in 30 minutes

Pain diminished/ adequately controlled

Pain diminished but not adequately controlled

Pain increases

Next time c/o similar pain

☐

Next time c/o pain

☐

Seek order to give

☐
now

Reassess pain level in 30 minutes

If effective

Not effective

☐

☐

---

2. What information should be assessed regarding his pain and pain control in addition to the rating of pain on the pain scale?

3. Assuming that Gordon reports minimal pain relief for 2 hours after receiving one Percocet, what is the most appropriate action to take?

CRITICAL THINKING CHALLENGE

Gordon continues to report severe pain with pain ratings of 8 or 9 using the visual analogue scale. You have switched to giving him morphine 10 mg every 3 hours. This dose reduces Gordon's pain, and he remains awake and alert. Gordon's roommate, Tyler, is also 20 years old. He also has severe pain, rating it at 8 on the visual analogue scale. Tyler had surgery 2 hours ago for a ruptured appendix. His medication orders read morphine 8 to 15 mg IM q 4 hours prn × 24 hours. You administer 10 mg of morphine to Tyler also. Thirty minutes later, Tyler is very lethargic and hard to arouse. His pulse rate has dropped from 88 to 68 per minute.

What can account for the difference in reaction to the same dose of analgesic?

CHAPTER 25

Drugs for Treating Fever and Inflammation

TOP TEN THINGS TO KNOW ABOUT DRUGS FOR TREATING FEVER AND INFLAMMATION

1. Prostaglandins modulate some components of inflammation, body temperature, pain transmission, platelet aggregation, and many other body actions. Prostaglandins are converted from arachidonic acid by the enzyme cyclooxygenase (COX). There are two forms of the COX enzyme, COX-1 and COX-2. COX-1 synthesizes prostaglandins involved in the regulation of normal cell activity; COX-2 produces prostaglandins mainly at sites of inflammation.
2. Nonsteroidal anti-inflammatories (salicylates and prostaglandin synthetase inhibitors [PSI]) and para-aminophenol derivatives (acetaminophen) work by inhibiting the synthesis of prostaglandins.
3. Most NSAIDs indiscriminately target both COX-1 and COX-2, and deplete the prostaglandins needed for normal cell function and protection. This is the cause of many of these drugs' adverse effects.
4. Aspirin, a salicylate, is used for analgesic, antipyretic (fever reduction), anti-inflammatory, and antiplatelet effects. It irreversibly inhibits COX and, therefore, inhibits the synthesis of prostaglandins. Therapeutic and most adverse effects are related to the inhibition of COX-1.
5. Most common adverse effects of aspirin are gastrointestinal (GI); renal and hepatic toxicities are possible although not common. Avoid use in children with flulike illness, pregnant women—especially third trimester, and in patients with pathophysiologic conditions that would be adversely affected by the action or adverse effects of aspirin.
6. Ibuprofen, a prostaglandin synthetase inhibitor, is used for anti-inflammatory, analgesic, and antipyretic effects. It reversibly inhibits COX. Therapeutic and most adverse effects are related to the inhibition of COX-1.
7. Most common adverse effects of ibuprofen are GI; renal and hepatic toxicities are possible although not common; long-term use increases the risk. Avoid use in third-trimester pregnancy (Category D) patients with active GI disease and in patients with pathophysiologic conditions that would be adversely affected by the action or adverse effects of ibuprofen.
8. Acetaminophen, a para-aminophenol derivative, is used for its antipyretic and analgesic effects. Often grouped with the NSAIDs because of some similarities in actions, it has no anti-inflammatory effects, and no effect on platelet aggregation. The exact mechanism of action is unknown.
9. Hepatic and renal toxicities are possible from acetaminophen. Overdosage produces hepatic and renal failure and is fatal if not treated. Antidote is acetylcysteine.
10. The COX-2 inhibitors, celecoxib and rofecoxib, reduce inflammation without removing the protective prostaglandins in the stomach and kidney made by COX-1. They don't have the GI adverse effects of other anti-inflammatories. They are used in treating osteoarthritis and rheumatoid arthritis.

KEY TERMS

Matching

Match the following key terms with their definitions.

1. _____ cyclooxygenase
2. _____ NSAID
3. _____ para-aminophenol derivative
4. _____ PSI
5. _____ prostaglandins
6. _____ Reye's syndrome
7. _____ salicylates
8. _____ salicylate poisoning
9. _____ salicylism

a. Life-threatening toxicity of salicylic acid
b. Drugs containing a salt or ester of salicylic acid
c. Umbrella term for anti-inflammatory drugs that are not steroids
d. Toxicity of salicylic acid or any of its compounds
e. Another term for a class of NSAIDs
f. Derived from arachidonic acid
g. Enzyme that produces prostaglandins from arachidonic acid
h. Acetaminophen is the only drug in this class
i. An acquired encephalopathy of young children that follows an acute febrile illness

PHYSIOLOGY AND PATHOPHYSIOLOGY: THE BODY HUMAN

Essay

1. What are the classic signs of local inflammation?

2. What occurs in the vascular response of acute inflammation?

3. What are the four phases of cellular response to acute inflammation?

4. Why are PSIs responsible for both decreasing inflammation and inducing adverse effects?

CORE DRUG KNOWLEDGE: JUST THE FACTS

Multiple choice

Circle the option that best answers the question or completes the statement.

1. Which of the following is NOT an action of aspirin?
   a. analgesic
   b. anti-inflammatory
   c. antipyretic
   d. antihistamine

2. In which of the following patients would aspirin be contraindicated?
   a. Mary with hypertension
   b. Judy with migraine headaches
   c. Constance with peptic ulcer disease
   d. Clair with chronic constipation

3. What is the usual adult dosage of aspirin?
   a. 325 mg q 8 hours
   b. 650 mg q 4 to 6 hours
   c. 325 mg q 4 hours
   d. 650 mg q 12 hours

4. Salicylate poisoning may occur in adults with a dose of
   a. 5 to 8 g.
   b. 10 to 30 g.
   c. 50 to 100 g.
   d. 40 to 60 g.

5. Salicylism is a form of mild aspirin toxicity with symptoms such as
   a. headache, tinnitus, GI distress.
   b. respiratory stimulation, constipation, GI distress.
   c. GI distress, diarrhea, respiratory depression.
   d. headache, hypervigilance, confusion.

6. The most common adverse effects to most prostaglandin synthetase inhibitors (PSI) are _____ in nature.
   a. CNS
   b. respiratory
   c. GI
   d. cardiovascular

7. Analgesic effects of ibuprofen occur within
   a. 30 minutes.
   b. 24 hours.
   c. 2 to 4 hours.
   d. 12 hours.

8. Which of the following statements is correct concerning PSIs?
   a. If one medication does not work, none will.
   b. A benefit of PSI therapy is a longer duration of action than salicylates.
   c. There is a cross-sensitivity between all PSIs.
   d. Unlike salicylates, PSIs do not have antiplatelet activity.

9. Which of the following PSIs has both oral and IM administration?
   a. ketoprofen (Orudis)
   b. mefenamic acid (Ponstel)
   c. phenylbutazone (Butazolidin)
   d. ketorolac (Toradol)

10. Which of the following PSIs has a decreased incidence of GI adverse effects?
   a. ketoprofen (Orudis), naproxen (Naprosyn, Anaprox)
   b. diclofenac sodium (Voltaren), etodolac (Lodine)
   c. celecoxib (Celebrex) and rofecoxib (Vioxx)
   d. mefenamic acid (Ponstel) and meclofenamate sodium (Meclomen)

11. Cox-2 selective PSIs
   a. do not have any antiplatelet activity.
   b. have an increased antiplatelet activity.
   c. have an increased risk for CNS depression.
   d. have an decreased risk for CNS depression.

12. Which of the following effects occur with acetaminophen therapy?
   a. analgesia and anti-inflammatory
   b. antipyretic and antiplatelet
   c. antiplatelet and anti-inflammatory
   d. analgesia and antipyretic

13. Which of the following adverse effects is associated with acetaminophen therapy?
   a. pulmonary edema
   b. urinary retention
   c. hepatotoxicity
   d. ototoxicity

14. Which of the following patients should NOT take acetaminophen?
   a. Kelly, age 30, who is pregnant
   b. Helen, age 16, who has a seizure disorder
   c. Mark, age 55, with a history of hepatitis
   d. John, age 40, who is an alcoholic

CORE PATIENT VARIABLES: PATIENTS, PLEASE

Multiple choice

Circle the option that best answers the question or completes the statement.

1. Jason Kennedy, age 60, has arthritis. Mr. Kennedy smokes one pack of cigarettes per day and drinks at least six beers each evening. Which of the following statements would be most appropriate during patient teaching for Mr. Kennedy?
   a. "Take the aspirin at least 4 times a day. If you have no relief, then take an additional dose."
   b. "Due to your age, you should limit your aspirin intake to only 6 times a day."
   c. "You have three predisposing factors for an increased risk to develop an ulcer with aspirin therapy. Let's start with trying to stop smoking."
   d. "You just can't take these pills because of your lifestyle. Get used to the discomfort."

2. Wendy Baker takes aspirin for chronic arthritis pain. She is currently hospitalized for treatment of a deep vein thrombosis and is prescribed warfarin. Which of the following interventions should be done with Mrs. Baker? Monitor
   a. daily PT
   b. urine output
   c. respiratory rate
   d. CBC every other day

3. Beverly Tappen is a steroid-dependent asthmatic. Mrs. Tappen also takes aspirin for bursitis. You would anticipate that Mrs. Tappen's aspirin dose may

   a. need to be increased.

   b. need to be decreased.

   c. remain unchanged.

4. Julia Barnard has nasal polyps and asthma. Because of her health status history, Ms. Barnard has an increased risk for aspirin-induced _____ with aspirin therapy.

   a. ototoxicity

   b. CHF

   c. GI bleeding

   d. bronchospasm

5. Jay Peterson, age 54, takes propranolol for hypertension. Mr. Peterson has chronic tendonitis from playing tennis. Which of the following interventions should be done for Mr. Peterson while he receives PSIs for his tendonitis?

   a. monitor renal output

   b. monitor for CHF

   c. monitor for loss of hypertension control

   d. monitor for constipation

6. Carmen Flores, age 55, has bipolar disorder and has taken lithium. Mrs. Flores also has arthritis, and her health care provider has prescribed ibuprofen. Mrs. Flores states she is concerned about taking other drugs with her lithium. Which of the following statements would be most appropriate?

   a. "Taking these drugs together is not a problem."

   b. "We will monitor your lithium level closely and make any adjustments necessary."

   c. "Call us if you have any adverse reactions. You should be OK."

   d. "I'm not sure why your provider has prescribed this—it's pretty dangerous."

7. Joanna Farmer has been taking ibuprofen 1 week for bursitis. She calls the clinic and states, "I just don't feel any better." Which of the following statements is most appropriate?

   a. "It may take up to 2 weeks to feel the benefit of this medication."

   b. "I guess you should make an appointment and get something else."

   c. "Your bursitis is obviously resistant to PSIs."

   d. "It might work better if you double the dose for a few days."

8. Louisa Parker, age 60, has been taking ibuprofen (Motrin) for 6 months. Her doctor has changed Mrs. Parker to rofecoxib (Vioxx). Because of her age, Mrs. Parker should be advised to

   a. increase the amount of fluids taken with her rofecoxib.

   b. take an additional 81 mg of aspirin daily.

   c. monitor her blood pressure closely.

   d. add green leafy vegetables to her daily diet.

9. Patient teaching for acetaminophen therapy should include

   a. take only the recommended dose.

   b. read the labels of OTC medications to avoid overdose.

   c. seek medical care immediately for accidental overdose.

   d. all of the above

10. Alex Carpenter takes acetaminophen daily for his chronic headaches. Mr. Carpenter should have which of the following lab tests done periodically?

   a. CBC

   b. liver function tests

   c. kidney function tests

   d. all of the above

NURSING MANAGEMENT: EVERY GOOD NURSE SHOULD . . .

Multiple choice

Circle the option that best answers the question or completes the statement.

1. Helen Gorsuch, 70 years old, is taking aspirin for her arthritis. Patient teaching should include

   a. take aspirin on an empty stomach.

   b. store aspirin in the bathroom medicine chest.

   c. return for laboratory tests every 6 months.

   d. crush the extended-release tablets for easier swallowing.

2. Patients receiving ibuprofen on a regular basis should be told to contact the physician or nurse practitioner immediately if they note

   a. unusual bruising.

   b. slow heartbeat.

   c. upset stomach.

   d. slight dizziness.

3. Terry Robochek, 16 years old, is brought to the emergency room after having attempted suicide by swallowing half of a bottle of acetaminophen. The nurse would expect to

a. draw blood work for platelet count.

b. administer acetylcysteine.

c. administer acetylsalicylic acid.

d. send Terry for an abdominal computed tomography (CT) scan.

4. Ashley Caprioti is 4 years old. Her mother calls the clinic to report that Ashley developed a sudden fever of 101.5° F orally, that she is listless, and complaining of muscle aches all over, a scratchy throat, and loss of appetite. Her mother asks what she should give Ashley to treat her fever and muscle aches. Ashley's medical record indicates that she has no allergies and has no chronic medical problems. The nurse practitioner should recommend

a. children's aspirin.

b. children's acetaminophen.

c. adult aspirin.

d. adult acetaminophen, cut in half.

5. Gina Scarpio, 67 years old, has a history of a gastric ulcer. She is to be started on celecoxib, a COX-2 inhibitor, for osteoarthritis. She asks you, the nurse, to explain why she has to have a prescription medicine and can't take aspirin or ibuprofen, which she can buy over the counter. The best reply of the nurse is

a. she can substitute either aspirin or ibuprofen if she doesn't want to use a prescription medicine.

b. aspirin and ibuprofen don't relieve arthritis pain.

c. celecoxib does not cause GI adverse effects like aspirin and ibuprofen.

d. celecoxib is prescription-strength aspirin.

CASE STUDY

Thomas Brooks, 72 years old, had a right hip replacement related to degeneration of his hip from arthritis. Postoperatively, he is started on ibuprofen 400 mg every 6 hours and oxycodone (an opioid analgesic) 5 mg every 6 hours.

1. Describe why Mr. Brooks was started on ibuprofen postoperatively.

2. Is it safe for Mr. Brooks to receive both ibuprofen and oxycodone? (Need help? See Chapter 24.)

3. Why were these drugs ordered to be given every 6 hours (around the clock) as opposed to prn?

CRITICAL THINKING CHALLENGE

On the second postoperative day, the nurse notices that Mr. Brooks' urine output has decreased and he has not made 30 mL of urine during each of the last 2 hours, although his intake has been adequate. His blood pressure this morning is 150/90 compared to 136/84 previously.

1. What is your assessment of Mr. Brooks' current condition?

2. What core patient variables may have contributed to his current condition?

3. What actions would you take?

CHAPTER 26

Drugs for Treating Arthritis and Gout

TOP TEN THINGS TO KNOW ABOUT DRUGS FOR TREATING ARTHRITIS AND GOUT

1. Auranofin, a disease-modifying antirheumatic drug (DMARD), is a gold salt used in the treatment of rheumatoid arthritis. It is used as a second-line drug, used after nonsteroidal anti-inflammatory drugs (either prostaglandin synthetase inhibitors or salicylates) have been ineffective.

2. Auranofin slows or halts the progression of rheumatoid arthritis by an unknown mechanism.

3. The most common adverse effects of auranofin are gastrointestinal (GI). Serious blood dyscrasias, including fatal bone marrow suppression, can occur from auranofin; these adverse effects can even occur several months after therapy is stopped.

4. Colchicine, an antigout drug, is used in treating acute gout attacks. It acts through inhibition of leukocyte migration, resulting in an interruption of the inflammatory response. It does not affect uric acid clearance.

5. Teach patients receiving colchicines to take these drugs at the first sign of a gout attack.

6. Colchicine causes GI effects (nausea, vomiting, or diarrhea) in the majority of patients. Long-term use may cause bone marrow depression.

7. Patients receiving auranofin or colchicine need to have their complete blood count measured periodically to check for abnormalities.

8. Probenecid, a uricosuric, prevents resorption of uric acid in the kidney, preventing the formation and deposit of urate crystals. It is used to prevent acute gout attacks.

9. Probenecid should not be taken if an acute attack of gout occurs, because it will prolong inflammation. Acute attack may occur when therapy is first started.

10. Probenecid is also used to potentiate the effect of penicillin because it delays the renal clearance of the antibiotic, increasing serum drug levels.

KEY TERMS

Matching

Match the following key terms with their definitions.

1. _____ antigout drugs
2. _____ chrysotherapy
3. _____ cytokine
4. _____ DMARDs
5. _____ nitritoid crisis
6. _____ pannus
7. _____ tophi
8. _____ tumor necrosis factor
9. _____ uricosuric drugs

a. Drugs that slow the progression of rheumatoid arthritis
b. Drugs that increase the excretion of uric acid
c. Lysosomal nodules found along the extensor surface of the forearm
d. Administration of gold salts
e. Severe reaction following administration of gold salts
f. Drugs that abate gout
g. Mediates inflammation and joint destruction
h. Type of cytokine
i. Destructive granular tissue that damages the articular cartilage

PHYSIOLOGY AND PATHOPHYSIOLOGY: THE BODY HUMAN

Essay

1. How does rheumatoid arthritis destroy joint cartilage?

2. What clinical signs may indicate the presence of rheumatoid arthritis?

3. Explain the etiology of gout.

CORE DRUG KNOWLEDGE: JUST THE FACTS

Multiple choice

Circle the option that best answers the question or completes the statement.

1. The most SERIOUS adverse effects to auranofin (Ridaura) therapy affect the _____ system.
   a. central nervous system (CNS)
   b. GI
   c. hematopoietic
   d. renal

2. The most COMMON adverse effects to auranofin (Ridaura) therapy affect the _____ system.
   a. CNS
   b. GI
   c. hematopoietic
   d. renal

3. Fifty percent of patients receiving auranofin (Ridaura) therapy may experience
   a. proteinuria.
   b. hirsutism.
   c. cardiac arrhythmias.
   d. constipation.

4. In general, auranofin (Ridaura) should not be coadministered with other medications that may
   a. increase the blood pressure.
   b. cause sedation.
   c. increase intracranial pressure.
   d. induce blood dyscrasias.

5. Which of the following lab tests must be completed before IM aurothioglucose (Solganal) therapy?
   a. CBC and renal function
   b. hepatic and renal function
   c. UA and hepatic function
   d. CBC and UA

6. Before administration of aurothioglucose (Solganal), the nurse should
   a. warm blankets in case the patient feels cold after the injection.
   b. have an ice pack ready to place over the injection site.
   c. have resuscitation equipment available in the room.
   d. have an emesis basin at the bedside.

7. Which of the following medications used in the management of rheumatoid arthritis has a unique mechanism of action that allows for its use in combination with other DMARDs?

   a. leflunomide (Arava)

   b. aurothioglucose (Solganal)

   c. penicillamine (Cuprimine)

   d. methotrexate (Rheumatrex)

8. How do tumor necrosis factor (TNF)-inhibitors, such as etanercept (Enbrel), work?

   a. They decrease the amount of neutrophils that circulate in the serum.

   b. They block the ability of the cytokine to attach to its receptor.

   c. They block the release of macrophages.

   d. They increase the number of neutrophils in the joint space.

9. Which of the following drugs is indicated for treatment of acute exacerbations of gout?

   a. acetaminophen (Tylenol)

   b. probenecid (Benemid)

   c. colchicine

   d. allopurinol (Zyloprim)

10. During colchicine therapy, patients may experience

    a. constipation, flatulence, or cramps.

    b. headache, flatulence, constipation.

    c. nausea, vomiting, or diarrhea

    d. foot cramps, headache, blurred vision

11. Allopurinol (Zyloprim) is used in the treatment of

    a. bursitis.

    b. chronic gout.

    c. rheumatoid arthritis.

    d. acute gout.

12. In addition to gout, probenecid is used to

    a. enhance renal excretion of copper.

    b. enhance bioavailability of antiretroviral agents.

    c. delay renal excretion of antibiotics.

    d. enhance renal excretion of diuretics.

CORE PATIENT VARIABLES: PATIENTS, PLEASE

Multiple choice

Circle the option that best answers the question or completes the statement.

1. Beverly Cass, age 60, has been receiving auranofin (Ridaura) for rheumatoid arthritis for the past 3 months. She states, "This has helped me so much. Why did I have to wait so long to get it?" Which of the following responses is most accurate?

   a. "This medication is very expensive, and we try the less expensive medications first."

   b. "Gold salts have many serious adverse effects. Less toxic drugs are used early in the disease."

   c. "Some doctors just don't like using this drug."

   d. "This is an experimental drug and is not approved by the FDA."

2. Valerie Burton, age 66, is receiving auranofin (Ridaura) therapy. Mrs. Burton should be advised to expect which of the following adverse reactions to auranofin?

   a. diarrhea

   b. constipation

   c. rash

   d. cough

3. Henry Taylor, age 60, has rheumatoid arthritis. He is being prescribed auranofin (Ridaura) today. While doing patient education, Mr. Taylor states, "I'm not coming back for those lab tests. Just give me a year-long prescription." What is your best action?

   a. administer the medication and schedule the lab tests anyway

   b. notify the health care provider of the potential for nonadherence

   c. administer the medication, then notify the health care provider of Mr. Taylor's statement

   d. administer only half of the dose and tell Mr. Taylor he can receive the other half after he has the lab test completed

4. Jessica James, age 70, has been receiving auranofin (Ridaura) for her arthritis for the past 2 months. She comes to the clinic today and states, "I just don't feel any better—are you sure this drug works?" What is your best response?

   a. "You seem a little cranky today, Mrs. James."

   b. "Are you sure you are taking the medication correctly?"

   c. "You are right—you should be feeling much better by now."

   d. "This drug can take up to 6 months for you to feel its effects."

5. Leon Grimes is receiving aurothioglucose (Solganal) for rheumatoid arthritis. After administration, Mr. Grimes complains of feelings of warmth and light-headedness. You note facial flushing and hypotension. You suspect

   a. anaphylaxis.

   b. drug interaction.

   c. nitritoid crisis.

   d. this is an expected reaction to IM therapy.

6. Mary Turner, age 65, comes to the clinic today for her monthly aurothioglucose (Solganal) injection. The nurse should assess Mrs. Turner for

   a. easy bruising or bleeding.

   b. severe headaches.

   c. constipation.

   d. muscle pains.

7. Susan Hill, age 6, has been receiving methotrexate for her juvenile rheumatoid arthritis. Today, the doctor suggests that etanercept (Enbrel) be added to her treatment. Before the initiation of etanercept therapy, the nurse should ensure that Susan

   a. does not have a history of migraine headaches.

   b. is up-to-date on all immunizations.

   c. understands the mechanism of action of her drugs.

   d. does not have an aversion to needles.

8. Joe Fayer, age 45, has acute gout and is prescribed colchicine. He tells you his brother takes allopurinol (Zyloprim) for his gout and wonders why it was not prescribed for him. Which of the following is the best response?

   a. "At this time, allopurinol may make your attack worse."

   b. "Different health care providers use different drugs."

   c. "I'll see if your health care provider will change the prescription."

   d. "At your age, allopurinol is contraindicated."

9. Cindy Barq has brought her mother, Clair Smith, age 74, to the clinic for treatment of acute gout. Mrs. Smith is prescribed colchicine. When Mrs. Barq asks why she needs to bring her mother back to the clinic, you explain that Mrs. Smith needs to be monitored for cumulative toxicity to colchicine due to her age. Mrs. Barq states, "That's interesting, does anyone else have a possibility for toxicity?" What other patients are at risk for cumulative toxicity?

   a. debilitated patients

   b. severe renal and hepatic disease patients

   c. severe cardiac disease patients

   d. all of the above

10. Mr. Young, age 50, is experiencing his first gout attack. He is prescribed colchicine. Which of the following is appropriate patient teaching?

   a. "Decrease your intake of spinach, asparagus, cauliflower, and mushrooms."

   b. "Decrease your alcohol intake to only three glasses of wine a day."

   c. "Decrease your fluid intake to only four glasses of water a day."

   d. "Decrease your intake of dairy products."

11. Melvin Burke is receiving radiation therapy for a tumor. He has a history of hypertension, atrial fibrillation, and gout. His medications include clonidine, atenolol, digoxin, and probenecid (Benemid). Which of his medications should be discontinued while he is receiving radiation therapy?

   a. clonidine (Catapres)

   b. probenecid (Benemid)

   c. digitalis (Digoxin)

   d. atenolol (Tenormin)

12. Jennifer Wilson has diabetes and gout. She takes probenecid (Benemid) for prophylaxis of her gout. What instructions should be given to Mrs. Wilson?

    a. Monitor for ketones in her urine.

    b. Monitor blood glucose with Clinitest strips.

    c. Monitor for dehydration from diarrhea.

    d. Monitor blood glucose with blood monitoring system.

4. Tim Greenley is being treated with colchicine for acute gout. He asks you, the nurse, if there is anything he can do to decrease his levels of uric acid. You recommend that he avoid eating, or minimize his consumption of

    a. organ meats and oily fish.

    b. lettuce and apples.

    c. chicken and wheat products.

    d. dairy products.

NURSING MANAGEMENT: EVERY GOOD NURSE SHOULD . . .

Multiple choice

Circle the option that best answers the question or completes the statement.

1. Rita Grempler, 59 years old, is to start auranofin, a DMARD, for her rheumatoid arthritis. Teaching related to this drug therapy should include which of the following?

    a. Take with food or milk if GI upset occurs.

    b. Diarrhea may occur initially.

    c. Full therapeutic effect is not seen immediately.

    d. all of the above

    e. none of the above

2. Gary Franklin has been given a prescription for colchicine because he has attacks of gout periodically. Teaching regarding appropriate dosing of this drug includes taking the drug

    a. every day to prevent gout attacks.

    b. at the first sign of a gout attack.

    c. when the gout attack is resolving.

    d. when the gout attack is most severe.

3. George Sheely has been prescribed probenecid to treat his chronic gout. Patient education regarding diet, lifestyle, and habits should include which of the following?

    a. Take the probenecid with cranberry juice.

    b. Take the probenecid with milk.

    c. Drink two or three glasses of water a day.

    d. Drink two or three alcoholic drinks a day, if desired.

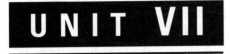

UNIT VII

Cardiovascular and Renal System Drugs

CHAPTER 27

Drugs for Treating Congestive Heart Failure

TOP TEN THINGS TO KNOW ABOUT DRUGS FOR TREATING CONGESTIVE HEART FAILURE

1. Cardiac output is the product of stroke volume and heart rate (CO = SV × HR). Stroke volume is affected by three factors: preload (amount of blood that has filled the ventricles by end of diastole), contractility (force of squeezing achieved by ventricles), and afterload (amount of pressure ventricles must overcome to eject blood; pressure is controlled by peripheral resistance).

2. In congestive heart failure (CHF), there is increased preload, increased afterload, and decreased cardiac output from the left ventricle. Drug therapy for CHF alters one or more of these factors to improve the functioning of the heart.

3. Angiotensin converting enzyme (ACE) inhibitors, diuretics, and cardiac glycosides are the three primary drug groups used to treat CHF.

4. The combined use of ACE inhibitors and diuretics has been found to decrease mortality from CHF. Cardiac glycosides do not decrease mortality, but they treat the symptoms of CHF and improve quality of life.

5. Digoxin, a cardiac glycoside, is used to manage the symptoms of CHF and to treat atrial fibrillation or flutter. It strengthens the force of contraction (positive inotropic effect), slows conduction (negative dromotropic effect), and slows heart rate (negative chronotropic effect) with a net effect of increasing cardiac output and controlling atrial rhythm.

6. The most common adverse effects of digoxin are cardiotoxicity, gastrointestinal (GI) disturbances, and central nervous system (CNS) toxicity. Antidote for overdose is digoxin immune FAB.

7. Always check apical pulse for 1 minute before administration of digoxin. Hold the dose if less than 60 beats/minute.

8. Monitor electrolyte levels, especially potassium, while on digoxin. Also assess drug blood levels when starting therapy, changing dose, or if toxicity is suspected.

9. Two drugs, inamrinone and milrinone, are used for short-term treatment of CHF in patients who are not responding to other drug therapy. They are given IV. They are not cardiac glycosides.

10. One beta blocker, carvedilol, is used in treating mild to moderate CHF. It is used as an adjunct to other therapy. Carvedilol decreases force of contraction and cardiac output (which may make CHF worse initially), and increases vasodilation and decreases peripheral resistance (which is helpful in CHF). Because of possible negative effects, dose is started small and gradually increased. Increased diuretic dosage may be needed to offset negative effects.

KEY TERMS

Word find exercise

Answer the questions below and find the correct key terms in the following:

```
D Z H A F T E R L O A D R T M D
G D P V Y N O I T C E J E A I Y
B C R C P D I A S T O L E G H B
P I E S U B T F G M O I I T E Y
T P L T U P T U O C B T A Z T R
T O O R B H J I G B A P R I O O
R R A O N H H D N L O V L L I R
E T D K H G F K I Y N I T O J G
S O G E G B B Z M A T M J G O P
I N F N V D A O B C S K U G H P
S I G F E T I D A H J T M N V F
T G B L I D N R S Y S T O L E M
A M C O R V T G N I D A O L R J
N Y N A V N W E T A R T R A E H
C N C D O C I P O R T O M O R D
E W V C H R O N O T R O P I C Z
```

1. Blood is circulated throughout the body by a coordinated sequence of chamber contractions and valve openings and closings known as the cardiac _____.
2. During _____, blood is pumped into the aorta and pulmonary artery.
3. Blood flows into the atria during _____.
4. Cardiac _____ is the volume of blood that leaves the left ventricle in 1 minute.
5. The amount of blood that leaves the left ventricle with each contraction is called the _____ volume.
6. _____ is the passive stretching force exerted on the ventricular muscle created by the amount of blood that has filled the heart by the end of diastole.
7. The force of the squeezing that the ventricle is able to achieve to eject the blood into the systemic circulation is called _____.
8. _____ is the amount of pressure the ventricular muscles must overcome to eject the blood into the systemic circulation.
9. The diameter of the vessel and the pressure within the vessel control peripheral _____.
10. The amount of blood leaving the ventricle with contraction compared with the total amount in the ventricle before contraction is called the _____ fraction.
11. Disorder in which the heart muscle enlarges.
12. The number of times the heart beats in a minute is called _____.
13. Drugs that affect the contractility of the heart are called _____ agents.
14. Drugs that affect the heart rate are called _____ agents.
15. Drugs that affect the rate of conductivity of the heart are called _____ agents.
16. _____ is the administration of a cardiac glycoside to treat symptoms rapidly.
17. A _____ dose is used to increase a serum drug level quickly.

PHYSIOLOGY AND PATHOPHYSIOLOGY: THE BODY HUMAN

Essay

1. Describe blood flow from the vena cava to the aorta.

2. What three factors influence stroke volume?

3. Compare and contrast the symptoms of right vs left heart failure.

CORE DRUG KNOWLEDGE: JUST THE FACTS

Multiple choice

Circle the option that best answers the question or completes the statement.

1. The management of congestive heart failure includes all of the following classes of medications EXCEPT
   a. positive inotropic agents
   b. diuretics.
   c. angiotensin converting enzyme inhibitors.
   d. antiarrhythmic agents.

2. The appropriate dose of digoxin is based on
   a. age.
   b. weight.
   c. lean body mass.
   d. hepatic enzyme levels.

3. Digoxin has which of the following actions on the heart?
   a. positive inotropic, positive dromotropic, negative chronotropic
   b. positive inotropic, negative dromotropic, negative chronotropic
   c. negative inotropic, positive dromotropic, positive chronotropic
   d. negative inotropic, negative dromotropic, negative chronotropic

4. Which of the following electrolyte imbalances is NOT associated with inducing digoxin toxicity?
   a. hyperkalemia
   b. hypokalemia
   c. hypomagnesemia
   d. hypercalcemia

5. Which of the following drugs may be used to treat digoxin toxicity?
   a. colestipol
   b. activated charcoal
   c. digoxin immune FAB
   d. all of the above

6. In general, the therapeutic margin for digoxin is
   a. 0.5 to 2.0 ng/mL.
   b. 0.5 to 20 ng/mL.
   c. 5 to 20 ng/mL.
   d. 0.05 to 0.2 ng/mL.

7. In addition to their inotropic effect, inamrinone and milrinone are used in the treatment of CHF because of their ability to
   a. increase conductivity through the heart.
   b. vasodilate.
   c. vasoconstrict.
   d. increase heart rate.

CORE PATIENT VARIABLES: PATIENTS, PLEASE

Multiple choice

Circle the option that best answers the question or completes the statement.

1. Elliott has CHF and is being started on digoxin. He also has a history of Graves' disease and has undergone thyroidectomy and takes levothyroxine. You have assessed Elliott's thyroid function tests and noted they are all within normal limits. Because of the status of Elliott's thyroid disease, his dose of digoxin should be
   a. increased.
   b. decreased.
   c. unchanged.

2. Judith Crane, age 88, is hospitalized for a fractured hip. She has a history of CHF and takes digoxin and furosemide. Before administering medications, you evaluate her lab results. You note a digoxin level of 2.96 ng/mL. You should
   a. give the medication as directed.
   b. take an apical pulse and give the medication if the pulse is normal.
   c. hold the medication and contact the provider.
   d. question Mrs. Crane about her symptoms, and give the medication unless there are cardiac abnormalities.

3. Karen Yates, age 55, is taking digoxin 0.125 mg QD for CHF. Mrs. Yates comes to the clinic today and states, "I've lost 5 lb. I can breath better and my heart rate is only 70." What is your assessment of these facts?

   a. The drug is working well.

   b. The dosage should be decreased.

   c. The dosage should be increased.

   d. The drug should be discontinued.

4. You are administering digoxin 0.125 mg to Mr. Kline. Before administering this drug, you should

   a. take the radial pulse 30 seconds and multiply by 2.

   b. take the apical pulse 15 seconds and multiply by 4.

   c. take the carotic pulse 1 full minute.

   d. take the apical pulse 1 full minute.

5. Mr. Smith takes digoxin 0.25 mg QD with furosemide (Lasix) 40 mg QD. This morning, Mr. Smith complains of anorexia and nausea. He vomited one time yesterday. What is your best action?

   a. Contact the physician and obtain an order for a nutritional supplement.

   b. Contact the physician for an order to keep Mr. Smith NPO for 24 hours.

   c. Contact the physician for an order to obtain a serum digoxin and electrolyte levels.

   d. Contact the physician for an order to obtain a potassium level.

6. Your patient is being discharged from the hospital with a prescription for digoxin. Which of the following should be OMITTED from your patient teaching?

   a. how to take a pulse

   b. avoidance of OTC antihistamines

   c. keep out of the sunlight

   d. do not stop this medication

NURSING MANAGEMENT: EVERY GOOD NURSE SHOULD . . .

Complete the decision tree on page 141.

Justine Banks , 81 years old, is admitted at 7 AM with acute CHF. She has right- and left-sided failure. Her pulse on admission is 122 beats/ minute. Her blood pressure is 166/110.

Her medication orders are:

furosemide (a loop diuretic) 20 mg IV push STAT; may repeat the dose in 2 hours if urine output is 30 cc/ hour or less or if respiratory symptoms worsen

captopril (an ACE inhibitor) 25 mg PO TID

hydrochlorothiazide (a thiazide diuretic) 50 mg PO BID

digoxin 0.375 mg PO STAT as loading dose

digoxin 0.125 mg PO 6 hours after loading dose, and 12 hours after loading dose

digoxin 0.25 mg PO daily beginning 24 hours after the loading dose

The night nurse tells you in report that she has administered the STAT dose of furosemide and the STAT dose of digoxin. You will be caring for Mrs. Banks today until 7 PM. At 9 AM, you complete a physical assessment to learn if the drug therapy is being effective in managing Mrs. Banks' CHF.

CASE STUDY

Mrs Banks wants to know why she is getting so many different medicines. Describe the patient education you will provide regarding the rationale for her drug regimen. (Need more help? See chapters 28, 30, and/or 31.)

CRITICAL THINKING CHALLENGE

After 24 hours Mrs. Banks still has crackles and wheezes in her lungs, 3+ edema in her hands and feet, a pulse of 96, and blood pressure of 150/96. You consult with her physician regarding these findings.

What additional orders might you seek, or might expect the physician to order?

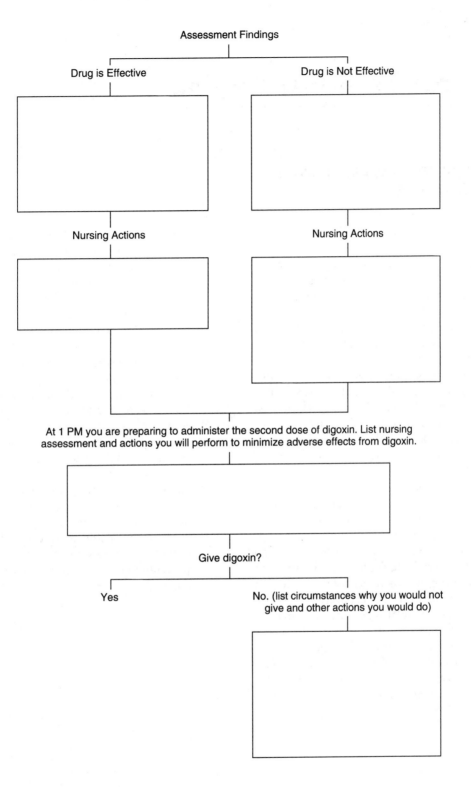

Assessment Findings

Drug is Effective

Drug is Not Effective

Nursing Actions

Nursing Actions

At 1 PM you are preparing to administer the second dose of digoxin. List nursing assessment and actions you will perform to minimize adverse effects from digoxin.

Give digoxin?

Yes

No. (list circumstances why you would not give and other actions you would do)

CHAPTER 28

Drugs for Treating Angina

TOP TEN THINGS TO KNOW ABOUT DRUGS FOR TREATING ANGINA

1. Three groups of drugs are used to treat angina: beta blockers, calcium channel blockers, and nitrates.
2. Beta blockers prevent the beta receptors of the heart from being stimulated; this alters cardiac function. Beta blockers slow the heart rate, depress atrioventricular (AV) conduction, decrease cardiac output, and reduce blood pressure. These effects decrease the oxygen demands of the heart and, thereby, decrease angina.
3. Calcium channel blockers inhibit calcium from moving across cell membranes. This also alters cardiac function. Calcium channel blockers slow heart rate, depress impulse formation (automaticity), and slow the velocity of conduction. These effects decrease the oxygen needs of the heart.
4. Calcium channel blockers are used in chronic stable angina when the patient cannot tolerate beta-blockers or nitrates, or if the symptoms are not adequately controlled while on these therapies.
5. Nitroglycerin relaxes vascular smooth muscle and dilates both arterial and venous vessels, although more effect is on venous vessels. Venous dilation decreases peripheral resistance, decreasing blood pressure. Arteriolar dilation reduces systemic vascular resistance and arterial pressure, thus reducing afterload. Myocardial oxygen consumption is decreased because of these effects. Nitroglycerin also redistributes blood flow in the heart, improving circulation to ischemic areas.

6. Nitroglycerin is used to treat acute angina (sublingually, transmucosal or translingual spray), to prevent chronic recurrent angina (topical, transdermal, translingual spray, and transmucosal or oral sustained-release), and significant hypertension (intravenously [IV]).
7. Tolerance to the vascular and antianginal effects may develop. To minimize this, start with as small a dose as possible and remove the nitroglycerin (paste or transdermal patches) from the patient for 10 to 12 h a day.
8. Nitroglycerin loses potency if exposed to light, humidity, heat, and plastic IV bags of fluid.
9. Assess the patient's blood pressure and pulse before administration and throughout therapy because nitroglycerin may cause hypotension and reflex tachycardia.
10. Adjunct drug therapy used with patients who have angina include aspirin, heparin, lipid-lowering agents, and morphine. These therapies do not decrease oxygen demands on the heart, but slow down the progression of coronary artery disease or prevent/treat complications that may arise with angina.

KEY TERMS

Matching

Match the following key terms with their definitions.

1. _____ angina

2. _____ chronic stable

3. _____ microvascular

4. _____ MI

5. _____ Prinzmetal's

6. _____ unstable

7. _____ variant

a. Cessation of oxygenation to a portion of the heart

b. Pain resulting from vasospasms in the coronary arteries

c. Pain resulting from decreased O_2 to the heart

d. Critical phase of coronary heart disease

e. Another term for Prinzmetal's angina

f. Chest pain without discernible coronary blockage

g. Predictable pain that results when O_2 demand exceeds O_2 supply

PHYSIOLOGY AND PATHOPHYSIOLOGY: THE BODY HUMAN

Essay

1. What is the etiology of angina?

2. What serum coronary markers can be found in patients with unstable angina?

3. What three classes of drugs are useful in the management of angina?

4. How do antianginal drugs relieve angina?

CORE DRUG KNOWLEDGE: JUST THE FACTS

Multiple choice

Circle the option that best answers the question or completes the statement.

1. What is the pharmacodynamics of nitrates such as nitroglycerin?
   a. decrease the contractility of the heart
   b. vasodilate arterial and venous vessels
   c. block the body's ability for an action potential
   d. thin the blood

2. Which of the following routes of administration would be appropriate for an acute angina attack?
   a. transdermal
   b. topical
   c. sustained-release tablet
   d. sublingual tablet

3. After administration of nitroglycerin, the nurse should expect to see
   a. increased blood pressure and decreased pulse.
   b. increased blood pressure and increased pulse.
   c. decreased blood pressure and decreased pulse.
   d. decreased blood pressure and increased pulse.

4. What action should be taken by the nurse to safely and effectively administer IV nitroglycerin?
   a. Use pressure-sensitive tubing.
   b. Use non-PVC IV administration tubing.
   c. Use blood tubing and attach to a D_5W main line.
   d. No special action is needed.

5. How frequently can the nurse administer sublingual nitroglycerin to the patient with acute chest pain?
   a. one tablet every 5 min, to a maximum of three
   b. one tablet every 3 min, to a maximum of five
   c. one tablet every 15 min, to a maximum of three
   d. one tablet every 30 min, to a maximum of two

6. Which of the following may occur in response to sublingual nitroglycerin?
   a. hyperglycemia
   b. sedation
   c. orthostatic hypotension
   d. rash

CORE PATIENT VARIABLES: PATIENTS, PLEASE

Multiple choice

Circle the option that best answers the question or completes the statement.

1. Mrs. Grey has been experiencing tolerance to her transdermal nitroglycerin. Which of the following suggestions would be appropriate?
   a. "You should use the patch only when you have pain."
   b. "You should take the patch off when you go to bed and put a new one on in the morning."
   c. "You should stop the patch and use only the sublingual tablet for pain."
   d. "You should change the patch every other day."

2. Which of the following patients should not use nitroglycerin for angina?
   a. Mabel, with high blood pressure
   b. Susan, with hypothyroidism
   c. Dennis, with a small cerebral aneurysm
   d. Larry, with renal stenosis

3. Mr. Kierney had a myocardial infarction last night. What is the most appropriate route of administration for nitroglycerin for this patient?
   a. intravenous
   b. sublingual
   c. topical
   d. sustained-release tablets

4. Mrs. Exter has newly diagnosed angina and has been prescribed sublingual nitroglycerin PRN. Which of the following instructions would you give Mrs. Exter?
   a. "Increase your fluids every day."
   b. "Be sure to sit or lie down after taking a pill in case you get dizzy."
   c. "Throw the bottle away if you get a burning sensation under your tongue."
   d. "If you have problems getting the pill out of the bottle, just put it in an envelope in your purse."

5. Kelly Reyes, age 61, has been prescribed transmucosal nitroglycerin. The nurse recognizes that Mrs. Reyes needs additional patient teaching when the patient states
   a. "I'll place this in the pouch between my cheek and gum."
   b. "I won't drink any coffee or tea when it's in my mouth."
   c. "It will be difficult, but I'll remember not to play with it with my tongue."
   d. "After an hour, I can swallow the pill."

6. Mr. Lee, age 57, has been prescribed nitroglycerin transdermal patch. The nurse should include which of the following in Mr. Lee's patient teaching?
   a. Keep the patch out of the reach of children.
   b. Wear the patch in the same area of the body for a week at a time.
   c. Change the patch daily at the same time.
   d. Wear the patch on the distal arm or leg so it can be removed quickly if needed.

NURSING MANAGEMENT: EVERY GOOD NURSE SHOULD . . .

Multiple choice

Circle the option that best answers the question or completes the statement.

1. Your patient is admitted with a diagnosis of chest pain, rule out MI. He has an order for nitroglycerin 0.3 mg SL PRN for chest pain. When he complains of chest pain, you should
   a. administer a tablet into his mouth every 3 min.
   b. administer three tablets under his tongue.
   c. administer a tablet under his tongue; if no relief, repeat in 5 min, and then again in 5 min.
   d. contact the physician immediately.

2. In addition to administering nitroglycerin SL for acute chest pain for the patient listed above, what other actions or assessments should the nurse make?
   a. Listen for lung sounds.
   b. Check pulse.
   c. Check pulse and blood pressure.
   d. Determine urinary output.

3. Your patient, Sally Morgan, is admitted with a history of chronic stable angina. Her medication orders include: 1 inch Nitrol ointment topically every 6 h and Nitrostat tablets 0.4 mg SL PRN. Her last dose of Nitrol ointment was given 2 h ago. She calls you into her room and tells you that she has developed chest pain. You should

    a. administer the next regularly scheduled dose of Nitrol ointment now, and hold the next dose.

    b. administer an additional dose of Nitrol ointment now to her left foot.

    c. administer nothing now, but repeat the Nitrol ointment when it is next due.

    d. administer a Nitrostat tablet now.

4. Margarita Lopez is being sent home with a new prescription for transdermal nitroglycerin patches. She has told you, the nurse, how she cares for her grandchildren 3 days a week. In your patient education for Ms. Lopez, you should include information on

    a. measuring the correct dose of nitroglycerin.

    b. the importance of wearing the patch 24 h a day.

    c. applying the patch at the first sign of acute chest pain.

    d. safe disposal of the used patches.

5. Carol Denny is to be started on sublinguinal nitroglycerin tablets. She is to use them as needed at home. Patient education for this drug therapy should include

    a. keep the tablets in the original brown bottle.

    b. keep the cap off of the bottle so the tablets can be easily accessed.

    c. continue activity, such as walking, during acute chest pain.

    d. dall 911 before taking any SL nitroglycerin.

6. Which of the following should the nurse keep in mind before starting a hypertensive patient on an ordered IV infusion of nitroglycerin?

    a. The patient should be monitored in the ICU during infusion.

    b. The IV tubing provided by the manufacturer should be used.

    c. Glass bottles should be used to hold the diluted nitroglycerin.

    d. all of the above

CASE STUDY

Rob Thomlinson is 40 years old. He has a family history of coronary artery disease (both parents died in their fifties of MI). He is an insulin-controlled diabetic. He had angina for 3 months, before being admitted to the hospital with MI. He is stabilized now and is to be discharged on transdermal nitroglycerin, worn 14 h a day; sublinguinal nitroglycerin PRN; propranolol, an oral beta blocker, twice a day; and aspirin, orally, daily.

Discuss the rationale for this combination drug therapy.

CRITICAL THINKING CHALLENGE

If Rob Thomlinson also had asthma, in addition to his other health problems, would you expect any variation from the drug therapy prescribed above? If yes, what drugs would be added or subtracted?

CHAPTER 29

Drugs Affecting Cardiac Output and Rhythm

TOP TEN THINGS TO KNOW ABOUT DRUGS AFFECTING CARDIAC OUTPUT AND RHYTHM

1. Contractions of the heart depend on a specialized electrical conduction system. An action potential is started in the sinoatrial (SA) node and travels through the heart causing the atria to contract. The impulse is slowed at the atrioventricular (AV) node, and then spreads through the ventricles causing them to contract. Calcium is needed for the creation of the action potential.

2. Changes in the ionic currents (sodium, potassium, and calcium) through ion channels of the myocardial cell membrane are the main cause of cardiac arrhythmias (abnormal rhythm). These ionic changes allow arrhythmias to develop in one of three ways: through a disorder with impulse formation (the automaticity of the heart), through a disorder of the impulse conduction system, or through a combination of both.

3. Any drug used to treat an arrhythmia (or dysrhythmia) can also cause an arrhythmia.

4. Quinidine, a class IA antiarrhythmic is used to treat atrial arrhythmias. It suppresses phase 0 of the action potential; decreases myocardial excitability, conduction velocity, and contractility; and prevents reentry phenomenon. Indirect anticholinergic effects also occur. The most common adverse effect is gastrointestinal (GI) disturbance, but serious cardiac changes and hepatic toxicity can occur. Monitor electrocardiogram (ECG), serum drug levels, liver and renal function, CBC, and potassium while on quinidine.

5. Class IB drugs, such as lidocaine, also depress phase 0 (although not as much as IA drugs). They also suppress automaticity. They are used primarily with ventricular arrhythmias. Lidocaine's most common adverse effects affect the cardiovascular system (arrhythmias and hypotension) and the central nervous system (dizziness/light-headedness, fatigue, and drowsiness). Excessive levels of lidocaine can produce confusion and seizures. Monitor ECG continuously while on lidocaine and switch to another antiarrhythmic as soon as stable.

6. Class IC drugs (flecainide and propafenone) depress phase 0 considerably, have a slight effect on repolarization, and decrease conduction significantly. Use of these drugs is usually limited to life-threatening ventricular arrhythmias due to an increased risk of mortality.

7. Class II antiarrhythmics are beta blockers, such as propranolol. Propranolol depresses the cardiac action potential to control arrhythmias. Propranolol also slows heart rate and decreases cardiac output and is used to treat angina and hypertension.

8. Amiodarone, a class III antiarrhythmic, produces a prolonged phase 3 (repolarization). Amiodarone is used in life-threatening arrhythmias that have not responded to other drug therapies. Amiodarone has unique pharmacokinetics and pharmacodynamics; these have an effect on dosing, therapeutic effect, and adverse effects. Amiodarone has three potentially fatal adverse effects: pulmonary toxicity (most common), exacerbation of the arrhythmia being treated, and liver disease (rare). Monitor patients carefully for adverse effects.

9. Class IV antiarrhythmic drugs are calcium channel blockers, such as verapamil. Verapamil inhibits movement of calcium ions across the cardiac and arterial muscle cell membranes. It slows conduction, depresses automaticity, depresses myocardial contractility, and dilates coronary arteries and peripheral arterioles. It is used to control ventricular rate in chronic atrial flutter or fibrillation, prophylactically (with digoxin) to treat repetitive paroxysmal supraventricular tachycardia, and to treat supraventricular tachyarrhythmias. It is also used to treat angina and hypertension. The most common adverse effect is constipation.

10. Sodium polystyrene sulfonate (Kayexalate) is a potassium-removing resin used to lower serum potassium levels to prevent serious or life-threatening arrhythmias. It is given orally or by enema. Effective lowering of potassium may take several hours; avoid use in severe hyperkalemia, where a more rapid effect is needed.

KEY TERMS

True/false

Mark true or false for each of the following statements. If the statement is false, replace the underlined word with the words that will make the statement correct.

1. _____ <u>Arrhythmia</u> is the term used to describe an abnormality of cardiac rhythm.
2. _____ Absence of electrical activity is called a <u>dysrhythmia</u>.
3. _____ <u>Systole</u> is the resting phase of the cadiac cycle.
4. _____ The blood exits the ventricles during <u>diastole</u>.
5. _____ A cycle of systole and diastole is called the <u>cardiac cycle</u>.
6. _____ There is an electrical gradient across the membrane of the cell called an <u>action potential</u>.
7. _____ Phase 0 of the action potential is called <u>repolarization</u>.
8. _____ <u>Ventricular fibrillation</u> is one of the lethal arrhythmias.
9. _____ The ability to generate an impulse spontaneously is called <u>proarrhythmia</u>.
10. _____ The movement of the transmembrane potential away from a positive value and toward the negative resting potential is called <u>depolarization</u>.
11. _____ <u>Resting membrane potential</u> causes repetitive cardiac stimulation, firing, and arrhythmias.
12. _____ The most common arrhythmia seen in clinical practice is <u>atrial flutter</u>.
13. _____ An arrhythmia produced by the use of antiarrhythmic agents is called an <u>action potential</u>.
14. _____ <u>Automaticity</u> means that the electrical impulse originated outside the SA node.
15. _____ Electrical changes that occur during an entire cycle of contraction and relaxation are called the <u>resting membrane potential</u>.
16. _____ <u>Atrial fibrillation</u> frequently converts to ventricular fibrillation.
17. _____ <u>Atrial flutter</u> can cause the heart to beat at 300 beats per minute.

PHYSIOLOGY AND PATHOPHYSIOLOGY: THE BODY HUMAN

Essay

1. Describe the normal electrical conduction through the heart.

2. Describe the phases of an action potential.

3. What is the purpose of the plateau phase of the action potential in cardiac muscle?

4. Differentiate between the absolute and relative refractory periods.

5. Identify the etiology of electrolyte-induced arrhythmias.

CORE DRUG KNOWLEDGE: JUST THE FACTS

Multiple choice

Circle the option that best answers the question or completes the statement.

1. What is the purpose of antiarrhythmic drugs?
   a. to change the flow of blood through the heart
   b. to substitute for implantable cardio defibrillators
   c. to prevent, suppress, or treat a disturbance in cardiac rhythm
   d. to increase or decrease the contractility of the heart muscle

2. What is the prototype for class IA antiarrhythmic agents?
   a. quinidine (Quinora, Cardioquin)
   b. flecainide (Tambocor)
   c. lidocaine (Xylocaine)
   d. propranolol (Inderal)

3. What is the mechanism of action of class I antiarrhythmic agents?
   a. They block adrenergic receptors, affecting phase 4.
   b. They block sodium channels, affecting phase 0.
   c. They lengthen the action potential duration, affecting phase 3.
   d. They block calcium channels, affecting phase 4 depolarization and phases 1 and 2 of repolarization.

4. Quinidine (Quinora, Cardioquin) can be used in the management of
   a. atrial arrhythmias.
   b. ventricular arrhythmias.
   c. both atrial and ventricular arrhythmias.
   d. heart block only.

5. Class IB drugs, such as lidocaine (Xylocaine) are most often used in the management of
   a. atrial arrhythmias.
   b. ventricular arrhythmias.
   c. both atrial and ventricular arrhythmias.
   d. heart block only.

6. What is the prototype for class II antiarrhythmic agents?
   a. quinidine (Quinora, Cardioquin)
   b. flecainide (Tambocor)
   c. lidocaine (Xylocaine)
   d. propranolol (Inderal)

7. What is the mechanism of action of class II antiarrhythmic agents?
   a. They block beta-adrenergic receptors, affecting phase 4.
   b. They block sodium channels, affecting phase 0.
   c. They lengthen the action potential duration, affecting phase 3.
   d. They block calcium channels, affecting phase 4 depolarization and phases 1 and 2 of repolarization.

8. Amiodarone (Cordarone, Pacerone) is used only in the treatment of documented life-threatening recurrent ventricular arrhythmias because of its
   a. prohibitive cost.
   b. extremely long half-life.
   c. potential adverse effects.
   d. ability to interact with any other medication.

9. A unique feature of amiodarone (Cordarone, Pacerone) is that its mechanism of action affects
   a. phases 0 and 1 of the action potential.
   b. phases 1 and 2 of the action potential.
   c. phases 0, 2, and 3 of the action potential.
   d. all four phases of the action potential.

10. What is the prototype for class IV antiarrhythmic agents?
    a. quinidine (Quinora, Cardioquin)
    b. verapamil (verapamil hydrochloride, Calan, Isoptin)
    c. lidocaine (Xylocaine)
    d. amiodarone (Cordarone, Pacerone)

11. What is the mechanism of action of class IV antiarrhythmic agents?
    a. They block beta-adrenergic receptors, affecting phase 4.
    b. They block sodium channels, affecting phase 0.
    c. They lengthen the action potential duration, affecting phase 3.
    d. They block calcium channels, affecting phase 4 depolarization and phases 1 and 2 of repolarization.

12. What is the most common adverse effect to verapamil (verapamil hydrochloride, Calan, Isoptin) therapy?
    a. constipation
    b. headache
    c. diarrhea
    d. muscle aches

CORE PATIENT VARIABLES: PATIENTS, PLEASE

Multiple choice

Circle the option that best answers the question or completes the statement.

1. Which of the following patients SHOULD NOT receive quinidine (Quinora, Cardioquin)?
   a. Henry, with migraine headaches
   b. Calvin, with hypothyroidism
   c. Molly, with myasthenia gravis
   d. Leslie, with diabetes

2. Mrs. Taylor comes to the clinic for a recheck of her cardiac status. She takes quinidine (Quinora, Cardioquin). During your assessment, you note on her ECG an increased PR and QT interval, 50% widening of the QRS complex, and a short run of ventricular tachycardia. With your knowledge of this drug, what do you anticipate Mrs. Taylor needs?
   a. an increase in the dose of quinidine
   b. a decrease in the dose of quinidine
   c. an immediate cessation of the drug
   d. an immediate cessation of the drug, and hospitalization

3. Audrey Reese, age 60, takes quinidine (Quinora, Cardioquin) for her arrhythmias. Which of the following electrolytes should be closely monitored while Mrs. Reese is taking this medication?

   a. potassium

   b. sodium

   c. magnesium

   d. chloride

4. Mrs. Olson came to the Emergency Department and was noted to have a ventricular arrhythmia. The arrhythmia was stopped with an intravenous (IV) bolus of lidocaine (Xylocaine). The nurse should prepare to

   a. administer quinidine (Quinora, Cardioquin) if the arrhythmia recurs.

   b. double the initial IV dose of lidocaine if the arrhythmia recurs.

   c. hang an IV piggyback of lidocaine (Xylocaine).

   d. hang an IV piggyback of tocainide (Tonocard).

5. Which of the following patients SHOULD NOT take propranolol (Inderal) for cardiac arrhythmias?

   a. Henry, with migraine headaches

   b. Susan, with severe asthma

   c. John, with tachycardia

   d. Nancy, with hypertension

6. Steven James, age 54, has ventricular arrhythmias despite use of multiple antiarrhythmic agents and is being prescribed amiodarone (Cordarone, Pacerone). Identification of which of the following comorbid states would preclude the use of amiodarone for Mr. James?

   a. hypertension

   b. myasthenia gravis

   c. Parkinson's disease

   d. thyroid disease

7. Mrs. Kennedy is being prescribed IV amiodarone (Cordarone, Pacerone). Which body system should be CAREFULLY monitored during this therapy?

   a. respiratory system

   b. integumentary system

   c. GI system

   d. hematopoietic system

8. To ensure appropriate administration of IV amiodarone, the nurse should

   a. use non–polyvinyl chloride administration tubing and an in-line filter.

   b. use polyvinyl chloride administration tubing, an in-line filter, and a volumetric infusion pump.

   c. use polyvinyl chloride administration tubing and a volumetric infusion pump.

   d. use non–polyvinyl chloride administration tubing and a volumetric infusion pump.

9. Which of the following patients may receive verapamil (verapamil hydrochloride, Calan, Isoptin) therapy?

   a. Marjorie, with sick sinus syndrome

   b. Hilary, with severe CHF

   c. Kimberly, with hypertension

   d. Gina, with third-degree heart block

10. Leonard Kramer, age 67, has been started on verapamil (verapamil hydrochloride, Calan, Isoptin) therapy. Patient teaching should include management of potential

    a. sedation.

    b. constipation.

    c. hypertension.

    d. headache.

NURSING MANAGEMENT: EVERY GOOD NURSE SHOULD . . .

Multiple choice

Circle the option that best answers the question or completes the statement.

1. A sustained-release form of quinidine is being administered to Sheila Mathews to treat recurrent premature atrial contractions. Patient education regarding quinidine should include

   a. taking the drug on an empty stomach.

   b. limiting dietary intake of potassium.

   c. the need for periodic blood tests.

   d. chewing the drug thoroughly before swallowing.

2. Doug Jones has ventricular fibrillation. He was treated with lidocaine, a class IB antiarrhythmic. However, the lidocaine failed to control the ventricular fibrillation. Mr. Jones is ordered an IV infusion of amiodarone, a class III antiarrhythmic. Nursing management in this drug therapy includes

a. helping the patient to ambulate.

b. monitoring blood pressure throughout therapy.

c. thorough diluting of doses given by intramuscular (IM) injection.

d. encouraging fluids to prevent constipation.

3. The nurse should not administer IV verapamil, a class IV antiarrhythmic and calcium channel blocker, within a few hours of administering

a. digoxin.

b. beta blockers.

c. potassium.

d. diuretics.

4. Richard Guiseppe's potassium level is elevated at 5.5, and he is to receive sodium polystyrene sulfonate (Kayexalate) via an enema as treatment. The nurse should

a. administer a cleansing enema first.

b. administer the drug using an infusion pump.

c. monitor the patient's blood pressure during treatment.

d. monitor the patient's liver enzymes after treatment.

5. Louis Rappaport is to be started on propranolol, a beta blocker, for treatment of his cardiac arrhythmia. Before administering the first dose of the drug, the nurse should assess his health status and determine that he does not have

a. hypertension.

b. angina.

c. severe chronic obstructive pulmonary disease (COPD).

d. all of the above.

CASE STUDY

Kenny Thomas is to receive oral verapamil, a calcium channel blocker, class IV antiarrhythmic, to treat recurrent paroxysmal supraventricular tachycardia. He also has a history of renal disease.

1. What physical parameters need to be assessed before each dose of verapamil?

2. What is the impact of renal disease on verapamil therapy?

CRITICAL THINKING CHALLENGE

Kenny Thomas returns to the clinic for a follow-up appointment 6 weeks after beginning verapamil. During assessment, it is discovered that he has developed an atrial tachycardia.
What possible explanations related to drug therapy may explain this finding?

CHAPTER 30

Drugs Affecting Blood Pressure

TOP TEN THINGS TO KNOW ABOUT DRUGS AFFECTING BLOOD PRESSURE

1. Blood pressure is achieved from cardiac output multiplied by peripheral resistance (BP = CO × PR). Drug therapy to reduce hypertension is designed to reduce either cardiac output or peripheral resistance or both.

2. There are four steps to hypertension treatment. The first step is lifestyle changes. Steps 2 through 4 include lifestyle changes and the addition of one or more drugs. Patients are "stepped up" in treatment if hypertension is not controlled, or possibly "stepped down" if they demonstrate good control over time.

3. Diuretics or beta blockers are most frequently used as drugs of first choice in treating hypertension because they decrease mortality from hypertension. Calcium channel blockers are also used to treat hypertension and may be used as first-line drugs or (more frequently) when drug therapy is to include at least two different types of drugs.

4. Captopril, an angiotensin-converting enzyme (ACE) inhibitor, blocks the formation of angiotensin II. This prevents sodium and water retention, decreases peripheral vascular resistance, and lowers blood pressure. Significant adverse effects include chronic cough and first-dose hypotension.

5. Losartan, an angiotensin II receptor antagonist, blocks the vasoconstricting and aldosterone-secreting effects of angiotensin II by preventing angiotensin II from binding to receptors in many tissues. Peripheral resistance is reduced, lowering blood pressure. Losartan does not cause the "ACE cough," but upper respiratory infections are common adverse effects.

6. Labetalol is an adrenergic-blocking drug that blocks both beta-1 and beta-2 sites in addition to selective alpha-1 sites. Alpha blocking causes peripheral vasodilation that reduces blood pressure. Beta blocking prevents reflex tachycardia.

7. Clonidine is an alpha-2 stimulator. It inhibits sympathetic nervous system response and reduces sympathetic outflow from the central nervous system (CNS). This decreases heart rate, blood pressure, vasoconstriction, and renal vascular resistance. Clonidine can be used to control withdrawal symptoms from abused substances because of the sympatholytic effects; it can also be misused by substance abusers when they are unable to obtain a "fix."

8. Hydralazine is a direct-acting vasodilator that causes peripheral vasodilation. Peripheral resistance and arterial blood pressure are then decreased. Hydralazine is usually used as an adjunct drug to other antihypertensive drug therapy. It is used with beta blockers (preferably) or clonidine to prevent reflex tachycardia from the peripheral vasodilation, and with diuretics to offset fluid retention from the increased production of angiotensin II.

9. Nitroprusside is used to treat hypertensive crisis (BP 210/120). It directly relaxes vascular smooth muscle, dilates veins more than arteries thus decreasing preload and afterload, and lowers blood pressure dramatically. Administer nitroprusside by way of an infusion pump and monitor blood pressure constantly. Cyanide poisoning is possible from the metabolism of nitroprusside. Avoid overdosage.

10. Dopamine is a vasopressor used in treating shock. It increases cardiac output and peripheral resistance, thus increasing blood pressure. Because it increases renal perfusion, the drug's correct dose is often determined by the dose required to increase urinary output to adequate levels. The most common adverse effects involve the cardiovascular system. Administer dopamine by IV only in acute care settings where continuous monitoring of the patient's cardiovascular status can occur.

KEY TERMS

Fill in the blanks and word find exercise

Read each statement carefully and, using the chapter's key terms, write your answer in the space provided. Then locate the term in the puzzle below.

```
H  Y  P  E  R  T  E  N  S  I  O  N  O  C  Y  O
H  C  S  T  E  P  P  E  D  C  A  R  E  X  V  Y
V  A  I  S  T  Q  P  L  A  V  E  A  I  J  R  D
B  N  D  T  I  W  S  M  R  R  J  I  W  A  S  I
D  G  J  G  E  S  E  T  T  B  F  P  M  Y  P  A
E  I  R  B  C  M  I  Y  M  C  W  I  M  S  T  S
N  O  J  Z  O  Q  I  R  C  A  R  P  L  H  F  T
O  T  C  I  E  P  S  M  C  P  A  D  J  O  N  O
R  E  I  E  J  B  Y  J  O  T  V  D  Q  C  O  L
E  N  L  T  Q  T  N  R  H  H  G  M  W  K  D  I
T  S  O  Q  I  E  E  O  A  G  T  B  A  G  D  C
S  I  T  J  A  N  L  V  Z  U  M  A  P  D  Q  U
O  N  S  Z  I  Y  M  O  H  E  D  W  P  K  E  Z
D  H  Y  N  T  G  T  O  N  D  M  L  F  M  A  B
L  C  S  I  F  E  S  S  E  N  T  I  A  L  Y  N
A  Z  C  K  R  N  Y  R  A  D  N  O  C  E  S  S
```

1. Denoting mimicking of action of the sympathetic nervous system _____

2. Denoting antagonism to or inhibition of adrenergic nerve activity _____

3. The highest blood pressure measured when the heart contracts and ejects blood into the circulation _____

4. The lowest blood pressure measured when the heart relaxes _____

5. The type of hypertension responsible for 90% to 95% of all cases of hypertension _____

6. Another term for primary hypertension _____

7. Systolic blood pressure exceeding 210 mmHg and diastolic blood pressure exceeding 120 mmHg _____

8. Defined as a blood pressure greater than 140/90 _____

9. Systematic approach to the treatment options for hypertension _____

10. Characterized by low blood pressure _____

11. Type of hypertension that occurs because of another condition _____

12. System controlled by the kidneys that increases blood pressure _____

PHYSIOLOGY AND PATHOPHYSIOLOGY: THE BODY HUMAN

Essay

1. Which phase of the cardiac cycle is occurring when you are able to palpate the patient's pulse?

2. For a patient with a decreased cardiac output, what type of blood pressure would you expect?

3. In the adrenergic system, stimulation of alpha-1 would generate what type of response? Alpha-2? Beta-1? Beta-2?

4. What is the primary location of the adrenergic receptors?

5. What are the effects of the renin-angiotensin-aldosterone system?

CORE DRUG KNOWLEDGE: JUST THE FACTS

Multiple choice

Circle the option that best answers the question or completes the statement.

1. Which of the following adverse reactions may occur with ALL antihypertensive medications?
   a. cardiac arrhythmias
   b. volume depletion
   c. hypokalemia
   d. orthostatic hypotension

2. In addition to hypertension, captopril (Capoten), an ACE inhibitor, may be useful in the treatment of
   a. congestive heart failure (CHF).
   b. cardiac arrhythmias.
   c. reentry phenomena.
   d. pulmonary emboli.

3. Due to the action of captopril (Capoten), which of the following electrolytes should be monitored?
   a. calcium and chloride
   b. chloride and sodium
   c. potassium and sodium
   d. magnesium and calcium

4. Which of the following adverse reactions is associated with ACE inhibitors?
   a. bradycardia
   b. cough
   c. hypertension
   d. ankle edema

5. Which of the following cultural groups may have a decreased response to captopril (Capoten) when used as monotherapy?
   a. Black
   b. White
   c. Asian
   d. Mexican American

6. Losartan (Cozaar), an angiotensin II blocking agent, works by blocking the
   a. conversion of angiotensin I to angiotensin II.
   b. release of renin.
   c. binding of angiotensin II to the AT 1 receptors.
   d. sympathetic response to alpha-1 receptors.

7. Patient education for FEMALE patients receiving ACE inhibitors or angiotensin II blocking agents MUST include
   a. dietary restrictions.
   b. potential harm to a fetus or infant child.
   c. need for supplemental potassium.
   d. risk for increased menstrual bleeding.

8. Labetalol (Normodyne) is classified as a(an)
   a. beta blocker.
   b. ACE inhibitor.
   c. alpha-beta blocker.
   d. alpha blocker.

9. Maximum therapeutic effect of labetalol is achieved within
   a. 5 minutes.
   b. 2 to 3 weeks.
   c. 1 hour.
   d. 24 to 72 hours.

10. How does labetalol (Normodyne), an alpha-beta blocking agent, work?
    a. specifically blocks alpha-1 and nonspecifically blocks beta-1 and beta-2
    b. specifically blocks alpha-2 and specifically blocks beta-1
    c. specifically blocks alpha-1 and specifically blocks beta-2
    d. nonspecifically blocks alpha-1 and alpha-2 and specifically blocks beta-1

11. How does clonidine (Catapres), an alpha-2 agonist, work?
    a. Stimulation of alpha-2 inhibits the release of norepinephrine.
    b. Blocking alpha-2 inhibits the release of norepinephrine.
    c. Stimulation of alpha-2 inhibits the release of acetylcholine.
    d. Blocking alpha-2 inhibits the release of acetylcholine.

12. Pharmacotherapeutics for clonidine (Catapres) are derived from its
    a. parasympathetic inhibition effects.
    b. sympathetic stimulant effect.
    c. sympathetic inhibition effects.
    d. parasympathetic stimulant effect.

13. Clonidine (Catapres) by transdermal application is expected to maximize its effect within
    a. 30 to 60 minutes.
    b. 2 to 3 days.
    c. 3 to 5 hours.
    d. 24 hours.

14. Abrupt discontinuation of clonidine (Catapres) may result in
    a. increased drowsiness.
    b. rebound hypertension.
    c. orthostatic hypotension.
    d. constipation.

15. In addition to hypertension, alpha-1 blockers may be useful in the treatment of
    a. benign prostatic hypertrophy.
    b. diverticulitis.
    c. asthma.
    d. peptic ulcer disease.

16. Hydralazine (Apresoline), a direct-acting vasodilator, works by
    a. blocking the beta-1 receptors in the heart, decreasing cardiac output.
    b. interrupting the renin-angiotensin-aldosterone system.
    c. blocking the calcium channels, resulting in vasodilation.
    d. directing smooth muscle relaxation of the arterioles.

17. When administered as monotherapy, hydralazine (Apresoline) may induce
    a. decreased stroke volume.
    b. tachycardia.
    c. decreased cardiac output.
    d. hypertension.

18. Which of the following cultural groups are most likely to develop hydralazine-induced lupus?
    a. Black
    b. White
    c. Native American
    d. Mexican American

19. In addition to hypertension, minoxidil is useful in the treatment of
    a. male pattern baldness.
    b. peptic ulcer disease.
    c. psoriasis.
    d. hyperaldosteronism.

20. Nitroprusside (Nitropress) is the drug of choice in the management of
    a. rebound hypotension.
    b. hypertensive crisis.
    c. rebound tachycardia.
    d. bradycardia.

21. Maximum therapeutic effects of nitroprusside (Nitropress) occur within
    a. 2 to 3 days.
    b. 1 to 2 days.
    c. 24 hours.
    d. 1 to 2 minutes.

22. Dopamine (Intropin), a vasopressor, is used in the management of
    a. hypertensive crisis.
    b. rebound tachycardia.
    c. shock.
    d. acute respiratory failure.

23. Dopamine (Intropin) works by
    a. stimulation of alpha-2, beta-2, and a dopaminergic effect.
    b. inhibition of alpha-1, beta-1, and a dopaminergic effect.
    c. stimulation of alpha-1, beta-1, and a dopaminergic effect.
    d. inhibition of alpha-2, beta-2, and a dopaminergic effect.

24. Major differences between dopamine (Intropin) and dobutamine (Dobutrex) include which of the following?
    a. Dobutamine is more effective than dopamine at increasing the rate at the sinoatrial (SA) node.
    b. Dobutamine increases blood pressure whereas dopamine decreases blood pressure.
    c. Dopamine does not cause vasoconstriction or the release of endogenous norepinephrine.
    d. Dobutamine does not cause vasoconstriction or the release of endogenous norepinephrine.

CORE PATIENT VARIABLES: PATIENTS, PLEASE

Multiple choice

Circle the option that best answers the question or completes the statement.

1. Rich Goodman, age 45, has been diagnosed with hypertension and takes captopril (Capoten). His blood pressure has remained elevated despite his compliance with captopril and lifestyle changes. The provider decides to add a diuretic to Mr. Goodman's regimen. Which of the following classes of diuretics would be INAPPROPRIATE for Mr. Goodman?
    a. thiazide
    b. loop
    c. potassium-sparing
    d. osmotic

2. Julie Bright, age 33, takes captopril for hypertension. Which of the following instructions should be given to Ms. Bright?
    a. "It is better to use a salt substitute containing potassium instead of adding salt to your food."
    b. "If you decide to become pregnant, please make an appointment and discuss your medications with your health care provider."
    c. "You may experience more adverse effects, such as constipation, if you exercise while taking this medication."
    d. "Cough is a common adverse effect to this medication, but you have less than ½ of 1% chance to develop it because you are female."

3. Joyce Henson, age 55, has hypertension and is being started on medication. When reviewing Ms. Henson's health status history you note she has asthma and arthritis. Which of the following drugs would be INAPPROPRIATE for Ms. Henson?
    a. captopril (Capoten)
    b. clonidine (Catapres)
    c. hydralazine (Apresoline)
    d. labetalol (Normodyne)

4. Jack Palmer, age 61, is admitted to your unit with a hypertensive crisis. The health care provider orders IV labetalol (Normodyne). Because this medication is being administered by the IV route, the nurse should routinely evaluate Mr. Palmer for the development of
    a. CHF.
    b. hemorrhage.
    c. constipation.
    d. sedation.

5. Esther Karnes, age 40, has been prescribed labetalol (Normodyne) at her clinic visit today. Which of the following instructions would be INAPPROPRIATE?
    a. "You should change positions slowly to avoid hypotension."
    b. "Do not stop this medication abruptly because it may cause some severe problems."
    c. "Take this medication on an empty stomach to increase its absorption."
    d. "It is important to let us know if you become pregnant."

6. Jennifer Clinton has hypertension, and clonidine (Catapres) has been prescribed. Which of the following comorbid states may contraindicate the use of clonidine?

   a. chronic renal failure

   b. Parkinson's disease

   c. diverticulitis

   d. asthma

7. Kenny James is prescribed clonidine for his hypertension. Which of the following educational points should be made with Mr. James?

   a. "Stop the medication and make a new appointment if you are having adverse effects."

   b. "You need to stop the medication at least 4 weeks before you have any surgery."

   c. "It is very important that you do not stop this medication abruptly."

   d. "Take the full dose early in the morning."

8. Ralphe Uribe, age 55, has hypertension and benign prostatic hypertrophy. Because of these comorbid states, Mr. Uribe may benefit from the use of

   a. clonidine (Catapres).

   b. prazosin (Minipress).

   c. losartan (Cozaar).

   d. captopril (Capoten).

9. Philip Olson takes hydralazine (Apresoline) and propranolol (Inderal) for his hypertension. Propranolol is given concurrently with hydralazine to decrease the possibility of reflex tachycardia. Because of this combination, Mr. Olson should be instructed to

   a. eat green leafy vegetables.

   b. monitor his blood pressure for efficacy of treatment.

   c. monitor his weight for fluid retention.

   d. take the medication every other day.

10. Murray Thompson, age 72, is in the coronary care unit for hypertensive crisis. He is receiving nitroprusside (Nitropress). Mr. Thompson complains of abdominal pain, headache, and palpitations. You note that he appears apprehensive and restless. Which of the following actions would be appropriate?

    a. Medicate with morphine.

    b. Call the health care provider to respond STAT.

    c. Slow the infusion rate.

    d. Administer thiosulfate according to hospital protocol.

11. Eleanor Thomas is experiencing a hypertensive crisis. The provider has ordered intravenous nitroprusside (Nitropress). Before administration, the nurse should take action to

    a. protect the solution from light.

    b. use pressurized tubing for administration.

    c. administer by IV bolus only.

    d. use lidocaine as the diluent.

12. Nancy James, age 55, is admitted to your unit due to shock and has received fluid resuscitation. Dopamine (Intropin) is ordered to increase renal blood flow. With your knowledge of this drug, you expect the dopamine to be administered

    a. within the low dosage range.

    b. within the moderate dosage range.

    c. within the high dosage range.

    d. within any of the above ranges.

13. Throughout therapy with dopamine (Intropin), the nurse should carefully monitor all of the following EXCEPT

    a. cardiac output.

    b. pulmonary capillary wedge pressure.

    c. urinary output.

    d. arterial blood gases.

NURSING MANAGEMENT: EVERY GOOD NURSE SHOULD . . .

Multiple choice

Circle the option that best answers the question or completes the statement.

1. Bob Brenner is seen in the outpatient center today for evaluation of his hypertension. He is to be started on Captopril, an ACE inhibitor. He tells you he hates to take medicine because he always gets adverse effects. To minimize adverse effects experienced by Mr. Brenner with the initial dosing of Captopril, the nurse should recommend

   a. taking the drug with meals.

   b. taking the drug at bedtime.

   c. changing positions rapidly.

   d. increasing dietary sodium.

2. Gordon Schneider is receiving labetalol, a mixed alpha and beta adrenergic-blocking agent, for hypertension. In addition to hypertension, he also has diabetes and a history of ischemic heart disease. Patient teaching about labetalol for this patient should include advice to

   a. increase intake of dietary sugars.

   b. take hot baths or showers to promote pharmacotherapeutic effects.

   c. monitor blood glucose levels more closely.

   d. discontinue drug immediately if orthostatic hypotension occurs.

3. Val Gerber is to be started on transdermal clonidine, a centrally acting alpha-2 agonist, to treat hypertension. To maximize the therapeutic effect of the drug, the nurse should

   a. apply a new patch every 7 days.

   b. apply patch to an area that has a great deal of hair.

   c. always use the same application site.

   d. avoid using extra adhesives over the patch.

4. Wilma Wynnings has been started on hydralazine, a direct-acting vasodilator, for hypertension. She has also been started on atenolol, a beta blocker, and hydrochlorothiazide, a diuretic. She asks why she needs three new medicines. What is the most appropriate patient teaching that should be done regarding these drug therapies?

   a. Severe hypertension requires multiple drug therapies.

   b. Hypertension is always controlled by multiple drug therapies.

   c. Only hydralazine is used to treat hypertension.

   d. Atenolol and hydrochlorothiazide help to reduce blood pressure and to offset adverse effects of the hydralazine.

5. Donnell Johns has been ordered nitroprusside to treat a hypertensive crisis. As his nurse, you are to prepare this medication. You take out of the stock drug cabinet a vial of nitroprusside. After you reconstitute the powder with 3 mL of sterile water, the solution has a blue-green appearance. You should

   a. run the vial under warm water to clarify the solution.

   b. withdraw the solution and administer by IV push.

   c. further dilute in D5W and expose to sunlight.

   d. discard and use another vial of drug.

6. Shawanda Alexander is 28 years old, and she is to be started on losartan, an angiotensin II receptor antagonist for hypertension that is resistant to other drug therapy. Patient education for Ms. Alexander should include

   a. the need to prevent pregnancy while on this drug.

   b. the importance of a high-sodium diet.

   c. that fluid loss is an adverse effect.

   d. that hypertension is an adverse effect.

CASE STUDY

David Mohammed was admitted to the intensive care unit in a hypertensive crisis. His blood pressure is 220/170. He is started on a nitroprusside infusion. The orders read to start the infusion at 0.3 µg per kilogram of weight per minute and titrate upward until blood pressure is no greater than 130/80, the patient's previous known blood pressure. After the first 15 minutes, the blood pressure is 200/160, and the nurse increases the rate of the infusion. After another 15 minutes, the blood pressure is 190/156. The nurse again increases the rate of infusion. In 15 minutes, the blood pressure is 126/70. Mr. Mohammed is now complaining of abdominal pain and nausea.

1. What nursing actions would be most appropriate at this time?

2. Why?

CRITICAL THINKING CHALLENGE

Mr. Mohammed continues to require nitroprusside to keep his blood pressure under control. He remains on drug therapy of 7 µg per kilogram per minute of nitroprusside for 6 hours. At this time, the nurse needs to start a second IV line so labetalol, another antihypertensive drug that is longer acting, can also be administered. While inserting the line, the nurse notes that the venous blood appears brighter red than usual. Mr. Mohammed seems confused now as to why he is in the hospital; previously he knew his blood pressure was high.

1. What assessment would the nurse make?

2. What actions would be appropriate?

CHAPTER 31

Drugs Affecting Diuresis

TOP TEN THINGS TO KNOW ABOUT DRUGS AFFECTING DIURESIS

1. Diuretics are used to reduce fluid volume in the body. Reduction of fluid volume is useful in treating conditions such as hypertension, congestive heart failure (CHF), cirrhosis, renal disease, increased intracranial pressure, and increased intraocular pressure.

2. Diuretics work along the renal tubule of the nephron in the kidney to decrease reabsorption of sodium and water and, therefore, increase urine output. The degree of diuresis depends on which part of the tubule is affected by the drug.

3. Diuretics also affect the excretion and reabsorption of other electrolytes, especially potassium. The site of action in the tubule determines which electrolytes are lost and how great is the loss. Electrolyte imbalance is a major adverse effect of diuretic therapy. Thiazide and loop diuretics are the two classes of diuretics most frequently used.

4. Hydrochlorothiazide (HCTZ), a thiazide diuretic, acts in the distal tubule and increases the excretion of sodium, chloride, potassium, and water, although it is a weak diuretic (most water is reabsorbed before the distal tubule). It can reduce the glomerular filtration rate, so should not be used if the patient has preexisting renal disease. Hydrochlorothiazide is widely used alone or with other drugs to treat hypertension and edema.

5. Adverse effects of hydrochlorothiazide are related to fluid and electrolyte loss. Monitor patient's blood pressure, pulse, weight, intake and output, and serum electrolyte levels during therapy.

6. Furosemide, a loop diuretic, works in the loop of Henle to promote the excretion of sodium, chloride, potassium, and water. It has a strong diuretic effect. It is used to treat edema from CHF, pulmonary edema, and hepatic and renal disease. It may be used to treat hypertension, especially if preexisting renal disease is present.

7. Adverse effects of furosemide are related to fluid and electrolyte loss, especially potassium. Monitor patient's blood pressure, edema, breath sounds, weight, intake and output, and serum electrolyte levels. Encourage diet high in potassium or give supplements if indicated.

8. Triamterene, a potassium-sparing diuretic, works in the distal tubule to promote sodium and water excretion, but promotes reabsorption of potassium. It has the weakest diuretic effect of the diuretics if given alone, but works synergistically with other diuretics. Major electrolyte imbalance is hyperkalemia (high potassium); risk is highest in older adults.

9. Mannitol, an osmotic diuretic, is a sugar that draws water into the vascular space through osmosis. It is filtered in the kidney but not reabsorbed, and thus allows diuresis. It is used to treat acute renal failure, increased intracranial pressure, and increased intraocular pressure. Adverse effects include serious fluid and electrolyte imbalances. Mannitol crystallizes easily; warm drug in water before administering to dissolve crystals.

10. Acetazolamide, a carbonic anhydrase inhibitor diuretic, inhibits hydrogen ion secretion in the tubule and increases the loss of sodium, potassium, bicarbonate, and water. Inhibition of carbonic anhydrase also prevents formation of aqueous humor and decreases intraocular pressure. Acetazolamide is used primarily in treating chronic, open-angle glaucoma.

KEY TERMS

Anagrams

Using the following definitions, unscramble each of the following sets of letters to form a word. Write your response in the spaces provided.

1. movement across capsular membrane

   R L G M E R U L A O
   T I F L A R T N I O

2. molecules move from peritubular blood into tubule

   L U B T A R U
   C E S E N O I T R

3. abnormally reduced renal output

   A G I I R L U O

4. fluid shifts into interstitial spaces

   M E A D E

5. process of ridding the body of fluids

   S I D U R E S I

6. abnormal increase in circulating blood volume

   P O L E R Y E H M A I V

7. molecules move into peritubular blood

   R U B U L A T
   P A E R S O B N O I T R

8. chronically elevated blood pressure

   N Y E R N S O H P T E I

9. abnormally low potassium level in the blood

   P Y K A L E H O A I M

10. concentration of urine

    L O M O S I A L Y T

11. drug that causes diuresis

    C D I R U E I T

12. abnormally high potassium level in the blood

    K E I M A P E Y H R A L

PHYSIOLOGY AND PATHOPHYSIOLOGY: THE BODY HUMAN

Essay

1. What are the functions of the renal system?
2. Name the components of the renal system.
3. What processes are required for the formation of urine?
4. How much urine is usually produced in 24 hours?
5. What action by the kidney influences regulation of acid–base balance?
6. What action by the kidney influences regulation of blood pressure?
7. What action by the kidney influences the production of red blood cells?
8. What action by the kidney influences calcium deposition in bones?

CORE DRUG KNOWLEDGE: JUST THE FACTS

Multiple choice

Circle the option that best answers the question or completes the statement.

1. Maximum effect from hydrochlorothiazide (HCTZ) therapy occurs in
   a. 3 to 6 hours.
   b. 2 to 4 weeks.
   c. 1 to 2 days.
   d. 30 to 60 minutes.

2. Which of the following patients should refrain from HCTZ therapy?
   a. Julie, with CHF
   b. Anthony, with hypertension
   c. Justin, with renal impairment
   d. Stephanie, with kidney stones

3. Which of the following statements concerning HCTZ is correct?

   a. There are very few drug–drug interactions, and they are insignificant.

   b. There are numerous drug–drug interactions, but none are significant.

   c. There are numerous drug–drug interactions, and many are very significant.

   d. There are very few drug–drug interactions, and a couple may be significant.

4. Thiazide diuretics may cause hypersensitivity in patients with a known history of

   a. sulfa allergy.

   b. penicillin allergy.

   c. nasal polyps.

   d. asthma.

5. Loop diuretics, such as furosemide (Lasix), are called "high-ceiling" diuretics because

   a. the minimum dosage needed to affect diuresis is very high.

   b. the maximum dosage available for use is very high.

   c. the maximum diuretic effect is much higher than with other diuretics.

   d. all of the above.

6. In addition to diuresis, what effects does furosemide (Lasix) have on body processes?

   a. decreases blood glucose

   b. decreases low-density lipoprotein

   c. decreases excretion of uric acid

   d. decreases triglyceride levels

7. Long-term therapy with furosemide (Lasix) may

   a. increase glucose.

   b. decrease glucose.

   c. increase potassium.

   d. decrease uric acid.

8. Which of the following drugs should not be coadministered with drugs that may cause hyperkalemia?

   a. triamterene (Dyrenium)

   b. furosemide (Lasix)

   c. hydrochlorothiazide (HCTZ)

   d. ethacrynic acid (Edecrin)

9. Which of the following symptoms may indicate hyperkalemia?

   a. anorexia, nausea, diarrhea, constipation

   b. irregular pulse, muscle weakness, constipation

   c. nausea, diarrhea, weak pulse, cardiac arrhythmias

   d. elevated LDH and triglycerides, muscle cramps

10. Which of the following diuretics is the drug of choice in the treatment of cerebral edema?

    a. triamterene (Dyrenium)

    b. mannitol (Osmitrol)

    c. furosemide (Lasix)

    d. acetazolamide (Diamox)

11. Which of the following is a contraindication for the use of mannitol (Osmitrol)?

    a. pulmonary edema

    b. asthma

    c. hypertension

    d. diabetes

12. To maximize therapeutic effects of mannitol (Osmitrol), which of the following interventions may be done?

    a. refrigerate the solution until administration

    b. shield the medication from light

    c. warm the medication to 100°F

    d. infuse with an in-line filter

13. Chronic open-angle glaucoma is treated with

    a. bumetanide (Bumex).

    b. amiloride (Midamor).

    c. acetazolamide (Diamox).

    d. glycerin (glycerol).

14. Which of the following statements concerning the potential adverse effects of acetazolamide (Diamox) is correct?

    a. There are very few adverse effects, and they are insignificant.

    b. There are numerous adverse effects, but none are significant.

    c. There are numerous adverse effects, and many are very significant.

    d. There are very few adverse effects, and a couple may be significant.

CORE PATIENT VARIABLES: PATIENTS, PLEASE

Multiple choice

Circle the option that best answers the question or completes the statement.

1. Molly Kincade has hypertension and is being treated with hydrochlorothiazide (HCTZ). On her next clinic visit, you would anticipate obtaining which of the following lab tests?
   a. CBC
   b. sed rate
   c. electrolyte panel
   d. hepatic enzymes

2. Mrs. Harrelson takes HCTZ for ankle edema. She states she is compliant with her medication, yet continues to have swelling. Before changing her medication, which of the following assessments should be made?
   a. diet, especially sodium intake
   b. time of day medication is taken
   c. smoking history
   d. amount of water ingested each day

3. Madelyn Lin takes several medications including HCTZ, pancrelipase, and levothyroxine. Mrs. Lin comes to the clinic with a complaint of irregular pulse, muscle weakness, constipation, and abdominal pain. Which of the following abnormalities would you suspect may be the cause of these symptoms?
   a. hypercalcemia
   b. hypermagnesemia
   c. hyponatremia
   d. hypokalemia

4. Ginger Kane, age 88, is admitted to your unit for CHF. She is ordered intravenous (IV) furosemide (Lasix). Mrs. Kane has an increased risk for which of furosemide's many adverse effects?
   a. hyperuricemia
   b. vascular thrombosis or embolism
   c. headache
   d. photosensitivity

5. Terri Whitt is prescribed furosemide (Lasix) 40 mg IVP. You should administer this medication
   a. within 30 seconds.
   b. over 1 to 2 minutes.
   c. over 5 to 10 minutes.
   d. over 1 hour.

6. Leonard Froley takes furosemide (Lasix) daily for his hypertension. Mr. Froley should have which of the following tests done periodically?
   a. HbA_{1C}
   b. CBC
   c. ophthalmologic exam
   d. chest x-ray

7. Which of the following instructions should be given to a patient taking triamterene (Dyrenium), a potassium-sparing diuretic?
   a. "Be sure to eat lots of green leafy vegetables."
   b. "Drink at least 3 glasses of orange juice a day."
   c. "Eat liver at least twice a week."
   d. "Limit your intake of potassium-rich foods."

8. Evelyn Newson takes triamterene and HCTZ (Dyazide) daily. Instructions should include
   a. "take at bedtime."
   b. "take TID with meals."
   c. "take in the AM."
   d. "take every other day."

9. Hal Holland, age 72, has been involved in an auto accident and has blunt head trauma. He is receiving IV mannitol (Osmitrol). When reviewing Mr. Holland's health status history, you note he has a history of CHF and arthritis. Due to his history, the nurse should monitor
   a. his weight.
   b. lung sounds.
   c. temperature.
   d. extremity movement.

10. Frank Harvey has been admitted to your unit with a closed head injury and has an order for IV mannitol (Osmitrol). Before administration, the nurse should
    a. insert an indwelling catheter.
    b. shield the medication from heat.
    c. dilute with lidocaine (Xylocaine).
    d. contact the on-call physician to insert a central line.

11. Hal Morris, age 70, is receiving acetazolamide (Diamox) for chronic open-angle glaucoma. He is scheduled for knee surgery in the morning. His presurgical labs have returned. You would expect his UA to indicate

    a. acidic urine.

    b. alkaline urine.

    c. normal results.

12. Which of the following patients should NOT receive acetazolamide (Diamox) for chronic open-angle glaucoma?

    a. Patty, with hypertension

    b. Susan, with migraine headaches

    c. Carole, with hypothyroidism

    d. Janice, with adrenal insufficiency

NURSING MANAGEMENT: EVERY GOOD NURSE SHOULD . . .

Complete the decision tree on page 164

Marjorie Holmes, 80 years old, was admitted to your unit with congestive heart failure yesterday. Her symptoms were shortness of breath and mild edema in both feet. She also has a history of diabetes and chronic renal failure. She received 20 mg of furosemide when she was first admitted, which decreased the shortness of breath and edema exhibited. She is to receive this same dose daily. This is a new drug therapy for her. Complete the decision tree for Ms. Holmes based on your findings from your assessment. List parameters you will examine in your physical assessment, nursing diagnoses related to positive or negative findings from your assessment, actions to promote therapeutic effects and minimize adverse effects, and patient teaching required.

CASE STUDY

Tim Buttons, 70 years old, was in a car accident and hit his head on the interior side of the car. He is admitted to the hospital with increased intracranial pressure from cerebral edema. He is to be started on mannitol 1.5 g/kg of weight, infused over 60 minutes. When the vial of mannitol is taken from the medication cart, the nurse notices many clear crystals in the solution.

1. What actions of the nurse would be appropriate to prepare the mannitol for infusion?

2. Why is this drug administered by an IV route?

3. How will the nurse determine whether the drug therapy is effective?

CRITICAL THINKING CHALLENGE

Before the mannitol infusion is started, the nurse learns that Mr. Buttons has an elevated creatinine level, a sign that renal impairment may be present.

1. How should the nurse proceed?

2. What patient-related variables placed Mr. Buttons at risk for impaired kidney function?

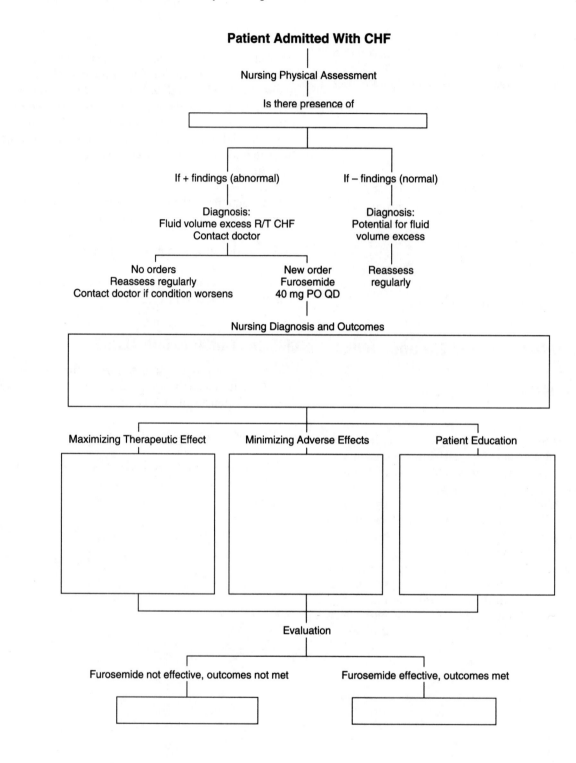

Patient Admitted With CHF

Nursing Physical Assessment

Is there presence of

If + findings (abnormal)   If − findings (normal)

Diagnosis:
Fluid volume excess R/T CHF
Contact doctor

Diagnosis:
Potential for fluid
volume excess

No orders
Reassess regularly
Contact doctor if condition worsens

New order
Furosemide
40 mg PO QD

Reassess
regularly

Nursing Diagnosis and Outcomes

Maximizing Therapeutic Effect   Minimizing Adverse Effects   Patient Education

Evaluation

Furosemide not effective, outcomes not met   Furosemide effective, outcomes met

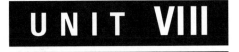

UNIT VIII

Blood and Immune System Drugs

CHAPTER 32

Drugs Affecting Coagulation

TOP TEN THINGS TO KNOW ABOUT DRUGS AFFECTING COAGULATION

1. Anticoagulants prevent blood clots from forming. They do not break down existing clots.
2. Heparin, an anticoagulant, prevents the conversion of prothrombin to thrombin and prevents the formation of a stable clot. Heparin is administered intravenously (IV) or subcutaneously (SC). It is safe in pregnancy. Monitor the active partial thromboplastin time (aPTT) to determine patient's response to therapy; therapeutic aPTT levels are one and a half to two times the control level. The most common adverse effect is bleeding. Antidote to overdosage is protamine sulfate.
3. Warfarin, an anticoagulant, blocks vitamin K and prevents activation of prothrombin and other factors. Warfarin is given orally. Avoid use in pregnancy because fetal warfarin syndrome will occur. Maximum anticoagulant effect takes 3 to 4 days after dosing begins. Monitor the prothrombin time (PT) or the international normalized ratio (INR) to determine patient's response to therapy; PT should be about one and one half times the control; INR should be equal to 2 or 3. Vitamin K is the antidote. Teach patients not to greatly increase dietary vitamin K intake while on warfarin.
4. Ticlopidine is an antiplatelet and inhibits platelet aggregation. It is used to prevent cerebrovascular accident (CVA; stroke) when aspirin is not tolerated. Most common adverse effect is diarrhea. A rare, but life-threatening, adverse effect is neutropenia. Complete blood count (CBC) should be monitored.
5. Pentoxifylline is a hemorrheologic drug used to manage symptoms of intermittent claudication from peripheral vascular disease. It reduces blood viscosity and increases flexibility of the red blood cells (RBC). Full therapeutic effects are not felt until 4 to 8 weeks of therapy. Smoking limits the effectiveness of drug therapy.

6. Thrombolytic drugs break down formed blood clots. They are used to treat evolving acute myocardial infarction (MI); pulmonary embolism (PE); acute, extensive deep vein thrombosis (DVT); and arterial thrombosis. In lower doses, they are used to open occluded arteriovenous catheters.
7. Streptokinase, a thrombolytic drug, activates plasminogen and dissolves fibrin, fibrinogen, and other clot-forming proteins. It changes fibrin throughout the body, not only at the site of the clot. Streptokinase can produce life-threatening bleeding. Transfusion may be needed. Aminocaproic acid is antidote. Fever occurs in 30% of patients.
8. Use an IV pump to administer streptokinase. Avoid invasive procedures. Monitor patient closely for vital sign changes, signs of bleeding, blood work abnormalities (hematocrit, hemoglobin, platelets, PT, thrombin time, aPPT), arrhythmias (in MI), and respiratory difficulties (in PE). Recombinant alteplase, which produces fewer systemic effects than streptokinase, is becoming the thrombolytic of choice.
9. Antihemophilic factor (AHF) is factor VIII and is used to temporarily treat or prevent bleeding in hemophilia. It is made from pooled human sources and carries a slight risk of hepatitis and human immunodeficiency virus (HIV) transmission. Dosage is individualized to meet patient needs. Teach patient to avoid injury and carry identification of hemophilia.
10. Aminocaproic acid is a systemic hemostatic drug that stops blood loss by enhancing coagulation. It is used only in life-threatening situations. Administer with an IV pump. Place patient on cardiac monitor to detect arrhythmias.

KEY TERMS

Crossword puzzle

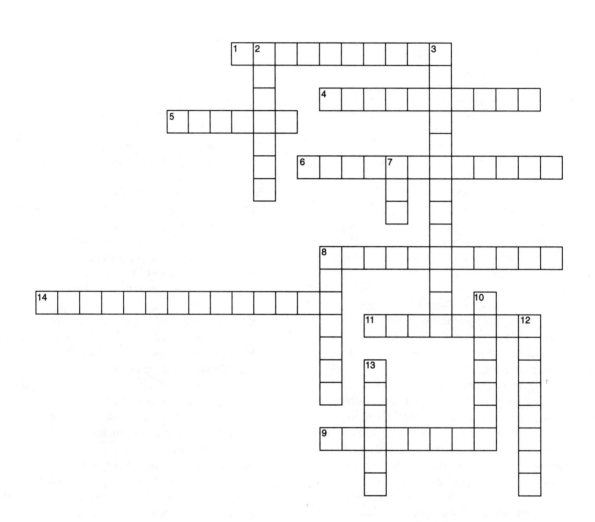

Across

1. Inherited disorder of blood coagulation
4. The arrest of bleeding
5. Plasma proteins that cause blood clotting
6. Hydrolysis of fibrin
8. Transformation of solution into a gel or semisolid mass
9. Enzyme that converts fibrinogen into fibrin
11. Thrombocyte
14. Dislodged portion of a thrombus that is floating in the bloodstream

Down

2. Any undissolved matter carried in a blood or lymph vessel to another location where it lodges and occludes the vessel
3. Drug that prevents clotting of blood
7. Monitoring test for anticoagulation
8. Fibrin is the end product of the clotting _____
10. When activated, it is the substance that lyses the blood clot
12. Attached clot in the cardiovascular (CV) system formed from constituents of blood
13. Insoluble protein product of the clotting cascade

PHYSIOLOGY AND PATHOPHYSIOLOGY: THE BODY HUMAN

Essay

1. How do anticoagulants, antiplatelet agents, hemorrheologics, and thrombolytic agents affect homeostasis?

2. What is the role of the clotting cascade?

3. What is a "factor"?

4. What is plasmin?

CORE DRUG KNOWLEDGE: JUST THE FACTS

Multiple choice

Circle the option that best answers the question or completes the statement.

1. Anticoagulants, such as heparin, work by
   a. preventing the synthesis of factors dependent on vitamin K.
   b. lysing plasmin.
   c. inhibiting platelet synthesis.
   d. inactivating Factor X.

2. The most useful test to monitor the effectiveness of heparin is
   a. aPTT.
   b. PT.
   c. bleeding time.
   d. CBC.

3. Heparin has many potential drug–drug interactions. In general, what is the most common potential adverse effect from these interactions?
   a. bleeding
   b. headache
   c. decreased effectiveness of heparin
   d. hypertension

4. When assessing the results of heparin anticoagulation, the aPTT should be
   a. 2 to 3 times the control.
   b. 1.5 to 2 times the control.
   c. 15 to 20 times the control.
   d. 0.2 to 0.3 times the control.

5. Which of the following statements accurately reflects the differences between traditional heparin and low-molecular-weight heparin?
   a. Low-molecular-weight heparin has decreased bioavailability.
   b. Traditional heparin interacts less with platelets.
   c. Low-molecular-weight heparin yields a very predictable dose response.
   d. Traditional heparin does not require monitoring of aPTT.

6. Anticoagulants, such as warfarin (Coumadin), work by
   a. preventing the synthesis of factors dependent on vitamin K.
   b. lysing plasmin.
   c. inhibiting platelet synthesis.
   d. preventing conversion of fibrinogen to fibrin.

7. When assessing the results of warfarin (Coumadin) anticoagulation, the PT should be
   a. 2 to 3 times the control.
   b. 0.2 to 0.3 times the control.
   c. 1.4 to 1.7 times the control.
   d. 20 to 30 times the control.

8. Maximum effects of warfarin (Coumadin) occur within
   a. 30 minutes.
   b. 6 hours.
   c. 24 hours.
   d. 3 to 4 days.

9. Which of the following drugs is NOT classified as an antiplatelet?
   a. dipyridamole (Persantine)
   b. ticlopidine (Ticlid)
   c. aspirin
   d. pentoxifylline (Trental)

10. To increase the absorption of ticlopidine (Ticlid), the patient should be advised to take this drug
    a. 1 hour before or 2 hours after a meal.
    b. with food.
    c. with 1 ounce of alcohol.
    d. with antacids.

11. In the treatment of angina, dipyridamole (Persantine) works by
    a. dilating coronary arteries.
    b. inhibiting platelets.
    c. decreasing contractility of the heart.
    d. increasing oxygen consumption in the heart.

12. Glycoprotein IIb/IIIa inhibitors are frequently used after a/an
    a. acute gastrointestinal (GI) bleed.
    b. myocardial infarction.
    c. coronary artery bypass graft (CABG).
    d. percutaneous transluminal coronary angioplasty (PTCA).

13. Which of the following drugs would be effective for intermittent claudication?
    a. heparin
    b. warfarin (Coumadin)
    c. streptokinase (Streptase)
    d. pentoxifylline (Trental)

14. Maximal therapeutic effect with pentoxifylline (Trental) therapy takes
    a. 2 to 4 weeks.
    b. 1 to 2 days.
    c. 4 to 8 weeks.
    d. 30 to 60 minutes.

15. Pentoxifylline (Trental) is chemically related to theophylline; therefore, adverse effects are primarily _____ in nature.
    a. central nervous system (CNS)
    b. hematologic
    c. integumentary
    d. respiratory

16. The difference between anticoagulants and thrombolytics is that
    a. anticoagulants require an unsafe dose to dissolve clots.
    b. anticoagulants dissolve clots whereas thrombolytics prevent further clot formation.
    c. thrombolytics dissolve clots whereas anticoagulants prevent further clot formation.
    d. thrombolytics decrease the risk of hemorrhage during therapy.

17. Streptokinase (Streptase) therapy is most effective when administered within _____ hour(s) of the onset of symptoms.
    a. 1
    b. 6
    c. 12
    d. 24

18. Streptokinase works by
    a. activation of plasminogen.
    b. inhibition of platelets.
    c. activation of factor XIII.
    d. inhibition of fibrinogen.

19. Antihemophilic factor (AHF) is used to
    a. prevent deep vein thrombosis.
    b. treat pulmonary emboli.
    c. prevent and control excessive bleeding.
    d. treat CVA.

20. After dilution, antihemophilic factor (AHF) should be administered within _____ hour(s).
    a. 1
    b. 24
    c. 12
    d. 3

21. Hemostatic drugs are used in the management of
    a. prevention of DVT.
    b. hemophilia.
    c. life-threatening bleeding disorders.
    d. disseminated intravascular coagulation (DIC).

22. The most common adverse effects to aminocaproic acid therapy affect the
    a. GI system.
    b. CV system.
    c. genitourinary (GU) system.
    d. CNS.

CORE PATIENT VARIABLES: PATIENTS, PLEASE

Multiple choice

Circle the option that best answers the question or completes the statement.

1. Which of the following patients should be closely monitored during heparin therapy?
   a. Beverly, with a history of Raynaud's disease
   b. Constance, with a history of peptic ulcer disease
   c. Stanley, with a history of pancreatitis
   d. Leon, with a history of angina

2. Your patient is to receive heparin 5,000U SC BID. To appropriately administer this medication, you should
   a. aspirate the syringe but do not rub the area after administration.
   b. not aspirate the syringe, but you should rub the area after administration.
   c. not aspirate the syringe and do not rub the area after administration.
   d. aspirate the syringe and rub the area after administration.

3. Kimberly Taylor is receiving a continuous heparin infusion. You note bruising on her arms and her aPTT is 150 with a control of 30. You would anticipate administration of which of the following drugs?
   a. vitamin K
   b. aminocaproic acid
   c. AquaMEPHYTON
   d. Protamine sulfate

4. Elizabeth Cooper has mitral valve prolapse and a history of pulmonary emboli, and she took "some kind of blood thinner." She comes to the clinic today and states a health care provider has not seen her in several months because she lost her insurance benefits. Which of the following drugs do you anticipate Mrs. Cooper will be prescribed?
   a. heparin
   b. ticlopidine (Ticlid)
   c. warfarin (Coumadin)
   d. pentoxifylline (Trental)

5. Your patient had hip surgery today. The health care provider ordered enoxaparin (Lovenox) daily. With your knowledge of this drug, you would expect the patient's aPTT to
   a. increase.
   b. decrease.
   c. stay within the normal dosage range.

6. Elias Moore is taking warfarin (Coumadin) for prophylaxis for deep vein thrombosis. Mr. Moore should be scheduled for which of the following laboratory tests to monitor the effectiveness of therapy?
   a. aPTT
   b. PT
   c. INR
   d. either b or c

7. Lisa Elliott comes to the clinic for a recheck of her medical problems. Her current medications include ticlopidine (Ticlid), theophylline (Theodur), cimetidine (Tagamet), and digoxin (Lanoxin). Which of these drugs, if any, may increase Mrs. Elliott's risk for hemorrhage?
   a. theophylline
   b. cimetidine
   c. digoxin
   d. all of the above

8. James Reyes takes ticlopidine (Ticlid) for angina. Patient teaching should include the need for periodic laboratory testing of
   a. complete blood count.
   b. aPTT.
   c. PT.
   d. bleeding time.

9. Peter Harnes takes pentoxifylline (Trental) for peripheral vascular disease. While you are assessing Mr. Harnes' lifestyle, diet, and habits, he tells you he smokes 1½ packs of cigarettes a day. You would expect that Mr. Harnes' symptoms may be
   a. increased.
   b. decreased.
   c. the same.

10. Which of the following patients should NOT receive streptokinase (Streptase)?

    a. Louise, 10 days postpartum

    b. Naomi, with glaucoma

    c. Carolyn, with NIDDM

    d. Peter, with asthma

11. Nancy Reiser is receiving streptokinase (Streptase) for an acute MI. In addition to bleeding, the nurse should monitor for

    a. sedation.

    b. muscle cramps.

    c. hypertension.

    d. fever.

12. Brenda Hall is receiving streptokinase (Streptase). She complains of abdominal pain and vomits 100 cc of dark coffee ground emesis. Her blood pressure has dropped to 80/40. The nurse should anticipate administration of which of the following drugs?

    a. protamine sulfate

    b. vitamin K

    c. aminocaproic acid (Amicar)

    d. pentoxifylline (Trental)

13. Leon Kendry has been admitted to the emergency department with a CVA. The computed tomography (CT) scan indicates the stroke is hemorrhagic in nature. Which of the following drugs would be effective for this CVA?

    a. recombinant alteplase (Activase)

    b. urokinase (Abbokinase)

    c. streptokinase (Streptase)

    d. none of the above

14. Your patient has gone to the cardiac cath lab for a percutaneous transluminal coronary angioplasty with stent placement. Which of the following drugs do you anticipate will be ordered for this patient?

    a. warfarin (Coumadin)

    b. abciximab (ReoPro)

    c. streptokinase (Streptase)

    d. aminocaproic acid (Amicar)

15. Taylor Olson, age 55, has just been started on pentoxifylline (Trental) for intermittent claudication. Patient teaching should include:

    a. "Take on an empty stomach."

    b. "You may not see immediate results, but keep on taking the medication."

    c. "Be sure to stay out of the sunlight as much as possible."

    d. "Increase your daily intake of calcium."

16. Your patient has hemophilia and intermittently takes antihemophilic factor (AHF) at home. Patient teaching should include instructions to contact the health care provider if _____ occurs.

    a. headache

    b. blurred vision

    c. constipation

    d. red or orange urine

17. Your patient has cirrhosis of the liver and is suspected of having systemic hyperfibrinolysis. What drug do you anticipate will be ordered?

    a. warfarin (Coumadin)

    b. abciximab (ReoPro)

    c. streptokinase (Streptase)

    d. aminocaproic acid (Amicar)

NURSING MANAGEMENT: EVERY GOOD NURSE SHOULD . . .

Multiple choice

Circle the option that best answers the question or completes the statement.

1. Kathy Riggs is receiving heparin IV into a peripheral vein to treat a left DVT. Unfortunately, she has also developed pneumonia and requires IV antibiotics given every 6 hours. Each antibiotic infusion requires 30 minutes. To accomplish administration of these two drug therapies, the nurse should

    a. stop the heparin infusion every 6 hours to allow the antibiotic to be infused.

    b. piggyback the antibiotic onto the heparin line and administer both at the same time.

    c. add the antibiotic to the bag of heparin solution.

    d. use a separate IV insertion site to administer the antibiotic.

2. To prevent hematoma formation when administering subcutaneous heparin, the nurse should

    a. massage injection site vigorously.

    b. use a 3-cc syringe.

    c. aspirate before injecting drug.

    d. use the scapula as the preferred injection site.

3. Gina Lancaster, 26 years old, is to be discharged on warfarin, an oral anticoagulant, following a mitral valve replacement. Patient teaching for Gina regarding warfarin should include

    a. increase dietary intake of green leafy vegetables.

    b. avoid foods high in potassium.

    c. use birth control while on warfarin.

    d. take two doses at one time if a dose is accidentally missed.

4. Larry Hughes has been started on ticlopidine to prevent a stroke after several mild TIAs (transient ischemic attacks). Patient education regarding ticlopidine should include

    a. take this drug with food.

    b. blood work will be needed every 6 months.

    c. bleeding time will be shortened.

    d. all of the above.

    e. none of the above.

5. Christopher Lee is started on pentoxifylline, a hemorrheologic drug, to treat his intermittent claudication from peripheral vascular disease in both legs. A follow-up telephone call is made 1 week after starting therapy to see if Mr. Lee has any questions or problems with the drug therapy. Mr. Lee tells the nurse that he doesn't feel any better and wants to stop taking the drug. The best response of the nurse would be

    a. "Drug therapy doesn't always work for every patient."

    b. "The drug is helping you, but you just don't realize it."

    c. "Full therapeutic effect may take 4 to 8 weeks to occur."

    d. "The drug should be stopped because it is not effective."

6. Ray Miller is brought to the emergency room with an evolving MI. He is started on streptokinase, a thrombolytic agent. To minimize adverse effects during this drug therapy, the nurse should

    a. assess vital signs every 15 minutes during the first hour of therapy.

    b. increase the infusion if coffee ground emesis occurs.

    c. administer by gravity flow.

    d. give other ordered drugs by IM injection.

7. Jared Wilson, a 12-year-old hemophiliac, is brought to the emergency room for uncontrolled bleeding after falling off his bicycle. Antihemophyllic factor is ordered. Nursing management in this drug therapy should include

    a. rotate the vial of diluted drug gently to mix.

    b. monitor coagulation studies during therapy.

    c. administer drug by the IV route.

    d. all of the above.

    e. none of the above.

8. Joe Becker had a nephrectomy 1 hour ago. From the surgery, he has developed systemic hyperfibrinolysis and is experiencing severe hemorrhaging. Aminocaproic acid, a hemostatic drug, has been ordered. To minimize adverse effects from this therapy, the nurse should

    a. administer by way of an IM injection.

    b. check incision site for bleeding.

    c. add the drug to other current drug infusions.

    d. obtain an electrocardiogram (ECG) at the end of therapy.

CASE STUDY

Martina Lopez is 30 years old and pregnant. She develops a DVT in her right leg and is hospitalized. Her medication orders are as follows:

Heparin 35 units per kg of body weight IV push followed by 20,000 units per 24 hours per IV infusion

Additional orders read:

Bed rest

aPTT before starting heparin; repeat every 6 hours for 24 hours

Contact physician if aPTT is not in therapeutic range

1. Why is heparin used as the anticoagulant for Martina Lopez?

2. Why is some heparin ordered to be given by IV push and some heparin ordered to be given by IV infusion?

3. What is the purpose of the repeated drawing of the aPTT?

4. What is the rationale for bed rest while receiving heparin?

CRITICAL THINKING CHALLENGE

The nurse starts the heparin infusion and regulates it with an IV pump. The nurse checks the infusion rate hourly and assesses whether Ms. Lopez is having adverse effects from the heparin. Ms. Lopez tolerates the heparin infusion well. In 6 hours, her aPTT is repeated. The level is 1.25 times the control. The nurse obtains an order to increase the heparin infusion and continues to monitor Ms. Lopez hourly. Three hours later, the nurse realizes that Ms. Lopez has received four times the hourly rate in the last hour. The IV pump has apparently malfunctioned. Ms. Lopez shows no signs of bleeding and her vital signs are stable. What actions should the nurse take?

CHAPTER 33

Drugs for Modifying Biologic Response

TOP TEN THINGS TO KNOW ABOUT DRUGS FOR MODIFYING BIOLOGIC RESPONSE

1. The essential components of the immune system are hematopoietic cells, barrier defenses, the nonspecific immune response, the specific immune response, and immunity.

2. Epoetin alfa functions the same as endogenous erythropoietin and stimulates the production of red blood cells. It is used in the treatment of anemia associated with chronic renal failure, use of zidovudine with human immunodeficiency virus (HIV) infection, and use of antineoplastics in cancer.

3. Epoetin alfa takes up to 8 weeks for its full effect on the hematocrit to be determined. Monitor the patient's hematocrit twice a week, and adjust the dose upward after 8 weeks if needed.

4. Colony-stimulating factors (filgrastim, sargramostim, and oprelvekin [also known as interleukin 11]) stimulate the production of white blood cells. Oprelvekin also stimulates the formation of platelets. They are used to treat myelosuppression after antineoplastic use.

5. Cytokines are chemical mediators released by leukocytes to enhance and accelerate the inflammatory responses that will destroy an invading antigen. Cytokines are generally proinflammatory, but many also have antiviral, antiproliferative, and antineoplastic properties. Cytokines are interferons and interleukins.

6. Interferon alfa-2a is a cytokine. It inhibits the growth of tumor cells, prevents their multiplication, heightens host immune response to help protect the body from tumor cells, and blocks specific viral infection by preventing viral replication. Interferon alfa-2a is used to treat hairy cell leukemia, acquired immunodeficiency syndrome (AIDS)-related Kaposi's sarcoma, chronic myelogenous leukemia in chronic phase Philadelphia chromosome-positive patients, and various cancers. It is given by injection. Flulike adverse effects are common, and premedication (acetaminophen or diphenhydramine) is usually given.

7. Monoclonal antibodies can suppress one cell subtype or receptor site and can react with specific tumor receptor sites for diagnosis or treatment of cancer. Antitumor monoclonal antibodies include rituximab. There are also monoclonal antibodies that are used as immunosuppressant and they are considerably different.

8. Rituximab is used to treat non-Hodgkin's lymphoma. Rituximab binds specifically to an antigen found on non-Hodgkin's lymphoma cells; no receptor is found in normal bone marrow cells. When it binds, it causes cell lysis. Infusion-related effects occur in 80% of patients within 2 hours after beginning the first infusion. Premedication (antipyretics and antihistamines) will decrease the severity of the response.

9. Immune modulators appear to act directly on the function of T cells and B cells, and either stimulate or suppress the immune response from these cells. Some drugs stimulate certain functions of the cell response but suppress other functions.

10. Cyclosporine is an immune modulator that suppresses the immune system. It is used as adjunct treatment to prevent rejection after organ transplantation, and to prevent graft-versus-host disease in allogeneic bone marrow or stem cell transplants. Administer the oral form as soon as possible, but not with food or grapefruit juice. To protect the patient from infection, take immediate action at first sign of infection.

KEY TERMS

Matching

Match the following key terms with their definitions:

1. _____ active immunity

2. _____ anemia

3. _____ antibodies

4. _____ antigens

5. _____ aplastic

6. _____ B lymphocytes

7. _____ basophils

8. _____ biologic modifier

9. _____ biologic modulator

10. _____ cellular immune response

11. _____ chemotaxis

a. Contain chemical substances important for initiating and maintaining an immune response
b. Deficient cell production of all types of cells
c. Another term for biologic modulator
d. Found throughout the reticuloendothelial system in like groups called clones
e. Process to destroy a foreign cell, mark it for destruction by phagocytes, and elicit an inflammatory response
f. Condition of reduced circulating red blood cells
g. Complex proteins produced in response to the presence of antigens
h. Attraction of phagocytic cells to the area
i. Substances that induce the formation of antibodies
j. Process that involves B lymphocytes forming memory cells to an antigen
k. Biopharmaceuticals used to alter the body's hematologic or immunologic responses

Match the following key terms with their definitions:

1. _____ complement

2. _____ erythrocytes

3. _____ erythropoiesis

4. _____ erythropoietin

5. _____ granulocytes

6. _____ hematopoiesis

7. _____ HLAs

8. _____ immunoglobins

9. _____ interferon

10. _____ interleukins

11. _____ leukocytes

a. White blood cells
b. Most common leukocyte
c. Membrane-identifying antigens
d. Chemical secreted by cells that have been invaded by viruses
e. Red blood cells
f. New receptor site on an antibody that activates a series of plasma proteins in the body
g. Major peptide hormone that stimulates production of RBCs
h. Chemicals secreted by active leukocytes to influence other leukocytes
i. Process that stimulates the production of RBCs
j. Production of cellular components in blood
k. Circulate in the body and react with their specific "destiny" antigen when encountered

Match the following key terms with their definitions:

1. _____ lymphocytes

2. _____ lymphokines

3. _____ macrophages

4. _____ monocytes

5. _____ neutropenia

6. _____ neutrophils

7. _____ phagocytosis

8. _____ platelets

9. _____ T lymphocytes

10. _____ thrombocytopenia

11. _____ thrombopoietin

a. The formed element involved in blood coagulation
b. Decreased number of neutrophils in serum
c. Process of ingesting bacteria by a neutrophil
d. "Programmed" in the thymus gland to develop into at least three different cell types
e. Low platelet count in serum
f. Can be circulating phagocytes or can be fixed in specific tissues
g. Peptide responsible for platelet production.
h. Chemical that directly destroys a foreign cell or marks it for destruction
i. "First line of defense" against pathogens

j. Mature leukocyte

k. Differentiate into macrophages

PHYSIOLOGY AND PATHOPHYSIOLOGY: THE BODY HUMAN

Essay

1. What are the essential components of the immune system?

2. What are the three barrier defenses of the body against pathogens?

3. Identify the different types of leukocytes.

4. Identify the different types of lymphocytes.

5. What are the three types of T cells?

6. What hormone does the thymus gland release?

CORE DRUG KNOWLEDGE: JUST THE FACTS

Multiple choice

Circle the option that best answers the question or completes the statement.

1. A relative contraindication to the use of epoetin alfa (Epogen) is
    a. hyperthyroidism.
    b. uncontrolled hypertension.
    c. hypothyroidism.
    d. migraine headaches.

2. Which of the following types of anemia should NOT be treated with epoetin alfa (Epogen)?
    a. iron or folate deficiency
    b. hemolysis
    c. gastrointestinal (GI) bleeding
    d. all of the above

3. How frequently should the nurse schedule repeat laboratory testing for the patient beginning epoetin alfa (Epogen) therapy?
    a. two times a week until the target hematocrit is reached
    b. monthly until the target hematocrit is reached
    c. daily until the target hematocrit is reached
    d. weekly until the target hematocrit is reached

4. Filgrastim (Neupogen) works by
    a. increasing iron stores.
    b. increasing the RBC count.
    c. increasing the neutrophil count.
    d. increasing the platelet count.

5. Prevention of severe thrombocytopenia may be accomplished by use of
    a. filgrastim (Neupogen).
    b. epoetin alfa (Epogen).
    c. oprelvekin (Neumega).
    d. any of the above.

6. In addition to hairy cell leukemia, what other disorders may be treated with interferon alfa-2a (Roferon-A)?
    a. Kaposi's sarcoma
    b. breast cancer
    c. lung cancer
    d. Hodgkin's disease

7. What is the appropriate route(s) of administration of interferon alfa-2a (Roferon-A)?
    a. intravenous
    b. intramuscular
    c. subcutaneous
    d. both b and c

8. Patients receiving interferon alfa-2a (Roferon-A) should have monthly laboratory testing. Which of the following tests should be OMITTED?
    a. complete blood count (CBC)
    b. white cell differential
    c. liver and kidney function
    d. urinalysis

9. How frequently can rituximab (Rituxan) be administered?
    a. daily for 4 days
    b. weekly for 4 weeks
    c. monthly for 4 months
    d. every 4 hours for 24 hours

10. Palivizumab (Syangis) is used to
    a. reduce the number of viral organisms in the lower respiratory tract.
    b. decrease tumor size.
    c. inhibit platelet aggregation.
    d. increase circulating B lymphocytes.

11. Cyclosporine (Sandimmune, Neoral) works by suppressing
    a. T lymphocytes.
    b. B lymphocytes.
    c. cell-mediated immune reactions.
    d. phagocytosis.

12. A common, yet serious adverse effect to cyclosporine (Sandimmune, Neoral) affects the _____ system.
    a. GI
    b. genitourinary (GU)
    c. cardiovascular
    d. renal

CORE PATIENT VARIABLES: PATIENTS, PLEASE

Multiple choice

Circle the option that best answers the question or completes the statement.

1. Your patient has chronic renal failure and is being started on epoetin alfa (Epogen). The patient asks, "When will you see if this works?" Your best response is
    a. 10 days
    b. 2 to 6 weeks.
    c. 6 months.
    d. 24 hours.

2. Mr. Lindsey has chronic renal failure and has been receiving epoetin alfa (Epogen) for the past 6 months. As you begin to prepare his dose for today, you note that his CBC reflects a hematocrit of 40%. What is your best action?
    a. give the dose as ordered
    b. give half the dose and alert the health care provider of the CBC results
    c. hold the dose and contact the health care provider
    d. hold the dose and order a STAT CBC

3. Mr. Taylor is receiving chemotherapy. He has an order for filgrastim (Neupogen). To administer this medication appropriately, the nurse should
    a. dilute in 5% dextrose solution with albumin added to prevent absorption by plastic materials.
    b. not dilute in saline because it may precipitate.
    c. avoid shaking because this may damage the protein.
    d. do all of the above.

4. Mary Suto, age 27, is being treated for hairy cell leukemia with interferon alfa-2a (Roferon-A). Mary should be monitored for
    a. hypothyroidism.
    b. diabetes insipidus.
    c. constipation.
    d. GI bleed.

5. Jess Perez is receiving interferon alfa-2a (Roferon-A). As you prepare to give him diphenhydramine, he asks, "Why do I need that, and why do I get this med in the evening?" What is your best response?
    a. "This is the way your doctor ordered it."
    b. "The med is given in the evening with something to help you sleep so you will not feel the minor discomforts that the drug can cause."
    c. "The med is for the possible allergic response that you might have. I just haven't had the time to give it to you sooner."
    d. "It just came up from the pharmacy."

6. Leslie Uribe, age 16, is receiving rituximab (Rituxan) for the first time. After 1 hour of the infusion, she complains of fever, flushing, chills, and rigors. With your knowledge of this drug, you know
    a. this is an unexpected reaction and you need to stop the drug immediately.
    b. this drug does not cause these symptoms, and the patient is just anxious.
    c. these are expected symptoms that occur with approximately 80% of patients.
    d. this is the beginning of a potentially life-threatening reaction.

7. Jason Denny is receiving rituximab (Rituxan). He also has a history of hypertension. What special considerations should be taken for Mr. Denny?

   a. none are needed

   b. administer his antihypertensive medication just before the rituximab

   c. add a second type of antihypertensive medication to his regimen until he completes rituximab therapy

   d. do not administer the antihypertensive agent for 12 hours before rituximab administration, and for 12 to 24 hours afterward

8. Your patient is receiving abciximab (ReoPro) after a PTCA procedure. He states, "My friend was taking rituximab (Rituxan) for his tumor. They sure sound alike. Do I have a tumor they haven't told me about?" What is your best response?

   a. "You need to ask your doctor that question."

   b. "No, manufacturers just name the drugs any way they wish."

   c. "They are both from the same class of drugs, so the names sound alike, but the drugs are not used for the same purposes."

   d. "I've never heard of that other drug."

9. Dane Bullock is receiving cyclosporine (Neoral) to prevent rejection of his heart transplant. Which of the following instructions should be given to Mr. Bullock?

   a. "Wait at least 30 minutes after eating to take your med."

   b. "Mix the medication with grapefruit juice to disguise the taste."

   c. "Take the medication at bedtime only."

   d. "Stop the medication immediately if severe acne develops."

10. Your patient had a heart transplant 6 months ago. He is prescribed cyclosporine (Neoral) and prednisone daily. He comes to the clinic today for laboratory tests. He states, "I had a heart transplant, why are you guys so interested in my kidneys?" What is your best response?

    a. "You know how doctors are—they want to check out everything."

    b. "Cyclosporine can cause damage to your kidneys."

    c. "Prednisone can stop your kidneys from working."

    d. "I'll check—perhaps someone made a mistake."

NURSING MANAGEMENT: EVERY GOOD NURSE SHOULD . . .

Multiple choice

Circle the option that best answers the question or completes the statement.

1. Tyrone Williams, 22 years old, is to receive interferon alfa-2a to treat Kaposi's sarcoma related to his AIDS. What teaching should be done by the nurse?

   a. how to give a subcutaneous (SC) injection

   b. how to avoid infections

   c. when to return for blood tests

   d. all of the above

   e. none of the above

2. Lorraine Green, age 56, has chronic renal failure. Her hematocrit is 29, and she is to be started on epoetin alfa. When administering the first dose to her, you should

   a. shake the bottle vigorously after reconstituting.

   b. save any drug remaining in the single-dose 1-mL vial to use later.

   c. administer into the subcutaneous space.

   d. do all of the above.

   e. do none of the above.

3. Lorraine Green has been receiving epoetin alfa for 10 days. Her hematocrit is still 29. The nurse should

   a. administer the same dose.

   b. administer a larger dose, per protocol.

   c. administer a smaller dose, per protocol.

   d. contact the physician immediately.

4. Jamal Obologon has been prescribed filgrastim, a granulocyte colony-stimulating factor (G-CSF) to prevent febrile neutropenia secondary to antineoplastic therapy for his cancer. Patient education for Jamal should include

   a. filgrastim will be discontinued as soon as the neutrophil count begins to rise.

   b. filgrastim has no known adverse effects.

   c. the importance of being socially active to prevent depression.

   d. the importance of frequent hand washing to prevent infection.

5. You are to administer the first dose of rituximab to Tanya Silhan, 18 years old, after she has had a liver transplant. To minimize adverse effects from the rituximab, you should

   a. administer antipyretics after the first dose if needed.

   b. administer the drug by IV infusion using a pump.

   c. administer a high dose initially and then taper down the dose.

   d. do all of the above.

   e. do none of the above.

6. Within 1 hour of starting the rituximab infusion, Tanya Silhan has a fever of 101.4° F, is flushed, and is complaining of feeling cold. The best initial response of the nurse is to

   a. provide warm blankets and ice chips.

   b. seek order for acetaminophen.

   c. turn down the rate of rituximab infusion.

   d. turn off the rituximab infusion.

7. Cyclosporine, an immune modulator, has been prescribed for Kim Lee after he received a bone marrow transplant. Which of these findings should concern the nurse the most while Kim receives cyclosporine?

   a. slightly elevated serum potassium

   b. slightly low neutrophil count

   c. significantly elevated blood urea nitrogen

   d. none of the above would be a concern; they are all normal findings

CASE STUDY

Lydia Hamilton, 55 years old, is to be started on interferon alfa-2a for treatment of hairy cell leukemia. Lydia has poor eyesight from being a brittle type I diabetic since she was 12 years old. Lydia lives with her husband, Charles, 60 years old, who has arthritis in his hands. Their daughter lives about 20 minutes away.

1. To safely administer the interferon alfa-2a, what specific information does Lydia need?

2. What concerns might you have regarding Lydia and her drug therapy?

CRITICAL THINKING CHALLENGE

What questions regarding Lydia's environment should you ask before discharging her to take the drug at home?

CHAPTER 34

Drugs Affecting Lipid Levels

TOP TEN THINGS TO KNOW ABOUT DRUGS AFFECTING LIPID LEVELS

1. Hyperlipidemia is an elevation of serum lipid (fat) levels. The lipids include cholesterol, cholesterol esters (compounds), phospholipids, and triglycerides. They are transported in the blood as part of large molecules called lipoproteins.

2. Lowering serum lipid levels decreases the risk for cardiovascular disease (atherosclerosis, hypertension, and coronary heart disease).

3. Many people receiving antilipid drugs are not receiving enough to successfully lower their lipid levels into desired, targeted, therapeutic range; many more people with risk factors for cardiovascular disease who should be receiving antilipid therapy are not prescribed the drugs.

4. Limiting dietary fat intake is an important part of reducing serum lipid levels. Diet modifications are started before drug therapy and should continue with the use of antilipid drugs.

5. The lipid-lowering class of the statins (prototype lovastatin) is highly effective in reducing lipid levels and is the most prescribed class of antilipid drug. The statins all increase HDL and decrease LDL, total cholesterol, VLDL, and plasma triglycerides.

6. Adverse effects of lovastatin are generally mild and transient. Elevated liver enzymes may occur with lovastatin and all other antilipid drugs.

7. Lovastatin is metabolized by the hepatic enzyme CYP3A4; all drugs and substances (such as grapefruit juice) that inhibit this pathway may decrease lovastatin's metabolism and raise blood levels of lovastatin.

8. Fibric acid derivatives (gemfibrozil and clofibrate) lower triglyceride levels and increase HDL cholesterol. Unlike lovastatin and other statins, their effect on LDL cholesterol can be either to lower it slightly or to increase it slightly.

9. Nicotinic acid reduces triglycerides, reduces LDL cholesterol, and increases HDL cholesterol. The adverse effect of facial flushing often limits the ability to dose the drug appropriately to be completely therapeutic.

10. The bile acid sequestrants (cholestyramine and colestipol) are now used as second- or third-line therapy for reducing elevated serum cholesterol levels. These drugs are not orally absorbed; they bind with the bile acids in the intestine to make them nonreabsorbable, and excreted. The lowered bile acid level prompts cholesterol to be used to make more bile acid.

KEY TERMS

Essay

Define the following key terms.

1. atherosclerosis

2. arteriosclerosis

3. hyperlipidemia

4. lipids

PHYSIOLOGY AND PATHOPHYSIOLOGY: THE BODY HUMAN

Essay

1. Name the five major families of blood (plasma) lipoproteins.

2. Differentiate between the different types of cholesterol.

3. Why is an elevated triglyceride level an independent risk factor for coronary artery disease (CAD)?

4. What are the benefits of lowering serum lipid levels?

5. List the potential drug classes that may be beneficial in the management of hyperlipidemia.

CORE DRUG KNOWLEDGE: JUST THE FACTS

Multiple choice

Circle the option that best answers the question or completes the statement.

1. The action of lovastatin (Mevacor) is to
   a. inhibit peripheral lipolysis and decrease the hepatic extraction of free fatty acids.
   b. inhibit lipolysis in adipose tissue, decrease esterification of triglyceride in the liver, and increase lipoprotein lipase activity.
   c. promote the oxidation of cholesterol to bile acids.
   d. decrease the synthesis of cholesterol.

2. Patients taking lovastatin (Mevacor) should have periodic
   a. chest x-rays.
   b. liver function tests.
   c. ophthalmology exams.
   d. complete blood count (CBC).

3. Lovastatin (Mevacor) is a pregnancy category _____ drug.
   a. A
   b. B
   c. D
   d. X

4. The action of gemfibrozil (Gemcor, Lopid) is to
   a. inhibit peripheral lipolysis and decrease the hepatic extraction of free fatty acids.
   b. inhibit lipolysis in adipose tissue, decrease esterification of triglyceride in the liver, and increase lipoprotein lipase activity.
   c. promote the oxidation of cholesterol to bile acids.
   d. decrease the synthesis of cholesterol.

5. The action of nicotinic acid (niacin or vitamin B_3) is to
   a. inhibit peripheral lipolysis and decrease the hepatic extraction of free fatty acids.
   b. inhibit lipolysis in adipose tissue, decrease esterification of triglyceride in the liver, and increase lipoprotein lipase activity.
   c. promote the oxidation of cholesterol to bile acids.
   d. decrease the synthesis of cholesterol.

6. In addition to treating hyperlipidemia, cholestyramine (LoCHOLEST, Questran, Prevalite) is used to
   a. decrease peristalsis.
   b. increase peristalsis.
   c. relieve pruritus.
   d. relieve constipation.

7. The most common adverse effect to cholestyramine (LoCHOLEST, Questran, Prevalite) therapy is
   a. cough
   b. constipation.
   c. headache.
   d. sedation.

CORE PATIENT VARIABLES: PATIENTS, PLEASE

Multiple choice

Circle the option that best answers the question or completes the statement.

1. Michele Tooley takes lovastatin for hypercholesteremia. She has a history of alcohol and drug abuse. Which of the following interventions would be appropriate for Ms. Tooley?

   a. baseline and serial liver function tests

   b. monthly CBC

   c. monthly urine drug screen

   d. baseline renal function tests

2. Your patient is being prescribed lovastatin (Mevacor). Patient teaching should include to contact the health care provider IMMEDIATELY for

   a. severe muscle pain.

   b. diarrhea.

   c. intermittent headaches.

   d. nausea.

3. Your patient has hyperlipidemia, despite an aggressive lifestyle change. The health care provider has prescribed lovastatin (Mevacor). Patient teaching should include instructions to

   a. take this medication at bedtime.

   b. take this medication 1 hour before or 2 hours after eating.

   c. take this medication immediately after eating in the morning.

   d. take this medication 4 times a day.

4. Which of the following patients receiving gemfibrozil (Gemcor, Lopid) needs special patient education?

   a. Kim, with hypertension

   b. Allison, with diabetes

   c. Nancy, with asthma

   d. Susan, with bipolar disease

5. Your patient is taking nicotinic acid (niacin or vitamin B₃) for hyperlipidemia. Today, she comes to the clinic and complains of facial flushing. With your knowledge of this drug, what is your best response?

   a. "Stop taking this drug right away."

   b. "This is very unusual, I'll have to speak to the doctor."

   c. "You must be taking way too much."

   d. "This is normal and it usually goes away."

6. George Jameson takes cholestyramine (LoCHOLEST, Questran, Prevalite) for hypercholesteremia. He also takes vitamins daily. Which of the following instructions would be INAPPROPRIATE for Mr. Jameson?

   a. "Take you vitamins one hour before or 4 hours after your cholestyramine."

   b. "Take your vitamins with food to increase absorption."

   c. "You need to remain faithful to your low-cholesterol diet."

   d. "You need to drink plenty of water and continue exercising."

7. Patrick Frome takes clofibrate (Atromid-S) for hypercholesteremia. Mr. Frome should be monitored for the development of

   a. renal failure.

   b. hepatitis.

   c. cholelithiasis.

   d. pancreatitis.

NURSING MANAGEMENT: EVERY GOOD NURSE SHOULD . . .

Multiple choice

Circle the option that best answers the question or completes the statement.

1. Margaret Johnson has elevated LDL levels and low HDL levels. She has been on a fat-restricted diet for the last 6 months, but it has not significantly altered her blood levels. She is now to be started on lovastatin, a lipid-lowering statin, to treat her condition. She says to you, the nurse, that she won't mind starting the lovastatin because she "was tired of following that diet." Your best response to her would be

   a. "Yes, this therapy will be much simpler for you."

   b. "If you choose not to follow the diet, you will need to take a larger dose of the lovastatin."

   c. "Lovastatin will be much more effective when combined with a low-fat diet."

   d. "A slight increase in your dietary fat intake will help to prevent adverse effects from lovastatin."

2. Gregory Hudson, 84 years old, takes medication for hypertension, diabetes, peripheral vascular disease, and asthma. He is to be started on lovastatin, an antilipid drug, to treat his elevated cholesterol levels and atherosclerosis. The nurse knows that Mr. Hudson should be closely monitored for

    a. anaphylactic reactions.

    b. adverse effects.

    c. electrolyte imbalance.

    d. decreased therapeutic response.

3. Patient education for a patient who is to be started on lovastatin should include

    a. the need for periodic blood work to monitor liver enzymes.

    b. the importance of additional sun exposure while on lovastatin.

    c. that muscle aches and weakness are to be expected.

    d. that constipation should be reported at once to the prescriber.

CASE STUDY

Jared Chilcoat has a family history of cardiovascular disease. His LDL cholesterol levels are elevated (160), and he starts on lovastatin. His baseline AST is 15 (n = 7 to 27 U/L) and ALT is 10 (n = 1 to 21 U/L). After 6 weeks, he returns for follow-up blood work. His LDL levels are now 150. His AST is now 54, and his ALT is now 42. He is instructed to continue on the same dose of lovastatin and return in 6 weeks.

1. Why was he continued on the same dose of lovastatin?

2. What is the rationale for having him return for more blood work in another 6 weeks?

CRITICAL THINKING CHALLENGE

When Mr. Chilcoat returns in 6 weeks, his LDL level is 128. His AST is 89, and his ALT is 66.
What actions of the nurse would be appropriate now?

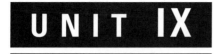

UNIT IX

Respiratory System Drugs

CHAPTER 35

Drugs Affecting the Upper Respiratory System

TOP TEN THINGS TO KNOW ABOUT DRUGS AFFECTING THE UPPER RESPIRATORY SYSTEM

1. The most common conditions affecting the upper respiratory system initiate an inflammatory response.

2. Antitussives are used to suppress the cough reflex, when chronic nonproductive coughing accompanies a disorder of the respiratory tract. Dextromethorphan, an antitussive, is often used in over-the-counter (OTC) products. Dextromethorphan has few adverse effects, although interaction with other central nervous system (CNS) depressants may exacerbate sedation. Avoid giving to patients who depend on their cough reflex to keep their airway clear (such as those with asthma or emphysema).

3. Decongestants decrease nasal congestion from inflammation secondary to upper respiratory infections. Pseudoephedrine, a decongestant, achieves nasal decongestion by mimicking the sympathetic nervous system causing vasoconstriction. The shrinkage reduces membrane size and allows for sinus drainage and improved air flow.

4. Adverse effects from pseudoephedrine are related to other sympathetic receptors being stimulated. The primary adverse effects are from sympathetic stimulation of the CNS and cardiovascular systems (e.g., anxiety, insomnia, tachycardia, and elevated blood pressure [BP]). Use caution in patients with conditions that may be adversely affected by these stimulation effects.

5. Antihistamines are used to treat symptoms associated with allergies. Histamine is released during the inflammatory response to an antigen invasion. Antihistamines block the H_1 receptor sites, preventing histamine action. Antihistamines restore normal air flow through the upper respiratory system. Many antihistamines are available over the counter.

6. Fexofenadine, an antihistamine, is used to relieve symptoms associated with seasonal and perennial allergic rhinitis, and some other conditions. It is most effective when given before symptoms occur.

7. Fexofenadine also has some anticholinergic effects and antipruritic effects. However, as a second-generation antihistamine, it causes less anticholinergic effects than first-generation drugs, like diphenhydramine (Benadryl).

8. Expectorants decrease the viscosity of secretions so they can be more easily coughed up, and improve air flow. As the cough becomes productive, less coughing is stimulated. They are available in many OTC preparations.

9. Guaifenesin, an expectorant, is used as symptomatic relief of respiratory conditions, such as colds, acute bronchitis, and influenza that have a dry, nonproductive cough. Available OTC, it is often combined with decongestants and antihistamines.

10. Assess the cause of the cough before using guaifenesin. A chronic cough from smoking will not be alleviated by guaifenesin. Long-term use should be avoided because it may mask a more serious condition. Teach patients to consult with physician if cough doesn't go away after a week's use of guaifenesin. Most oral solutions contain alcohol. Assess patients for alcohol abuse or the use of disulfiram (Antabuse; treatment for alcoholism).

KEY TERMS

True/false

Mark true or false for each of the following statements. If the statement is false, replace the underlined word with the words that will make the statement correct.

1. _____ Drugs that block the cough reflex are called <u>antihistamines.</u>
2. _____ <u>Dopamine</u> is a chemical released during the inflammatory process.
3. _____ Drugs that block the effects of histamine are called <u>antihistamines.</u>
4. _____ <u>Antitussives</u> are drugs that decrease the overproduction of respiratory secretions.
5. _____ The <u>sinuses</u> are in constant motion, moving the mucus and any trapped substance toward the throat.
6. _____ <u>Bronchodilators</u> increase a productive cough to clear the airways.
7. _____ <u>Influenza</u> is a viral infection that starts in the upper respiratory tract.
8. _____ <u>Laryngitis</u> is an inflammation or infection of the throat.
9. _____ Sinusitis occurs when the epithelial lining of the <u>oral</u> cavities becomes inflamed.
10. _____ <u>Influenza</u> is an infection caused by any of several strains of myxoviruses.
11. _____ Inflammation of the nose is known as <u>rhinitis.</u>
12. An inflammation of the voice box is called <u>pharyngitis.</u>

PHYSIOLOGY AND PATHOPHYSIOLOGY: THE BODY HUMAN

Essay

1. Identify the components of the upper respiratory system.

2. What is the purpose of goblet cells in the epithelial lining of the respiratory tract?

3. How are entrapped particles in the respiratory tract expelled from the body?

4. What are two mechanisms, stimulated by the CNS, that are initiated to clear airways?

CORE DRUG KNOWLEDGE: JUST THE FACTS

Multiple choice

Circle the option that best answers the question or completes the statement.

1. Dextromethorphan (Benylin) works by
   a. inhibition of the cough center in the medulla.
   b. inhibition of respiratory tract secretions.
   c. stimulation of opiate receptors.
   d. bronchodilation.

2. Which of the following statements concerning the adverse effects of dextromethorphan (Benylin) is correct?
   a. There are many adverse effects, but few are serious.
   b. There are many adverse effects, and many are serious.
   c. There are a few minor adverse effects.
   d. There are only a few adverse effects, but all of them are serious.

3. Pseudoephedrine (Sudafed) works by
   a. mimicking the action of the parasympathetic nervous system.
   b. mimicking the action of the sympathetic nervous system.
   c. blocking the action of the parasympathetic nervous system.
   d. blocking the action of the sympathetic nervous system.

4. Pseudoephedrine (Sudafed) is indicated for the treatment of which of the following?
   a. viral upper respiratory infection
   b. asthma
   c. bronchitis
   d. cerebral palsy

5. Which of the following adverse effects may occur during pseudoephedrine (Sudafed) therapy?
   a. urinary retention
   b. bradycardia
   c. tachycardia
   d. hunger

6. How does oxymetazoline (Afrin) differ from pseudoephedrine (Sudafed)?

    a. route and decreased incidence of adverse effects

    b. contraindications and increased dosing frequency

    c. route and increased adverse effects

    d. contraindications and decreased dosing frequency

7. Which of the following nasal sprays is a steroidal anti-inflammatory drug?

    a. oxymetazoline (Afrin)

    b. phenylephrine (Neo-Synephrine)

    c. ephedrine (Kondon's Nasal)

    d. dexamethasone sodium phosphate (Turbinaire)

8. Antihistamines, such as fexofenadine (Allegra), are the treatment of choice for

    a. viral upper respiratory infections.

    b. allergic rhinitis.

    c. influenza.

    d. asthma.

9. Fexofenadine (Allegra), a second-generation antihistamine, differs from first-generation antihistamines by

    a. increased adverse effect profile.

    b. decreased sedation.

    c. decreased incidence of allergy.

    d. increased anticholinergic effects.

10. An expectorant drug, such as guaifenesin (Robitussin), is used to relieve

    a. a dry, hacking cough.

    b. nasal congestion.

    c. chest congestion.

    d. sinus congestion.

CORE PATIENT VARIABLES: PATIENTS, PLEASE

Multiple choice

Circle the option that best answers the question or completes the statement.

1. James Anderson has been diagnosed with a viral upper respiratory infection and prescribed dextromethorphan (Benylin). You note that James is taking fluoxetine, a selective serotonin reuptake inhibitor (SSRI). You would advise Jim to

    a. refuse to take the medication at all.

    b. take the medication every other day.

    c. skip the PM dose and double the hs dose.

    d. call if symptoms such as fever, nausea, or hallucinations occur.

2. For the hospitalized patient, a priority nursing diagnosis for the patient receiving hydrocodone bitartrate is

    a. Risk for ineffective airway clearance.

    b. Risk for ineffective gas exchange.

    c. Risk for injury.

    d. Risk for constipation.

3. Which of the following patients should refrain from pseudoephedrine (Sudafed) therapy?

    a. Maria, with constipation

    b. Janice, with headaches

    c. Tyler, with severe hypertension

    d. James, with depression

4. Which of the following statements would be appropriate for patient teaching regarding pseudoephedrine (Sudafed) therapy?

    a. "You can take this medication for 30 days."

    b. "This medication does not have any major drug interactions."

    c. "This medication can make you really drowsy."

    d. "In addition to this medication, you should use a humidifier and drink at least 10 glasses of water a day."

5. Which of the following patients should refrain from fexofenadine (Allegra) therapy?

    a. Marilyn, who is breast-feeding

    b. Heather, who has Parkinson disease

    c. Evelyn, who has peripheral venous stasis

    d. Charlene, who has diabetes mellitus

6. Kendra, age 5, has allergic rhinitis. Which of the following drugs would be best for Kendra?

a. Cetirizine (Zyrtec)

b. fexofenadine (Allegra)

c. loratadine (Claritin)

d. diphenhydramine (Benadryl)

7. Lisa Lewis, age 46, calls the clinic to speak with the advice nurse. She complains of a cough for the past 4 weeks and has been self-treating with guaifenesin (Robitussin) from the local drug store. She states she has minimal relief with the guaifenesin and requests the name of a more efficacious cough syrup. Which of the following statements is most appropriate?

a. "This medication will work better if you stop smoking."

b. "Have you been drinking lots of water with this medication?"

c. "Because your cough has been with you for so long, it's best if you come to the clinic for a checkup."

d. "As long as you do not have a fever, I would just double the dose."

NURSING MANAGEMENT: EVERY GOOD NURSE SHOULD . . .

Multiple choice

Circle the option that best answers the question or completes the statement.

1. Lewis Rothgaber is seen in the outpatient center for a chronic cough, and he receives a prescription for dextromethorphan, an antitussive. Which of the following should the nurse include in patient education?

a. Do not drive until the effects of the drug on you are known.

b. Do not drink alcohol while on this drug.

c. Keep this medicine out of the reach of children.

d. all of the above

e. none of the above

2. What recommendations would you give a patient to maximize the therapeutic effect of pseudoephedrine, a nasal decongestant?

a. Eat a diet high in fiber.

b. Drink plenty of liquids.

c. Avoid taking hot, steamy showers.

d. Do not take for more than 14 days.

3. You are the nurse working a telephone hot line to answer questions about health problems. A patient calls and tells you that she has been taking fexofenadine, an antihistamine, for seasonal allergies. The drug is effective for her, but she complains of an upset stomach after taking it and wonders if she must stop taking the drug. What advice should you give her?

a. Stop taking the drug immediately.

b. Take half of the prescribed dosage.

c. Take the drug with food.

d. Take another antihistamine in addition to the fexofenadine.

4. Your next call, as the telephone advice nurse, is from a man who complains of a chronic nonproductive cough. He wants to know if it would be better for him to take guaifenesin, an expectorant, or dextromethorphan, an antitussive, for his cough, He has both at home. Which of the following questions would you include in your assessment to give him the best answer?

a. Do you have chronic asthma or emphysema?

b. Do you smoke?

c. What other medications do you take?

d. All of the above

e. None of the above

CASE STUDY

Gerald Fox, 72 years old, has been prescribed fexofenadine, an antihistamine, to treat his seasonal allergies.

To minimize adverse effects, and provide appropriate patient education, what questions about his lifestyle, diet, habits, and environment would you want to ask?

CRITICAL THINKING CHALLENGE

Mr. Fox has been on fexofenadine for about 2 months and does not have adverse effects from the drug. At this time, Mrs. Fox calls the outpatient department and speaks to the nurse. She is very concerned about her husband. She says, "He was working in the garden and got a rash from some weeds. He took some medicine for the rash and itching, and now I can't get him to stay awake."

1. What medicine do you think Mr. Fox took for his rash and itching?

2. What leads you to this belief?

CHAPTER 36

Drugs Affecting the Lower Respiratory System

TOP TEN THINGS TO KNOW ABOUT DRUGS AFFECTING THE LOWER RESPIRATORY SYSTEM

1. Acetylcysteine is a mucolytic used to break up thick, tenacious sputum in patients whose physical conditions make it difficult to cough up these secretions (e.g., chronic obstructive pulmonary disease [COPD], cystic fibrosis, pneumonia, tuberculosis [TB]). It is most frequently given by nebulizer, usually in an acute care setting. It is a fast-acting drug with onset of action within 1 minute. Main adverse effects are respiratory (bronchospasm, bronchoconstriction, chest tightness, burning in upper airway, rhinorrhea). Acetylcysteine is the antidote for severe acetaminophen overdosage.

2. Albuterol is a relatively selective beta-2 agonist used as a bronchodilator for patients with COPD and asthma. It may be given orally or inhaled by way of a metered-dose inhaler or nebulizer. Bronchodilation occurs quickly (in 15 minutes or less) after inhalation. Because of this, inhaled albuterol is considered a "rescue drug" when there is an acute attack of bronchoconstriction. It is the drug patients should use first when they begin to experience symptoms.

3. Although albuterol is relatively selective for beta-2 receptors, some stimulation of beta-1 receptors occurs. Adverse effects are related to these sympathomimetic effects, such as tachycardia, anxiety, and tremor. Oral doses are more likely to cause systemic adverse effects.

4. Ipratropium is an anticholinergic that decreases the formation of cyclic guanosine monophosphate (cGMP), creating relaxation of the smooth muscle in the bronchial tree. It is used as maintenance treatment for bronchospasm from chronic asthma, bronchitis, emphysema, or COPD. It is given by inhalation or intranasal spray.

5. Ipratropium is taken daily to decrease the frequency and severity of future asthmatic attacks. It will **not** provide "rescue relief" for an attack in progress. Patient education is important to achieve the full therapeutic effect.

6. Theophylline, a xanthine, has a direct effect on the smooth muscle of the respiratory tract and produces bronchodilation. It is used to treat or prevent bronchial asthma and bronchospasms in COPD. It is given orally. Aminophylline, a very similar drug that is water soluble, is given IV when oral theophylline is not appropriate.

7. Adverse effects of theophylline are gastrointestinal (nausea, vomiting, diarrhea) and central nervous system stimulation (headache, insomnia, irritability), and possibly CV (hypotension, arrhythmias). Adverse effects most frequently occur when serum levels are elevated above therapeutic range, although they may occur with therapeutic levels. Monitor serum levels throughout therapy.

8. Cromolyn sodium is a mast cell stabilizer that is used in prophylaxis for mild to moderate asthma. It prevents the mast cell from rupturing and spilling its contents (degranulation) after it has contact with an antigen. Thus, it has anti-inflammatory effects. It is administered by inhalation or intranasal spray. Cromolyn sodium must be taken daily as prophylaxis; it is not effective during an acute asthmatic attack. It may be used before exercise, however, to prevent exercise-induced bronchospasm.

9. Zafirlukast blocks the receptors for leukotrienes, which are potent bronchoconstrictors. This is how zafirlukast improves the wheezing, coughing, and dyspneic symptoms of asthma. Zafirlukast is used in the treatment of chronic asthma; it does not relieve the symptoms of an acute asthmatic attack. It is given orally. Food impairs the absorption of zafirlukast; give 1 hour before or 2 hours after eating.

10. Glucocorticoid steroids are the most effective anti-inflammatory drugs used in the management of respiratory disorders. They may be given orally, parenterally, or by inhalation. Inhaled glucocorticoids need to be used daily for their peak effect to occur. IV doses may be used in acute respiratory flare-ups, in combination with a xanthine or a beta-2 agonist. Inhaled glucocorticoids do not have the systemic adverse effects that occur with oral and parenteral forms. The adverse effects from inhaled steroids are localized in the respiratory tract (sore throat, hoarseness, cough).

KEY TERMS

Matching

Match the following key terms with their definitions:

1. _____ bronchodilators
2. _____ bronchospasm
3. _____ chemoreceptors
4. _____ CAL
5. _____ COPD
6. _____ mucolytics
7. _____ perfusion
8. _____ respiration
9. _____ ventilation

a. Delivery of blood to the alveoli
b. Act of breathing
c. Drugs that open the airways in the lungs
d. Umbrella term for a group of respiratory disorders
e. Muscle spasm that occurs in the airways
f. Current name for COPD
g. Exchange of gases at the alveolar level
h. Drugs that break down mucus in the airways
i. Neuroreceptors sensitive to CO_2 and acid levels

PHYSIOLOGY AND PATHOPHYSIOLOGY: THE BODY HUMAN

Essay

1. Identify the components of the lower respiratory system.

2. When assessing a patient, the nurse determines vital signs including blood pressure, pulse, temperature, and respirations. Is the term "respiration" accurate? Why or why not?

3. What is the action of the vagus nerve in the respiratory system?

4. In the respiratory system, what response is expected when stimulation of the sympathetic nervous system occurs?

CORE DRUG KNOWLEDGE: JUST THE FACTS

Multiple choice

Circle the option that best answers the question or completes the statement.

1. The action of acetylcysteine (Mucomyst) is to
   a. dilate the bronchioles.
   b. decrease inflammation in the bronchioles.
   c. break down mucoproteins in the airways that block airflow.
   d. stop the breakdown of the mast cell.

2. Acetylcysteine (Mucomyst) is the drug of choice in the treatment of
   a. viral upper respiratory diseases.
   b. cystic fibrosis.
   c. allergic rhinitis.
   d. sinusitis.

3. In addition to action on the respiratory system, acetylcysteine (Mucomyst) is used in the management of
   a. Tylenol overdose.
   b. migraine headaches.
   c. nephrotoxicity.
   d. pancreatitis.

4. The action of albuterol (Proventil) is to
   a. dilate the bronchioles.
   b. decrease inflammation in the bronchioles.
   c. break down mucoproteins in the airways that block airflow.
   d. stop the breakdown of the mast cell.

5. When albuterol (Proventil) is administered by inhalation, relief of symptoms should occur within
   a. 30 seconds.
   b. 1 hour.
   c. 30 minutes.
   d. 5 minutes.

6. Adverse effects associated with the use of albuterol (Proventil) include
   a. bradycardia and sedation.
   b. tachycardia and palpitations.
   c. constipation and bradycardia.
   d. sedation and constipation.

7. Ipratropium bromide (Atrovent) works by
   a. stimulating the action of the sympathetic nervous system.
   b. blocking the action of the sympathetic nervous system.
   c. stimulating the action of the parasympathetic nervous system.
   d. blocking the action of the parasympathetic nervous system.

8. Adverse effects of inhaled ipratropium bromide (Atrovent) include
   a. paradoxic acute bronchospasm.
   b. bronchodilation.
   c. tachycardia.
   d. headache.

9. In general, ipratropium bromide (Atrovent) should be used
   a. Every 2 hours as needed.
   b. 3 to 4 times a day.
   c. Only once a day.
   d. Not more than twice a day.

10. Theophylline (Theo-Dur) works by
    a. stimulating the sympathetic nervous system.
    b. blocking the rupture of a mast cell.
    c. directly affecting the smooth muscle of the respiratory tract.
    d. blocking the action of the parasympathetic nervous system.

11. The optimal therapeutic range for theophylline (Theo-Dur) is
    a. 10 to 20 μg/mL.
    b. 30 to 35 μg/mL.
    c. 2 to 5 μg/mL.
    d. 20 to 25 μg/mL.

12. Which of the following statements concerning theophylline (Theo-Dur) therapy is correct?
    a. There are very few drug–drug interactions with theophylline.
    b. Although there are many drug–drug interactions with theophylline, they are minor and require no special intervention.
    c. There are many drug–drug interactions with theophylline that may require dosage changes.
    d. CNS adverse effects rarely occur with theophylline.

13. Patients on theophylline (Theo-Dur) should avoid large amounts of
    a. milk.
    b. charcoal-broiled beef.
    c. chicken.
    d. green leafy vegetables.

14. Cromolyn sodium (Intal) works by
    a. blocking the action of the sympathetic nervous system.
    b. blocking the action of the parasympathetic nervous system.
    c. bronchodilation.
    d. preventing the release of chemicals that stimulate the inflammatory process.

15. Cromolyn sodium (Intal) is contraindicated for patients
    a. with hepatotoxicity.
    b. having an acute asthma attack.
    c. with nephrotoxicity.
    d. with chronic asthma.

16. Which of the following statements concerning cromolyn sodium (Intal) therapy is correct?
    a. There are no drug–drug interactions with cromolyn.
    b. Although there are many drug–drug interactions with cromolyn, they are minor and require no special intervention.
    c. There are many drug–drug interactions with cromolyn that may require dosage changes.
    d. CNS adverse effects rarely occur with cromolyn.

17. Zafirlukast (Accolate) works by
    a. blocking the rupture of a mast cell.
    b. blocking leukotriene receptor sites.
    c. blocking the action of the sympathetic nervous system.
    d. blocking the action of the parasympathetic nervous system.

18. Serious adverse effects to zafirlukast (Accolate) therapy include
    a. CNS obtundation.
    b. kidney failure.
    c. hepatic failure.
    d. respiratory depression.

19. Zafirlukast should not be given to children under the age of
    a. 18.
    b. 6.
    c. 12.
    d. 10.

20. Which of the following drugs is indicated for treatment of an acute asthma attack?
    a. beclomethasone (Beclovent)
    b. zafirlukast (Accolate)
    c. ipratropium bromide (Atrovent)
    d. albuterol (Proventil)

CORE PATIENT VARIABLES: PATIENTS, PLEASE

Multiple choice

Circle the option that best answers the question or completes the statement.

1. Alyssa Myers, age 7, has cystic fibrosis and is receiving acetylcysteine therapy. After completion of therapy, the nurse should anticipate the need for
   a. chest physiotherapy.
   b. the use of a cooling blanket.
   c. in and out catheterization.
   d. frequent vital sign checks.

2. After administration of nebulized acetylcysteine (Mucomyst), the nurse should wash the patient's face with
   a. betadine.
   b. alcohol.
   c. water.
   d. soap.

3. Kirby Taylor, age 16, has been diagnosed with asthma since age 11. Kirby uses an albuterol (Proventil) inhaler. Kirby comes to the clinic today and states, "This inhaler is worthless. I have to use it every 2 hours." With your knowledge of this drug, you suspect Kirby may be
   a. noncompliant.
   b. experiencing rebound bronchoconstriction.
   c. experiencing addiction.
   d. smoking.

4. Betty Hughes, age 27, comes to the clinic for a renewal of albuterol (Proventil). Betty states that the drug works well but she can feel her heart race, cannot sleep, and feels "wired" all the time. Which of the following core patient variables is important to assess at this time?
   a. health status
   b. culture
   c. lifespan and gender
   d. diet, lifestyle, and habits

5. Jason Ingles, age 21, has asthma and takes albuterol (Proventil) as needed. Jason is seen at the clinic today, and the health care provider adds ipratropium bromide (Atrovent) to his asthma regimen. It is important for the nurse to teach Jason to use this inhaler
   a. only when the albuterol is not helping.
   b. only when he is feeling poorly.
   c. twice a day, regardless of how he feels.
   d. twice a day, if he feels tightness in his chest.

6. Frank James, age 22, has asthma and an order for ipratropium bromide (Atrovent). Before the administration, the nurse should assess for allergies to
   a. eggs.
   b. milk.
   c. pasta.
   d. legumes.

7. Stephen Stone, age 42, has asthma. He states he hates to take his theophylline pills because "I'm up all night and nervous." Which of the following interventions would be most helpful to Stephen?
   a. Administer the medication every other day.
   b. Contact the health care provider for an order for a sympathomimetic by inhalation.
   c. Give the theophylline with milk.
   d. Break the pill in half and give each half 2 hours apart.

8. Which of the following patients should refrain from theophylline therapy?
   a. Jillian, with hypothyroidism
   b. Carlos, with peptic ulcer disease
   c. Tanya, with depression
   d. Louise, with a history of asthma

9. Despite a long history of asthma, Alex continues to smoke a pack of cigarettes per day. During theophylline therapy, you would expect to administer

   a. a higher dose of theophylline.

   b. a lower dose of theophylline.

   c. a dose that would be the same as that for a nonsmoker.

10. Mary Franklin has asthma. The health care provider has just prescribed cromolyn sodium (Intal) for Mary. Patient education should include instructions to

    a. use the inhaler at the first sign of an acute attack.

    b. use the inhaler only on days that you expect symptoms.

    c. use the inhaler 15 to 20 minutes before participating in anything known to cause bronchospasm in you.

    d. use the inhaler 4 times a day, regardless of how you feel.

11. Carson Hayes has severe persistent asthma. Use of which of the following inhalers should be followed by rinsing the mouth out to prevent overgrowth of fungi?

    a. albuterol (Proventil)

    b. ipratropium bromide (Atrovent)

    c. cromolyn sodium (Intal)

    d. beclomethasone (Beclovent)

12. Ben Crane has asthma and uses albuterol (Proventil), ipratropium bromide (Atrovent), and beclomethasone dipropionate (Beclovent) inhalers. Mr. Crane comes to the clinic for a routine checkup and states, "I can never remember which of these I should take first." Which of the following statements is most appropriate in response?

    a. "It really does not matter, just be sure to take them all 4 times a day."

    b. "Use the albuterol first. That will help the other two disperse further in your lungs."

    c. "Take the ipratropium first and then rinse your mouth. The other two can follow."

    d. "Use the beclomethasone first and then rinse your mouth. Take the ipratropium second and the albuterol last."

NURSING MANAGEMENT: EVERY GOOD NURSE SHOULD . . .

Multiple choice

Circle the option that best answers the question or completes the statement.

1. You are the nurse providing a nebulizer treatment of acetylcysteine for a patient with bilateral lower lobe pneumonia. Which of the following should you remember while administering drug therapy and caring for the patient?

   a. keep diluted acetylcysteine at room temperature

   b. the patient should avoid coughing after drug therapy

   c. nebulization of the drug initially produces a sweet smell

   d. a sticky residue may form on the patient's face from therapy

2. Juan Panchez has been started on an IV drip of aminophylline, a xanthine bronchodilator, for an acute COPD exacerbation. Which of the following should be included in the nursing care of Mr. Panchez while he receives IV aminophylline?

   a. assess breath sounds every 2 to 4 hours

   b. assess for insomnia, tachycardia, and irritability

   c. inform him that he will have blood drawn regularly while on the drug

   d. all of the above

   e. none of the above

3. Allen Gilchrist, 17 years old, has asthma. He has been prescribed zafirlukast (a mast cell stabilizer), beclomethasone (a glucocorticoid steroid) metered-dose inhaler, and albuterol (a beta-2 agonist) metered dose inhaler. He questions why he needs three medications, two of which are inhalers. Patient education for Allen should include

   a. the drugs work in different ways to provide better, more complete treatment.

   b. the zafirlukast and the beclomethasone work to prevent asthmatic attacks, and the albuterol works to provide quick relief of asthmatic attacks.

   c. giving beclomethasone and albuterol by inhalers helps to reduce their adverse effects.

   d. all of the above.

   e. none of the above.

4. Martha Ferral has been prescribed cromolyn sodium as part of the treatment for her asthma. She has a history of irregular menstrual periods and lactose intolerance. What teaching does Martha need regarding the cromolyn sodium?

   a. contact the provider if nausea, bloating, or abdominal cramps occur while on this drug

   b. use the inhaler whenever an asthmatic attack occurs

   c. use the inhaler by first inhaling deeply and then triggering the inhaler to release a dose

   d. all of the above

   e. none of the above

5. Mike Rosenbaum is to be started on theophylline. In your patient education, you'll need to tell him that he needs to avoid, or limit, the intake of which of these favorite foods and beverages?

   a. lemon meringue pie (eats once every 4 or 5 months)

   b. fettuccine alfredo (eats once every 6 weeks to 2 months)

   c. iced tea (drinks daily)

   d. Sprite soda (drinks daily)

   e. Cheerios cereal (eats 5 or 6 days in a row every 3 months)

6. Soo Han has been started on zafirlukast for her asthma. She returns for a checkup. Which of these findings would alarm you, the nurse, the most?

   a. absence of wheezing

   b. mild headache

   c. whites of the eyes are yellowed

   d. upset stomach

CASE STUDY

Jason March is an asthmatic patient who has a history of smoking one half pack of cigarettes a day. He is seen in the outpatient department and given a prescription for theophylline, a bronchodilator, to help control his asthma. His serum theophylline level after 1 week on the drug is checked and it is 15 μg/mL, which is within therapeutic range. He is told to continue on this dose but to stop smoking. He returns to the clinic for a visit 6 weeks after being started on theophylline for a checkup. His serum theophylline level is now 25 μg/mL, which is above the therapeutic range. He says to you, "I gave up smoking like they told me but, boy, now I feel rotten. I have a headache all the time and I can't sleep. I thought giving up smoking would make me feel better, not worse."

1. What explanations may account for Mr. March's complaints?

2. What actions might be necessary to correct these complaints?

CRITICAL THINKING CHALLENGE

Mr. March is stabilized on his theophylline. Nine months later, he is hospitalized for pneumonia and ordered 400 mg ciprofloxacin IV every 12 hours as treatment. He continues on his same dose of theophylline. On the third day of treatment with the ciprofloxacin, the nurse caring for Mr. March notes that he is very irritable, compared to his mood previously. He also is experiencing diarrhea and some nausea.

1. What do you think might be causing these problems?

2. What lab work is needed to confirm your assessment?

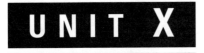

UNIT X

Gastrointestinal System Drugs

CHAPTER 37

Drugs for Treating the Upper Gastrointestinal Tract

TOP TEN THINGS TO KNOW ABOUT DRUGS FOR TREATING THE UPPER GASTROINTESTINAL TRACT

1. Peptic ulcers are caused by the bacteria *Helicobacter pylori*, not by smoking, caffeine use, or stress. To eradicate *H pylori*, a combination of antibiotics is used, usually with a proton pump inhibitor, or possibly with an H2 receptor antagonist.

2. Omeprazole is a proton pump inhibitor used in the treatment of duodenal ulcers associated with *H pylori*, and for treatment of heartburn and other symptoms of gastroesophageal reflux disease (GERD). Omeprazole suppresses the last phase of gastric acid production. Teach the patient to take omeprazole before meals, for the entire time prescribed, and not to crush or chew the medicine.

3. Cimetidine, an H2 receptor antagonist, blocks histamine action at the parietal cells in the stomach and, thus, inhibits all phases of gastric acid secretion. It is used in treating the symptoms of active peptic and duodenal ulcers, GERD, pathologic hypersecretory conditions, heartburn/acid indigestion, and in the prevention of upper GI bleeding in critically ill patients. Cimetidine is available in prescription and over-the-counter (OTC) strengths.

4. Cimetidine interacts with many drugs, often by decreasing their hepatic metabolism. Give 2 hours apart from other drugs to prevent interaction. Because of this, cimetidine is being replaced with therapy by other H2 receptor antagonists (ranitidine, famotidine), which do not have drug interactions. Assess for concurrent use of OTC forms of cimetidine and other H2 receptor antagonists.

5. Antacids are base salts that increase gastric pH. They relieve symptoms of hyperacidity, GERD, and the pain from duodenal ulcers. All antacids are closely related and used in various combinations. Aluminum hydroxide with magnesium hydroxide, like other antacids, interacts with many other drugs and may affect their pharmacokinetics and therapeutic effect. Give 2 hours after other drugs to prevent interactions. Assess patients for OTC use of antacids.

6. Aluminum antacids cause constipation, and magnesium antacids cause diarrhea. The combination of the two usually has no effect. Avoid using aluminum hydroxide with magnesium hydroxide (or other magnesium antacids) in patients with chronic renal failure; magnesium toxicity may occur. Aluminum carbonate is used in chronic renal failure because it binds with phosphorus and reduces hyperphosphatemia.

7. GI stimulants, such as metoclopramide, apparently increase the effect of acetylcholine in the GI tract, increasing peristalsis and gastric emptying, without stimulating gastric, pancreatic, or gallbladder secretions. Metoclopramide also is a dopamine receptor antagonist that produces antiemetic effects. It is used to treat diabetic gastroparesis and symptoms of GERD, and to prevent nausea and vomiting postoperatively and during chemotherapy. Serious adverse effects, related to the dopamine blocking effects, are not common but include depression, extrapyramidal symptoms, Parkinson-like symptoms, and tardive dyskinesia.

8. Digestive enzymes such as pancrelipase are a replacement for the body's intrinsic enzymes when the body produces too little (e.g., cystic fibrosis, chronic pancreatitis, after pancreatectomy). Administer pancrelipase with meals.

9. Orlistat inhibits the digestive enzyme lipase; this decreases the absorption of digested fat. Orlistat is used in the management of obesity in addition to a weight loss diet. GI adverse effects are common. Teach the patient to take orlistat with every meal that has fat in it; no dose should be taken if a meal is skipped or if it has no fat in it.

10. Ondansetron is a selective serotonin receptor antagonist (5-HT$_3$ receptor antagonist). It blocks stimulation of special serotonin receptors in the chemoreceptor trigger zone (CTZ), preventing nausea and vomiting. Ondansetron is used to prevent nausea and vomiting associated with chemotherapy, and postoperatively when nausea and vomiting must be avoided. Ondansetron should be administered before chemotherapy or induction into anesthesia.

KEY TERMS

Matching

Match the following key terms with their definitions.

1. _____ antiemetics
2. _____ chemoreceptor trigger zone
3. _____ digestive enzymes
4. _____ duodenum
5. _____ emetics
6. _____ GERD
7. _____ GI stimulants
8. _____ *H pylori*
9. _____ peptic ulcer
10. _____ peristalsis
11. _____ stress ulcer
12. _____ vomiting center
13. _____ Zollinger-Ellison syndrome

a. Stimulation of this area of the brain results in vomiting
b. Drugs that increase the transit time of gastric contents
c. Erosion of all layers of the wall of the stomach or duodenum
d. Bacterial organism found in 90% of patients with ulcers
e. Responsible for the breakdown of food
f. Drugs that stimulate vomiting
g. Drugs that inhibit vomiting
h. Peptic ulceration with gastric hypersecretion and non-beta cell tumor of the pancreatic islets
i. Waves of alternate circular contraction and relaxation of the intestine by which the contents are propelled onward
j. Located in the medulla of the brain
k. Part of the small intestine
l. Caused by acute or chronic stress
m. Characterized by chronic heartburn, dyspepsia, and ulceration of the mucosal lining

PHYSIOLOGY AND PATHOPHYSIOLOGY: THE BODY HUMAN

Essay

1. Name the components of the upper GI tract.

2. What are the four layers of the duodenum? What are their functions?

3. Name the cells in the stomach responsible for the production of "gastric juice."

4. What part of the autonomic nervous system (ANS) stimulates the production of gastric secretions?

5. Name the pancreatic enzymes. What are their functions?

CORE DRUG KNOWLEDGE: JUST THE FACTS

Multiple choice

Circle the option that best answers the question or completes the statement.

1. Omeprazole (Prilosec) is used in the management of
   a. diarrhea.
   b. constipation.
   c. GERD.
   d. nausea.

2. Omeprazole (Prilosec) works by
   a. neutralizing gastric acid.
   b. suppressing the H+/ K+/ATPase enzyme system.
   c. blocking histamine at the H_2 receptor site of parietal cells.
   d. adhering to the ulcer lesions and protecting them from stomach acids.

3. Which of the following statements concerning adverse effects to omeprazole (Prilosec) therapy is accurate?
   a. There are a few minor adverse effects.
   b. There are many potential adverse effects, but they are minor.
   c. There are few adverse effects, but they are potentially fatal.
   d. There are many potential adverse effects, and they are all serious.

4. Sucralfate (Carafate) works by
   a. neutralizing gastric acid.
   b. suppressing the H+/K+/ATPase enzyme system.
   c. blocking histamine at the H2 receptor site of parietal cells.
   d. adhering to the ulcer lesions and protecting them from stomach acids.

5. Cimetidine (Tagamet) is used in the management of
   a. nausea and vomiting.
   b. diarrhea.
   c. peptic and duodenal ulcers.
   d. constipation.

6. Cimetidine (Tagamet) works by
   a. neutralizing gastric acid.
   b. suppressing the H+/K+/ATPase enzyme system.
   c. blocking histamine at the H2 receptor site of parietal cells.
   d. adhering to the ulcer lesions and protecting them from stomach acids.

7. Which of the following statements concerning potential adverse effects of cimetidine (Tagamet) therapy is accurate?
   a. There are few potential adverse effects, and they are minor.
   b. There are few potential adverse effects, but they are all serious.
   c. There are many potential adverse effects, and they are all minor.
   d. There are many potential adverse effects, and some of them are serious.

8. Which of the following statements concerning potential drug–drug interactions during cimetidine (Tagamet) therapy is accurate?
   a. There are a few potential drug–drug interactions that are not significant.
   b. There are many potential drug–drug interactions, but they are not significant.
   c. There are few potential drug–drug interactions, and they are very significant.
   d. There are many potential drug–drug interactions, and many are very significant.

9. Misoprostol (Cytotec) is used to
   a. prevent gastric ulcer disease.
   b. treat gastric ulcer disease.
   c. prevent GERD.
   d. treat GERD.

10. Which of the following drugs is classified as an antacid?
    a. ranitidine (Zantac)
    b. misoprostol (Cytotec)
    c. sucralfate (Carafate)
    d. aluminum hydroxide

11. Which of the following adverse effects may occur with the use of aluminum-based antacids?
    a. diarrhea
    b. constipation
    c. anemia
    d. peptic ulceration

12. When taken after meals, aluminum- and magnesium-based antacids should be effective for approximately
    a. 30 to 60 minutes.
    b. 3 hours.
    c. 6 hours.
    d. 24 hours.

13. What is a major difference between aluminum hydroxide and sodium bicarbonate?
    a. There is no difference.
    b. Aluminum hydroxide may be systemically absorbed, resulting in metabolic alkalosis.
    c. Sodium bicarbonate may be systemically absorbed, resulting in metabolic alkalosis.
    d. Sodium bicarbonate has less acid rebound than aluminum hydroxide.

14. Metoclopramide (Reglan) is effective in the treatment of
    a. peptic ulcers.
    b. duodenal ulcers.
    c. diabetic gastroparesis.
    d. diarrhea.

15. Which of the following statements concerning potential drug–drug interactions of metoclopramide (Reglan) is accurate?

    a. There are only a few potential drug–drug interactions.

    b. There are many drug–drug interactions due to its ability to disrupt the metabolism of many drugs.

    c. There are many drug–drug interactions due to its ability to disrupt the absorption of many drugs.

    d. There are many drug–drug interactions due to its ability to disrupt the excretion of many drugs.

16. During metoclopramide (Reglan) therapy, elderly females have an increased risk for

    a. fatigue.

    b. tardive dyskinesia.

    c. mental depression.

    d. restlessness.

17. Which of the following drugs would be an effective replacement for digestive enzymes?

    a. pancrelipase (Pancrease, Viokase)

    b. sucralfate (Carafate)

    c. dexpanthenol (Ilopan)

    d. metoclopramide (Reglan)

18. Contraindications to the administration of pancrelipase (Pancrease, Viokase) include an allergy to

    a. sulfa.

    b. dairy products.

    c. pork.

    d. seafood.

19. Orlistat (Xenical) is used in the management of

    a. diabetes.

    b. pancreatic insufficiency.

    c. peptic ulcer disease.

    d. morbid obesity.

20. Adverse effects to orlistat (Xenical) therapy usually affect the _____ system.

    a. CNS

    b. GI

    c. cardiovascular

    d. respiratory

21. Ondansetron (Zofran) is used to prevent

    a. morbid obesity.

    b. peptic ulcer disease.

    c. GERD.

    d. nausea and vomiting.

22. Which of the following statements concerning the potential adverse effects of ondansetron (Zofran) is accurate?

    a. There are only a few potential adverse effects, and they are all serious.

    b. There are many potential adverse effects, and a few are serious.

    c. There are only a few potential adverse effects, and they are minor.

    d. There are many potential adverse effects, and they are minor.

CORE PATIENT VARIABLES: PATIENTS PLEASE . . .

Multiple choice

Circle the option that best answers the question or completes the statement.

1. Henry Thomas, age 55, comes to the clinic today for a renewal of omeprazole (Prilosec). Mr. Thomas states, "This drug really works for me. I'm concerned about what will happen when I reached the time limit for taking it. What will they do for me then?" What is your best response?

    a. "That's a question you need to ask the nurse practitioner."

    b. "You will have to go back to using antacids as needed."

    c. "You can take a combination of antacids and sucralfate (Carafate)."

    d. "Because your condition is chronic, you should be able to stay on this medication indefinitely."

2. Connie Arrow has a duodenal ulcer and takes sucralfate (Carafate). She states she continues to have gastric discomfort and asks if she may also take an antacid. The most appropriate response would be

    a. "Sure, that's no problem."

    b. "You can take the antacid, but you will probably have a real problem with constipation."

    c. "You can take the antacid, but it's important to take it at least 30 minutes after the sucralfate."

    d. "No, that would be two drugs that are increasing the pH and that would be dangerous."

3. Your patient has a hip fracture and is scheduled for surgery in the morning. You note an order for cimetidine (Tagamet) but are unable to find a history of GERD or ulcers. This medication is being given to prevent

   a. stress ulcers.

   b. diarrhea.

   c. constipation.

   d. vomiting.

4. Your patient has an order for cimetidine (Tagamet) IVP. What action should be taken by the nurse to administer this drug safely?

   a. dilute in 5 cc normal saline and administer over 30 seconds

   b. dilute in 20 cc NS and administer over 2 minutes

   c. contact the health care provider because this drug should not be administered IVP

   d. dilute in 2 cc sterile water and administer over 1 minute

5. Your patient has GERD and takes cimetidine (Tagamet). She states she continues to have gastric discomfort and asks if she may also take an antacid. Which of the following responses is correct?

   a. "No, that would be two drugs that are decreasing the pH and that would be dangerous."

   b. "You can take the antacid, but you will probably have a real problem with diarrhea."

   c. "Sure, that's no problem."

   d. "You can take the antacid, but it's important to take it at least 2 hours after the cimetidine."

6. Tommy Jenkins, age 7, has been taking cimetidine for over 2 years. What adverse effect may Tommy experience due to the duration of his therapy?

   a. gynecomastia

   b. muscle spasm

   c. increased gastric secretion

   d. impotence

7. Which of the following drugs would be an ABSOLUTE contraindication for your patient's peptic ulcer during pregnancy?

   a. aluminum hydroxide

   b. misoprostol (Cytotec)

   c. cimetidine (Tagamet)

   d. magnesium hydroxide

8. Nancy Jones states her 14-year-old son had an upset stomach after eating spicy food. She gave him an antacid. She asks, "How soon will it work?" What answer would you give? Within

   a. 5 minutes

   b. 3 hours

   c. 1 hour

   d. 6 hours

9. Daniel Uribe, age 50, has chronic renal failure and remembers being told something about reading the labels on antacids, but cannot remember what it was. What would you tell Daniel?

   a. Do not take an antacid that is aluminum based.

   b. Do not take an antacid that is magnesium based.

   c. Do not take an antacid.

   d. Take whatever type of antacid is available.

10. Which of the following patients should refrain from metoclopramide (Reglan) therapy?

    a. Jason, with hypertension

    b. Billy, with GERD

    c. Alex, with seizure disorder

    d. Bob, with asthma

11. Phyllis Ganz is taking metoclopramide (Reglan) for diabetic gastroparesis. Which of the following instructions for Mrs. Ganz is correct?

    a. "Take the medication 1 hour after eating."

    b. "Take the medication at bedtime."

    c. "Take the medication 30 minutes before meals."

    d. "Take the medication 2 hours before meals."

12. Kimberly Taylor, age 35, is receiving chemotherapy for breast cancer. To minimize the adverse effects of chemotherapy, the nurse should administer metoclopramide (Reglan)

    a. IV 30 minutes before chemotherapy.

    b. IM at bedtime.

    c. PO before each meal.

    d. IV 30 minutes after chemotherapy.

13. Your patient is receiving IV metoclopramide (Reglan). You note involuntary movements of the limbs, facial grimacing, and rhythmic protrusion of the tongue. You suspect the patient is experiencing

    a. parkinsonism.

    b. tardive dyskinesia.

    c. overdose.

    d. extrapyramidal effects.

14. Sally Uram, age 46, is hospitalized for acute pancreatitis. At home, Mrs. Uram takes pancrelipase. She states, "I'm worried that I'm not getting my pancrelipase. Do you know why?" What is your best response?

    a. "I'm not sure, but I will ask the doctor."

    b. "Pancrelipase should not be given until after your acute pancreatitis has subsided."

    c. "I'll get an order for it right away."

    d. "I'm sure the doctor knows what he is doing."

15. Orin Chase takes pancrelipase. He also takes albuterol for his asthma. What instructions should you give to Mr. Chase?

    a. Do not use your albuterol inhaler within 30 minutes of taking pancrelipase.

    b. Be careful not to inhale the pancrelipase because it may trigger an asthma attack.

    c. Use your inhaler just before taking pancrelipase.

    d. All of the above

16. Samantha Baker, age 43, has type 2 diabetes due to her morbid obesity. She has been prescribed orlistat (Xenical). After 6 weeks, Samantha has lost 15 pounds. You anticipate that her diabetic medication dose may need to be

    a. increased.

    b. decreased.

    c. left alone.

17. Patient education for patients receiving orlistat (Xenical) need to include instructions to

    a. take your vitamins 1 hour before or 4 hours after a meal.

    b. take your vitamins with meals.

    c. increase intake of fats.

    d. increase intake of cholesterol-rich foods.

18. Molly Rich has breast cancer and is receiving radiation therapy. Mrs. Rich has an order for ondansetron (Zofran). In this situation, how should ondansetron be administered?

    a. IV 30 minutes before the procedure

    b. PO 15 minutes before the procedure

    c. IV 1 to 2 hours before the procedure

    d. PO 1 to 2 hours before the procedure

NURSING MANAGEMENT: EVERY GOOD NURSE SHOULD . . .

Multiple choice

Circle the option that best answers the question or completes the statement.

1. Hunter Pugh is to start on liquid aluminum hydroxide with magnesium hydroxide to treat recurrent esophageal reflux. To maximize the therapeutic effect of the drug therapy, the nurse should teach him to

    a. shake the bottle well before measuring the dose.

    b. administer 1 hour before meals.

    c. mix the drug with water before administering.

    d. do all of the above.

    e. do none of the above.

2. John Gutzmer has GERD. He is to receive 30 mL of aluminum hydroxide with magnesium hydroxide PO every 4 hours while awake and cimetidine, an H2 receptor antagonist, 800 mg PO twice a day. To maximize therapeutic and/or minimize adverse effects, the nurse should

    a. stagger doses of the two drugs so they are given 2 hours apart.

    b. give the cimetidine immediately before meals and the aluminum hydroxide with magnesium hydroxide immediately after meals.

    c. crush the cimetidine and mix with the aluminum hydroxide with magnesium hydroxide.

    d. do all of the above.

    e. do none of the above.

3. Gwynn Hart had abdominal surgery 2 days ago. She is having nausea and vomiting every time she eats. She is started on metoclopramide 10 mg PO TID. For effective nursing management of this drug therapy, the nurse should

    a. administer the metoclopramide 30 minutes before each meal.

    b. monitor Gwynn for depression while on drug therapy.

    c. caution Gwynn that the drug may make her drowsy or fatigued.

    d. do all of the above.

    e. do none of the above.

4. Ashley Miller is one and a half years old and has been diagnosed with cystic fibrosis. She is to start on pancrelipase. What teaching would be important for Ashley's parents?

   a. The drug should be administered on an empty stomach.

   b. Avoid inhaling the powdered drug.

   c. Steatorrhea stools are an adverse effect of the drug.

   d. The drug should be taken once a day.

5. William Head has been diagnosed with a gastric ulcer. He is to start on a combined drug therapy of amoxicillin, metronidazole, and omeprazole, a proton pump inhibitor. He is known to be allergic to salicylates. He asks why he needs to take antibiotics for an ulcer and why he has to take three different drugs. As his nurse, your best response to him is

   a. "Infections of the stomach frequently occur secondary to gastric ulcers; all three drugs are needed to treat the infection."

   b. "The antibiotics are to prevent an infection; the omeprazole is to treat the gastric ulcer."

   c. "*H pylori* organisms are normally responsible for gastric ulcers; the antibiotics will eradicate the organisms. The omeprazole will decrease gastric acid, relieving pain and helping to eradicate the *H pylori* organisms."

   d. "*H pylori* organisms can multiply after a gastric ulcer is formed. The antibiotics will prevent infection from *H pylori*. The omeprazole will decrease pain from the gastric ulcer."

6. Samantha Ternansky has been prescribed orlistat to assist her in weight loss. You know from taking a diet history from her that she often skips breakfast, but has a snack, usually from the vending machine at work, at 4 PM. Currently, about 40% of her daily calories come from fat. Which of the following would you include in your teaching for her?

   a. Take the orlistat in the morning, at noon, and at dinnertime.

   b. Divide your fat intake evenly between the meals you eat.

   c. Keep the same amount of fat in your diet as you have now.

   d. This medication reduces your need for exercise.

7. Josh Meyers is to receive IV ondansetron to prevent nausea and vomiting from his chemotherapy. To maximize the therapeutic effect from the ondansetron, the nurse should

   a. give the drug 30 minutes before the start of chemotherapy.

   b. administer the drug quickly via IV push.

   c. avoid redosing after chemotherapy.

   d. do all of the above.

   e. do none of the above.

CASE STUDY

Milton Bernstein has a pathologic hypersecretory condition and has been started on cimetidine, an H2 receptor antagonist. He also smokes one pack of cigarettes per day and drinks two gin and tonics every night before dinner.
What teaching would be appropriate relevant to the cimetidine drug therapy?

CRITICAL THINKING CHALLENGE

Mr. Bernstein returns to the clinic for follow-up in 3 weeks. He appears to be doing well. He continues on the cimetidine for another 3 weeks. When he returns to the clinic this time, he complains of confusion, headaches, and dizziness.

1. What questions should you ask to help determine the cause of these adverse effects?

2. Are there any lab tests that would assist you to fully assess Mr. Bernstein and determine the cause of these problems?

CHAPTER 38

Drugs for Treating the Lower Gastrointestinal Tract

TOP TEN THINGS TO KNOW ABOUT DRUGS FOR TREATING THE LOWER GASTROINTESTINAL TRACT

1. Drugs used to treat disorders of the lower gastrointestinal tract include antiflatulents, antidiarrheals, and laxatives.
2. Simethicone, an antiflatulent, changes the surface tension of gas bubbles so they can be passed more easily. It is not systemically absorbed. Administer after meals. Tablets should be chewed well.
3. Diphenoxylate HCl with atropine sulfate, an antidiarrheal, acts on the smooth muscle of the intestine to slow intestinal motility, prolong transit time, and promote reabsorption of fluid. Diphenoxylate HCl is similar to a narcotic in structure; the dose is not high enough to provide pain relief. The atropine, an anticholinergic, is added to discourage deliberate abuse. Assess patients, especially children, for adverse effects from the atropine.
4. Locally acting antidiarrheals, such as kaolin, pectin, and bismuth salicylate, are sold over the counter. They are commonly used, but their efficacy is not well established.
5. Laxatives are used to treat constipation. They are for short-term use. Types of laxatives include saline, irritant, bulk forming, lubricating, surfactants, and miscellaneous.
6. Laxatives are contraindicated with patients who have severe abdominal pain that has not been diagnosed, are nauseated and vomiting, or have a bowel obstruction.

7. Magnesium hydroxide is a saline laxative. It attracts and retains water in the large intestine, resulting in an increase in peristalsis and a bowel movement. Repeated use may cause fluid and electrolyte imbalance. It is also used as an antacid. Avoid use in patients with renal failure.
8. Lactulose, a miscellaneous laxative, pulls water into the colon like magnesium sulfate. In the colon, it is metabolized into acids and carbon dioxide. The acids also pull ammonia into the stool; thus, lactulose is used to decrease the elevated blood ammonia levels found in hepatic coma and hepatic encephalopathy.
9. Bulk laxatives, such as psyllium and polycarbophil, increase the bulk of the fecal material, stimulating peristalsis and evacuation. Stimulants, such as bisacodyl, have a direct effect on the intestinal mucosa, stimulating peristalsis.
10. Mineral oil is a lubricant that coats the walls of the intestine and the fecal matter to ease passage of the stool. Stool softeners, such as docusate, promote the movement of water into the stool to promote easier passage. Stool softeners are used to prevent constipation, not treat it.

KEY TERMS

Word find exercise

Using the following definitions, unscramble the letters to form a word.

```
V U F C Z A E H R R A I D C P
C S N S O S I T I L O C H R C
K M K R Z J K C C U R K Y T
S X A T K L S B H B O N O G F
E I P H I L I Q P N O O A T R
I S S D D O K R W I R F T W E
H K K L B V Q L T W Q J A N V
F N K C A I X A H J I Z Y O I
I A P X R T P K B G K O Z I T
P E G E S I S S W W I F T A
X N P W T H L I U S X T I C R
F D Q S N G J O R T A A S A E
A G N P J L X X T E A S B P C
J O Z N A D Q Y T G P L I M L
C D U S V B P E V X Q G F I U
```

1. Wavelike muscular contraction of the intestine
2. Abbreviation for irritable bowel syndrome
3. Abbreviation for inflammatory bowel disease
4. Infrequent or incomplete passage of stool
5. Frequent, watery stools
6. Inability to pass hardened mass of feces
7. Byproduct of digestion that may be painful
8. Inflammatory disease characterized by inflammation extending into the deeper layers of the intestinal wall
9. Inflammatory disease of the large intestine
10. General term for inflammation of the colon

PHYSIOLOGY AND PATHOPHYSIOLOGY: THE BODY HUMAN

Essay

1. The large intestine consists of:

2. What are the four components of the colon?

3. The defecation reflex causes:

4. In a healthy person, fecal material consists of:

5. Bacteria in the colon produce which important vitamins?

CORE DRUG KNOWLEDGE: JUST THE FACTS

Multiple Choice

Circle the option that best answers the question or completes the statement.

1. Which of the following drugs is used to decrease gas production?
   a. magnesium hydroxide
   b. simethicone (Mylicon)
   c. diphenoxylate HCl (Lomotil)
   d. docusate (Colace)

2. Which of the following statements concerning the adverse effects of simethicone (Mylicon) is accurate?
   a. There are no potential adverse effects to its use.
   b. There are a few potential adverse effects, but they are minor.
   c. There are many potential adverse effects, but they are minor.
   d. There are a few potential adverse effects, and they are serious.

3. Which of the following drugs is NOT used in the treatment of diarrhea?
   a. magnesium hydroxide (Milk of Magnesia)
   b. loperamide (Imodium)
   c. kaolin
   d. diphenoxylate HCl (Lomotil)

4. Diphenoxylate (Lomotil) works by
   a. decreasing the absorption of fats and carbohydrates.
   b. increasing the water absorption from the bowel.
   c. slowing intestinal motility and prolonging intestinal transit time.
   d. decreasing water absorption from the bowel.

5. Administration of diphenoxylate (Lomotil) to a patient with diarrhea caused by a bacteria may result in
   a. impaction.
   b. prolongation of symptoms.
   c. headache.
   d. no known interaction.

6. Magnesium hydroxide (Milk of Magnesia) works by
   a. increasing the bulk of fecal material.
   b. stimulating peristalsis of the bowel.
   c. softening the stool for easy passage.
   d. retaining water in the intestinal lumen to increase pressure.

7. Potential adverse effects of long-term magnesium hydroxide (Milk of Magnesia) therapy include
   a. headaches.
   b. sedation.
   c. electrolyte imbalance.
   d. peptic ulcer.

8. Which of the following laxatives may also be used in the treatment of hepatic coma?
   a. magnesium hydroxide (Milk of Magnesia)
   b. polyethylene glycol-electrolyte solution
   c. lactulose (Cephulac)
   d. bisacodyl (Dulcolax)

9. Which of the following types of laxatives is the closest to a natural defecation?
   a. lubricants
   b. bulk forming
   c. stimulants
   d. stool softeners

10. What adverse effect is associated with long-term use of lubricant laxatives?
    a. headache
    b. hypertension
    c. decreased absorption of fat-soluble vitamins
    d. decreased absorption of fat and cholesterol

CORE PATIENT VARIABLES: PATIENTS, PLEASE

Multiple choice

Circle the option that best answers the question or completes the statement.

1. Alexis Frommelt is prescribed simethicone (Mylicon) as needed for flatus. Patient teaching should include instructions to
   a. swallow the tablet with a glass of water.
   b. chew the tablet thoroughly.
   c. take the medication only at bedtime.
   d. allow the suspension to separate before taking.

2. Alice Karris has diarrhea and is taking diphenoxylate (Lomotil). She also has a seizure disorder and is prescribed phenobarbital. You should monitor Alice for
   a. increased sedation.
   b. profound nausea.
   c. abdominal discomfort.
   d. headache.

3. Which of the following patients would have a high risk for atropine toxicity when taking diphenoxylate (Lomotil)?
   a. Lisa, with a history of migraine headache
   b. Susan, with Down syndrome
   c. Allison, with ulcerative colitis
   d. Francine, with peptic ulcer disease

4. Tom Jenkins, age 35, is hospitalized for diarrhea and dehydration. He has been prescribed diphenoxylate (Lomotil). After reviewing Tom's medical history, you note he has been taking Nardil, a monamine oxidase inhibitor. You should monitor Tom for
   a. tachycardia.
   b. hypertension.
   c. fever.
   d. blood dyscrasias.

5. Carey Leonard has frequent constipation and takes magnesium hydroxide (Milk of Magnesia). Additionally, she takes theophylline (Theo-Dur), beclomethasone (Beclovent), and phenytoin (Dilantin). Carey should be monitored for
   a. exacerbation of asthma symptoms.
   b. theophylline toxicity.
   c. seizure activity.
   d. diarrhea.

6. Which of the following patients should refrain from using psyllium, a bulk-forming laxative, for constipation?
   a. Julie, with a mental heath disorder
   b. Adam, with asthma
   c. Tom, with benign prostatic hypertrophy
   d. Dixie, with congestive heart failure

7. Beatrice Lovett, age 45, is taking psyllium (Metamucil) for constipation. Patient teaching should include instructions to
   a. increase intake of water to avoid further constipation.
   b. decrease intake of water to avoid further constipation.
   c. increase intake of dairy products.
   d. decrease intake of dairy products.

8. Lucy Rose, age 17, has irritable bowel syndrome (IBS). Which of the following drugs would you anticipate administering to Lucy?
   a. simethicone (Mylicon)
   b. magnesium hydroxide (Milk of Magnesia)
   c. dicyclomine (Bentyl)
   d. kaolin

NURSING MANAGEMENT: EVERY GOOD NURSE SHOULD . . .

Multiple choice

Circle the option that best answers the question or completes the statement.

1. Which of the following should be included in patient education for simethicone, an antiflatulent?
   a. Chew tablets before swallowing.
   b. Administer before meals or 2 hours after meals.
   c. Increase dietary intake of cabbage, cucumbers, and onions.
   d. Decreased belching is expected.

2. Sue Kim, 10 years old, is being treated with diphenoxylate HCl with atropine sulfate for severe diarrhea. At the beginning of your shift, you, the nurse, perform a physical assessment of Sue. You note the following findings: temperature 100°F orally, pulse 110, R 24. Suprapubic distention noted, with tenderness to palpation. No urine output for 8 hours recorded. Stools have decreased in frequency but are still loose. The patient is due for another dose of diphenoxylate HCl with atropine sulfate. How should you act based on these findings?

   a. Administer another dose of diphenoxylate HCl with atropine sulfate.

   b. Administer another dose of diphenoxylate HCl with atropine sulfate, acetaminophen (Tylenol), and extra fluids.

   c. Hold the next dose of diphenoxylate HCl with atropine sulfate and place an indwelling catheter in the patient to drain her bladder.

   d. Hold the next dose of diphenoxylate HCl with atropine sulfate and contact the doctor.

3. Greg Upton has chronic renal failure. He complains of being extremely constipated. You, the nurse, believe that more than one dose of a laxative may be necessary to correct his constipation. Which of the following laxatives would **not** be appropriate for Greg?

   a. senna (Senokot)

   b. lactulose (Cephulac)

   c. magnesium sulfate (Milk of Magnesia)

   d. bisacodyl (Dulcolax)

4. Ada Wells, 75 years old, complains of frequent constipation. She asks if she should take magnesium sulfate every day to prevent constipation. The best nursing response would be

   a. "Yes, this will help you be regular in bowel patterns."

   b. "Yes, the extra magnesium will correct any dietary deficiencies."

   c. "No, magnesium sulfate is not intended for long-term use."

   d. "No, magnesium sulfate has only antacid effects."

5. Martin Taylor has been ordered polyethylene glycol-electrolyte solution, also known as PEG-ES (GoLYTELY), before an x-ray of the lower GI tract. Teaching related to this drug therapy should include that PEG-ES will

   a. prevent constipation after the x-ray.

   b. induce diarrhea within 4 hours.

   c. stop diarrhea within 4 hours.

   d. reduce blood ammonia levels.

CASE STUDY

Ray Holmes is 65 years old. He was admitted to the hospital for a bleeding gastric ulcer. While he was hospitalized, he had a myocardial infarction. He is on bed rest, is on a low-fat, bland diet, and has medication orders for docusate (Colace) daily.

What patient-related variables are relevant to the order for docusate? Why?

CRITICAL THINKING CHALLENGE

Why are patients who have had myocardial infarctions ordered docusate routinely?

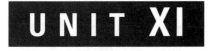

UNIT XI

Endocrine System Drugs

CHAPTER 39

Drugs Affecting Pituitary, Thyroid, and Parathyroid, and Hypothalamic Function

TOP TEN THINGS TO KNOW ABOUT DRUGS AFFECTING PITUITARY, THYROID, AND PARATHYROID, AND HYPOTHALAMIC FUNCTION

1. Drugs given to treat disorders of the pituitary, thyroid, or parathyroid glands either supply additional hormone because the gland does not produce enough, or prevent the release of additional hormone because the gland produces too much.

2. Somatropin, a synthetic human growth hormone (rGH), is used as treatment in hypopituitarism. It is used to treat children with growth failure due to a lack of adequate endogenous growth hormone; it is also used in adults with somatropin deficiency syndrome (SDS) and HIV catabolism.

3. Desmopressin is a synthetic form of the anti diuretic hormone (ADH), also known as vasopressin. It is given to treat central, or neurogenic, diabetes insipidus (a problem of excessive water loss due to partial or total deficiency in the production or secretion of ADH). The antidiuretic effect of desmopressin is longer acting than that from natural ADH. This synthetic form of the hormone has very little pressor effects (unlike naturally occurring ADH).

4. Patients taking desmopressin, especially young children and older adults, are at risk of water intoxication if they take excessive oral fluids. Caution patients only to drink enough to quench their thirst.

5. Levothyroxine, a synthetic salt of T_4, is used as replacement in hypothyroidism. It produces increased metabolic effects such as elevating pulse and blood pressure. Treatment is usually lifelong.

6. Adverse effects of levothyroxine (Synthroid) are usually signs of hyperthyroidism (hypertension, tachycardia, hyperreflexia, anxiety, increased sweating). If signs of hypothyroidism occur, the dose is insufficient and should be increased.

7. Propylthiouracil (PTU) blocks the formation of thyroid hormone and the conversion to the more potent hormone in peripheral tissue; it is used to treat hyperthyroidism. It must be taken around the clock. Excess propylthiouracil will cause signs of hypothyroidism; not enough will result in continued hyperthyroidism. Although it may cause fetal hypothyroidism and cretinism, it can be used in pregnancy if absolutely necessary.

8. Low doses of iodine are needed for the formation of thyroid hormone. High doses inhibit thyroid function. Strong iodide solutions are used for presurgical suppression of the thyroid or in acute thyrotoxicosis. Radioactive iodine is used to diagnose an overactive thyroid and to destroy thyroid tissue in severe Graves' disease.

9. Calcitonin, salmon is a synthesized form of naturally occurring calcitonin. It has a role in the regulation of calcium and bone metabolism. It increases the renal loss of phosphate, calcium, and sodium. It is used to prevent bone resorption in Paget's disease and postmenopausal osteoporosis, and in the early treatment of hypercalcemic emergencies (SC or IM only). Due to potential systemic allergic reaction, skin testing is often done before starting therapy.

10. Calcitriol is a fat-soluble vitamin that increases gastrointestinal (GI) absorption of calcium and increases serum calcium. It is used in the management of hypocalcemia, especially in patients on chronic renal dialysis. Common adverse effects are GI and central nervous system (CNS) in nature. If serum calcium levels increase too much, cardiac arrhythmias may occur. Monitor serum calcium levels.

KEY TERMS

Matching Exercise

Match the following key terms with their definitions:

1. _____ acromegaly

2. _____ bone resorption

3. _____ cretinism

4. _____ diabetes insipidus

5. _____ gigantism

6. _____ Graves' disease

7. _____ hyperthyroidism

8. _____ hypopituitarism

9. _____ hypothyroidism

10. _____ myxedema coma

11. _____ osmolarity

12. _____ Paget disease

13. _____ thyrotoxicosis

14. _____ thyrotoxic crisis

15. _____ SIADH

a. Concentration of osmotically active particles in solution

b. Impaired renal conservation of water

c. Inappropriate antidiuretic hormone secretion

d. Diminution or cessation of anterior pituitary function

e. Abnormality of the thyroid gland in which secretion of thyroid hormone is usually increased.

f. Diminished production of thyroid hormone, leading to clinical manifestations of thyroid insufficiency

g. Characterized by retardation of both physical and mental development

h. Disorder marked by progressive enlargement of peripheral parts of the body

i. Life-threatening condition manifested by coma, hypothermia, bradycardia, hypoglycemia, and hypoventilation

j. Condition of abnormal size or overgrowth of the entire body or of any of its parts

k. Generalized skeletal disease, frequently familial, in which bone resorption and formation are both increased, leading to thickening and softening of bones

l. Another term for hyperthyroidism

m. Type of hyperthyroidism thought to be an autoimmune disorder

n. Loss or destruction of bone tissue

o. Another term for thyroid storm

PHYSIOLOGY AND PATHOPHYSIOLOGY: THE BODY HUMAN

Essay

1. What is the master gland of the body?

2. What are the regulatory functions of the hypothalamus?

3. What are the releasing factors secreted by the hypothalamus?

4. What are the hormones released by the anterior pituitary?

5. What are the hormones released by the posterior pituitary?

6. Optimal production of thyroid hormones depends on what element in the body?

7. Why is thyroxine (T_4) thought to be the more important thyroid hormone?

8. What body processes are influenced by the thyroid hormones?

9. What hormone has the most influence of serum calcium in the body?

10. What body processes are influenced by calcium?

CORE DRUG KNOWLEDGE: JUST THE FACTS

Multiple choice

Circle the option that best answers the question or completes the statement.

1. Somatropin (Humatrope) is used in the management of
   a. Graves disease.
   b. hypopituitarism.
   c. gigantism.
   d. acromegaly.

2. Adverse effects associated with the use of somatropin (Humatrope) as an antiaging drug include
   a. renal failure.
   b. hepatic failure.
   c. cancer.
   d. pancreatitis.

3. Because of its potential adverse effects, children receiving somatropin (Humatrope) should have which of the following done before the start of therapy?
   a. electrocardiogram (ECG)
   b. pulmonary function tests
   c. urinalysis (UA)
   d. hip x-rays

4. Patients receiving somatropin should be monitored for which of the following disorders?
   a. hypertension
   b. hyperthyroidism
   c. hypothyroidism
   d. hypotension

5. Which of the following medications would be contraindicated in the management of growth hormone hypersecretion?
   a. somatropin (Humatrope)
   b. octreotide acetate (Sandostatin)
   c. bromocriptine mesylate (Parlodel)
   d. all of the above

6. Desmopressin (DDAVP) is used in the management of
   a. diabetes insipidus.
   b. diabetes mellitus.
   c. hyperthyroidism.
   d. hypothyroidism.

7. Desmopressin (DDAVP) can be administered by
   a. oral tablets.
   b. intranasal inhalation.
   c. IV or SC.
   d. all of the above.

8. Which of the following drugs is used in the management of hypothyroidism?
   a. somatropin (Humatrope)
   b. levothyroxine (Synthroid)
   c. propylthiouracil (PTU)
   d. calcitriol (Rocaltrol)

9. Maximal effect of levothyroxine (Synthroid) occurs in
   a. 6 to 7 weeks.
   b. 24 to 48 hours.
   c. 6 to 8 hours.
   d. 1 to 3 weeks.

10. Which of the following adverse effects is associated with levothyroxine (Synthroid) therapy?
    a. tachycardia
    b. bradycardia
    c. hypotension
    d. constipation

11. During pregnancy, the dose of levothyroxine (Synthroid) may need to be
    a. discontinued.
    b. increased.
    c. decreased.
    d. kept the same.

12. Which of the following drugs is used in the management of hyperthyroidism?
    a. somatropin (Humatrope)
    b. levothyroxine (Synthroid)
    c. propylthiouracil (PTU)
    d. calcitriol (Rocaltrol)

13. The onset of action of propylthiouracil (PTU) is
    a. 1 to 2 hours.
    b. 24 hours.
    c. 3 to 6 minutes.
    d. 10 to 21 days.

14. Common adverse effects of propylthiouracil (PTU) include
    a. headache.
    b. epigastric distress.
    c. diarrhea.
    d. rash.

15. In addition to propylthiouracil (PTU), what other drugs may be useful in the management of hyperthyroidism?
    a. levothyroxine (Synthroid)
    b. ^{131}I
    c. calcitriol (Rocaltrol)
    d. liothyronine (Cytomel)

16. ^{131}I is a pregnancy category _____ drug.
    a. A
    b. B
    c. D
    d. X

17. Calcitonin, salmon (Calcimar) is used in the management of
    a. Paget disease
    b. Graves disease
    c. hyperparathyroidism.
    d. a and c.

18. Which of the following statements concerning potential adverse effects to calcitonin, salmon (Calcimar) therapy is accurate?
    a. There are few potential adverse effects, and they are minor.
    b. There are few potential adverse effects, but they are serious.
    c. There are many potential adverse effects, but they are minor.
    d. There are many potential adverse effects, and they are serious.

19. Calcitriol (Rocaltrol) is used in the management of
    a. hypercalcemia.
    b. hypocalcemia.
    c. hyperthyroidism.
    d. hypothyroidism.

20. Calcitriol (Rocaltrol) is
    a. vitamin A.
    b. vitamin B.
    c. vitamin E.
    d. vitamin D.

CORE PATIENT VARIABLES: PATIENTS, PLEASE

Multiple choice

Circle the option that best answers the question or completes the statement.

1. Jennifer Gaines, age 7, is taking somatropin for growth deficiency. Throughout therapy, Jennifer should be monitored for
   a. cancer.
   b. hyperthyroidism.
   c. CNS depression.
   d. hypothyroidism.

2. Because of Jennifer's age, patient instructions are given to her mother. Which of the following statements is INAPPROPRIATE?
   a. "Be sure to wash your hands thoroughly before giving the injection."
   b. "Jennifer may develop a limp, but that is expected so don't worry about it."
   c. "If Jennifer complains of muscle discomfort, you may give her acetaminophen."
   d. "Call us immediately if you notice Jennifer drinking a lot of fluids and going to the bathroom more frequently."

3. Jackie Henry, age 3, is receiving somatropin (Humatrope) therapy. Which of the following lab values should be done periodically?
   a. CBC and liver function
   b. glucose and thyroid function
   c. hepatic and kidney function
   d. CBC and glucose

4. Kenny Tyler is being treated for diabetes insipidus with desmopressin (DDAVP). As you enter Mr. Tyler's room, you note that he is confused, drowsy, listless, and complains of a headache. Which of the following conditions would you suspect is the problem?
   a. water intoxication
   b. dehydration
   c. desmopressin allergy
   d. CHF

5. Which of the following patients has the highest risk for adverse effects from desmopressin (DDAVP) therapy?

   a. Kenneth, with hepatitis

   b. Julie, with asthma

   c. Carmen, with cardiovascular disease

   d. Henry, with bipolar disease

6. Carey Weeks, age 45, takes desmopressin (DDAVP). Which of the following laboratory tests should be done to evaluate the effectiveness of therapy?

   a. BUN and creatinine

   b. CBC

   c. chest x-ray

   d. Urine specific gravity

7. Barbara Belyea, age 24, has been diagnosed with hypothyroidism and is prescribed levothyroxine (Synthroid). Which of the following situations would contraindicate the use of this drug?

   a. pregnancy

   b. asthma

   c. osteoporosis

   d. breast-feeding

8. Julia Yearling, age 55, takes levothyroxine (Synthroid) for hypothyroidism and warfarin (Coumadin) for deep vein thrombosis prophylaxis. What is the possible interaction between these drugs?

   a. There is no interaction between these drugs.

   b. There is an increased risk for bleeding.

   c. There is a increased risk for cardiovascular effects from levothyroxine.

   d. The warfarin dose may need to be increased to anticoagulate the blood.

9. Samantha Yates, age 45, has primary hypothyroidism and is taking levothyroxine (Synthroid). Samantha asks, "Just how long do I need to take this medication?" You would respond

   a. "Generally, people with hypothyroidism need to take their medication for the rest of their life."

   b. "You should really ask the nurse practitioner that question."

   c. "Just until your thyroid function tests are in the normal range again."

   d. "Usually, they try to taper you off the drug after a year."

10. Which of the following instructions should be given to Sara who is beginning propylthiouracil (PTU) therapy?

    a. "Take small frequent meals to minimize GI distress."

    b. "Take the entire day's dose at breakfast."

    c. "Take the drug on an empty stomach."

    d. "Be sure to have your blood checked every couple of years."

11. Jillian Lewis, age 45, has just been diagnosed with hyperthyroidism and prescribed propylthiouracil (PTU). As you assess her health status, you note that Mrs. Lewis is also receiving warfarin (Coumadin). With this combination you should monitor for

    a. a decreased anticoagulation effect.

    b. an increased anticoagulation effect.

    c. There is no interaction between these drugs.

12. Kathy Wilson has hyperthyroidism and takes propylthiouracil (PTU). She called today and states, "I think I'm pregnant—at least my home pregnancy kit is positive." What instructions should you give Mrs. Wilson?

    a. "Stop the drug immediately."

    b. "You really will need to increase your dose now that you are pregnant."

    c. "You may need to stop or decrease your dose. Don't do anything until you see the nurse practitioner."

    d. "You can continue your medication. There is no problem with pregnancy and taking this drug."

13. John Zeller has been taking propylthiouracil (PTU) for the past year. What laboratory tests should be done?

    a. thyroid and parathyroid function tests

    b. CBC, thyroid function

    c. renal and parathyroid function tests

    d. ECG, thyroid and hepatic function tests

14. Judy Falk has drug-induced hypercalcemia. Which of the following labs should be done before initiating calcitonin, salmon (Calcimar)? Calcium and

    a. CBC

    b. renal function tests

    c. hormone status

    d. thyroid function tests

15. Your patient has Paget disease and takes intranasal calcitonin, salmon (Calcimar). Patient education should include instructions to
    a. maintain your intake of calcium and vitamin D every day.
    b. increase your intake of phosphorus and vitamin A every day.
    c. decrease your intake of calcium and vitamin D every day.
    d. decrease your intake of phosphorus and vitamin A every day.

16. Olive Turkel has post menopausal osteoporosis and is prescribed etidronate. Which of the following instructions to Mrs. Turkel would be APPROPRIATE?
    a. "Take your medication at bedtime."
    b. "Take your medication first thing in the morning and remain upright for 30 minutes before ingesting food or fluids."
    c. "Decrease your ingestion of calcium and vitamin D."
    d. "Call immediately if you have severe diarrhea or dark-colored urine."

17. Sharon Saunders, age 52, had a hysterectomy at age 30. During her recent clinic visit, she was diagnosed with osteoporosis. Which of the following drugs would you anticipate for Mrs. Pitts?
    a. alendronate (Fosamax)
    b. bromocriptine (Parlodel)
    c. calcitriol (Rocaltrol)
    d. levothyroxine (Synthroid)

18. Benny Fuer, a dialysis patient, takes calcitriol (Rocaltrol). Patient teaching for Mr. Fuer should include to refrain from taking antacids with a/an
    a. aluminum base.
    b. calcium base.
    c. magnesium base.
    d. sodium bicarbonate base.

NURSING MANAGEMENT: EVERY GOOD NURSE SHOULD . . .

Multiple choice

Circle the option that best answers the question or completes the statement.

1. Jenny Willoughby, 8 years old, has been started on somatropin, growth hormone, because of a deficiency of intrinsic growth factor. Patient teaching necessary for Jenny and her family includes
   a. how to administer an SC injection.
   b. proper storage is in a sunny location.
   c. adverse effects such as limping are not serious problems.
   d. all of the above.
   e. none of the above.

2. Lisa Wiggins, 55 years old, had a thyroidectomy yesterday due to hyperthyroidism. She is started on levothyroxine (Synthroid) as thyroid hormone replacement. The nurse should monitor Ms. Wiggins for
   a. bradycardia.
   b. hypertension.
   c. intolerance to heat or cold.
   d. all of the above.
   e. none of the above.

3. John Tillman is receiving propylthiouracil (PTU) for hyperthyroidism. He calls the advice nurse help line for his HMO and reports that he is having a great deal of nausea and abdominal pain. The nurse should advise him to
   a. take the propylthiouracil (PTU) on an empty stomach.
   b. eat small, frequent meals.
   c. take all propylthiouracil doses in the evening after dinner.
   d. stop taking the propylthiouracil at once.

4. Roberto Nunez has chronic renal failure and receives dialysis. He is receiving calcitriol, an antihypocalcemic drug. Lab values relevant to drug therapy for which the nurse should monitor include
   a. potassium.
   b. calcium.
   c. BUN.
   d. SGOT.
   e. all of the above.

5. You, the nurse, are to administer the first dose of calcitonin, salmon, and an antihypercalcemic drug to a patient with acute severe hypercalcemia. The drug is to be given IM. Before giving the first dose, you should

   a. administer calcium.

   b. administer vitamin D.

   c. perform a skin test with calcitonin, salmon.

   d. assess for bone deformities.

CASE STUDY

Hector Gonsalves, 66 years old, has been determined to be hyperthyroid and is to be started on propylthiouracil (PTU), an antithyroid drug before having a thyroidectomy. His medical history also shows that he has a history of a mitral valve replacement 5 years ago and takes 2.5 mg of warfarin for this daily.
Mr. Gonsalves wants to know why he cannot just have the surgery because he hates to take medicine. What teaching should you give him?

CRITICAL THINKING CHALLENGE

Mr. Gonsalves returns in 4 weeks to have his T_4 levels checked to determine if he is ready for surgery. At this time, he complains of bleeding gums when he brushes his teeth, and bruising easily.

1. What could be a possible cause of these problems?

2. What lab value should be evaluated?

CHAPTER 40

Drugs Affecting Hormone Levels: Corticosteroids and Their Antagonists

TOP TEN THINGS TO KNOW ABOUT CORTICOSTEROIDS AND THEIR ANTAGONISTS

1. The two types of corticosteroids are glucocorticoids and mineralocorticoids. Mineralocorticoids influence the regulation of sodium, potassium, and water balance. Glucocorticoids, released during the stress response, have a role in the inflammatory response, the immune response, and protein, fat, and carbohydrate metabolism.

2. Prednisone (Deltasone), a glucocorticoid, is used as replacement therapy in adrenal insufficiency, anti-inflammatory therapy for various inflammatory diseases and conditions, and as immunosuppressant therapy. The effects that prednisone has on the body account for its therapeutic uses but also its adverse effects.

3. Short-term treatment with prednisone may produce mild central nervous system (CNS) and gastrointestinal (GI) complaints, increased susceptibility to infections, poor wound healing, hyperglycemia, and suppression of pituitary adrenocorticotropic hormone (ACTH) release. Long-term treatment with prednisone may cause cushingoid characteristics, osteoporosis, fluid retention, electrolyte imbalance, glucose intolerance, hyperglycemia, obesity, hirsutism, and protein wasting, among other things.

4. Systemic adverse effects do not usually occur with inhaled or topical glucocorticoids.

5. Sudden withdrawal of prednisone, even if used only a short time, may bring about acute adrenal insufficiency, which may be fatal. Always withdraw glucocorticoids, such as prednisone, slowly by tapering down the dose over several days or weeks.

6. Dosage of prednisone, and other glucocorticoids, needs to be increased in times of stress to prevent drug-induced adrenal insufficiency.

7. Fludrocortisone has both mineralocorticoid and glucocorticoid effects but is used only for its mineralocorticoid activity as a replacement therapy in adrenocortical deficiency (Addison's disease). In small doses, the mineralocorticoid effects (urinary excretion of potassium, sodium retention, and an increase in blood pressure) predominate; larger doses result in predominance of glucocorticoid effects.

8. Adverse effects of fludrocortisone usually occur if the dose is too high (edema, hypertension, congestive heart failure (CHF), cardiomegaly, hypokalemic alkalosis). Rapid withdrawal will also precipitate adrenal crisis. Dosage needs to be increased in times of stress.

9. Aminoglutethimide (Cytadren) is used to treat hypercortisolism (Cushing's syndrome). It does not affect the underlying pathology and is used for less than 3 months. Orthostatic and persistent hypotension may occur. Monitor blood pressure carefully.

10. Patients receiving corticosteroids or their antagonists should carry a Medic-Alert card or wear a bracelet to alert medical personnel of special needs related to drug therapy in case of emergency.

KEY TERMS

Fill in the blanks

Read each statement carefully and, using the chapter's key terms, write your answer in the space provided.

1. Water and electrolyte balance of the body is mediated by _____ hormones.

2. Chronic adrenocortical insufficiency is also known as _____.

3. _____ is the formation of glucose from noncarbohydrates, such as protein or fat.

4. A congenital abnormality, _____, results in excess ACTH.

5. A general term encompassing both glucocorticoid and mineralocorticoid hormones is _____.

6. A disorder caused by excessive secretion of aldosterone is called _____.

7. The _____ hormones are potent anti-inflammatory agents.

8. Biologic variations or rhythms with a cycle are called _____.

9. _____ is a disorder resulting from increased adrenocortical secretion of cortisol.

PHYSIOLOGY AND PATHOPHYSIOLOGY: THE BODY HUMAN

Essay

1. What are the catecholamines secreted by the adrenal medulla?

2. What hormones are secreted by the adrenal cortex?

3. What is the major effect of aldosterone on the body?

4. List the factors that influence the regulation of ACTH.

5. What is the long-term effect of exogenous glucocorticoid therapy?

6. What is the major mineralocorticoid produced by the adrenal gland?

7. What are the major glucocorticoids produced by the adrenal gland?

CORE DRUG KNOWLEDGE: JUST THE FACTS

Multiple choice

Circle the option that best answers the question or completes the statement.

1. Which of the following steroids is the MOST potent?
   a. triamcinolone (Aristocort)
   b. prednisone (Deltasone)
   c. fludrocortisone (Florinef)
   d. hydrocortisone (Cortef)

2. Which of the following is NOT a primary use of prednisone (Deltasone)?
   a. replacement therapy for adrenal insufficiency
   b. maintainence of water and electrolyte balance
   c. anti-inflammatory therapy
   d. immunosuppressant effects

3. What is the most dangerous complication of prednisone (Deltasone) therapy?
   a. GI ulceration
   b. hyperglycemia
   c. immune system compromise
   d. vertigo

4. Which of the following body systems is UNAFFECTED by prednisone (Deltasone)?
   a. respiratory
   b. gastrointestinal
   c. integumentary
   d. every system of the body

5. To minimize GI ulceration, which of the following would be appropriate for the patient taking prednisone (Deltasone)? Take:
   a. only once a week.
   b. with H2 receptor antagonists.
   c. at bedtime only.
   d. with orange or cranberry juice.

6. Which of the following statements regarding drug–drug interaction with prednisone (Deltasone) therapy is correct?

    a. There are only a few drug–drug interactions and they are minor.

    b. There are only a few drug–drug interactions but many are serious.

    c. There are many drug–drug interactions and many are serious.

    d. There are many drug–drug interactions, some are serious and many are life-threatening.

7. Alternate day dosing of prednisone (Deltasone) may decrease

    a. potential drug–drug interactions.

    b. some adverse effects.

    c. sodium loss.

    d. GI distress.

8. Patients taking corticosteroids for a long period of time need to

    a. be tapered from the drug when discontinued.

    b. increase their intake of potassium-rich foods.

    c. take "drug holidays" at least once a week.

    d. take dietary supplements to counteract their weight loss.

9. Which of the following adverse effects is associated with the use of fludrocortisone (Florinef)?

    a. hypotension

    b. dehydration

    c. congestive heart failure (CHF)

    d. sedation

10. Patients on fludrocortisone (Florinef) therapy need to limit their intake of:

    a. potassium

    b. sodium

    c. magnesium

    d. chloride

11. Patients on fludrocortisone (Florinef) therapy need to increase their intake of:

    a. potassium.

    b. sodium.

    c. magnesium.

    d. chloride.

12. Which of the following drugs would be useful in the treatment of hypercortisolism?

    a. fludrocortisone (Florinef)

    b. methylprednisolone (Solu-Medrol)

    c. aminoglutethimide (Cytadren)

    d. spironolactone (Aldactone)

13. During aminoglutethimide (Cytadren) therapy, the nurse should closely monitor

    a. temperature.

    b. blood pressure.

    c. respiratory rate.

    d. pulse.

14. Which of the following baseline lab tests should be completed before initiating aminoglutethimide (Cytadren) therapy?

    a. CBC and arterial blood gas

    b. renal function and glucose tolerance

    c. thyroid function and CBC

    d. hepatic and thyroid function

CORE PATIENT VARIABLES: PATIENTS, PLEASE...

Multiple Choice

Circle the option that best answers the question or completes the statement.

1. Dr. Johe Morris, age 41, had a renal transplant today. She has been prescribed prednisone (Deltasone). Which of the following nursing actions is MOST important for Dr. Morris?

    a. Monitor for constipation.

    b. Take vital signs at least once a day.

    c. Assess for CNS depression.

    d. Monitor for signs of infection.

2. Melissa Young, age 6, has severe asthma. Melissa's mom states "She always feels so much better when she takes prednisone (Deltasone). Why can't she just stay on it?" Which of the following is your best response?

    a. "The cost of prednisone therapy is just too high."

    b. "Long term therapy could result in short stature for Melissa at her young age."

    c. "Melissa would come home crying because her face would be so puffy."

    d. "It would quit working if you gave it for a long time."

3. Noah Tyson, age 50, is on long-term prednisone (Deltasone) therapy. Which of the following diet restrictions should Mr. Tyson follow?

   a. limit carbonated beverages

   b. increase potassium intake

   c. decrease sodium intake

   d. decrease potassium intake

4. Eric Presley uses inhaled beclomethasone (Beclovent) for his asthma. Which of the following instructions should be given to Eric?

   a. "Rinse your mouth thoroughly after using to decrease the possibility of candidiasis."

   b. "Steroids given this way increase your risk of adverse effects. Be sure to call if any occur."

   c. "This inhaler is very powerful. Use it only when you have an asthma attack."

   d. "Use the inhaler without a spacer so you get better results."

5. Beverly Cass, age 66, takes prednisone (Deltasone) for chronic obstructive pulmonary disease (COPD). Mrs. Cass should have frequent follow-up clinic visits to assess for

   a. CHF and headaches.

   b. hyperglycemia and osteoporosis.

   c. weight loss and hypoglycemia.

   d. dermatitis and headaches.

6. Frank Failure, age 46, has adrenal insufficiency and is being placed on a daily dose prednisone (Deltasone). Which of the following instructions is appropriate?

   a. Take all of your medication at bedtime.

   b. Take one pill 6 times a day.

   c. Take 2/3 of your dose before 9 AM and the last third in the late afternoon.

   d. Take all of your medication in the early morning.

7. Susan Crawford takes prednisone (Deltasone) daily for adrenal insufficiency. Ms. Crawford is admitted to the hospital after a serious motor vehicle accident with multiple fractures and blunt head trauma. During her hospitalization Ms. Crawford's prednisone dose may need to

   a. increase.

   b. decrease.

   c. stay the same.

8. William Banks, age 60, is taking fludrocortisone (Florinef). After evaluating his baseline physical finding, you would expect his blood pressure to have

   a. increased.

   b. decreased.

   c. stayed the same.

9. Danuta Zakrzewski takes fludrocortisone (Florinef) for replacement therapy. Mrs. Zakrzewski calls the clinic and states she has occasional headaches and asks what type of analgesia she should take. Which of the following would be best for Mrs. Zakrzewski?

   a. meperidine

   b. aspirin

   c. acetaminophen

   d. any of the above

10. Your patient is taking fludrocortisone (Florinef) and complains of a 25-pound weight gain. You should assess for

    a. sodium intake.

    b. potassium intake.

    c. cigarette smoking.

    d. increased exercise regimen.

11. Florence Litner, age 66, has hypercortisolism and takes aminoglutethimide (Cytadren). Mrs. Litner was in an auto accident and sustained several fractured bones. While hospitalized, Mrs. Litner may need

    a. to increase her dose of aminoglutethimide.

    b. supplementation with a glucocorticoid.

    c. supplementation with a mineralocorticoid.

    d. b and c.

12. Your patient has just been diagnosed with hypercortisolism and is being started on aminoglutethimide (Cytadren). Patient teaching should include which of the following instructions?

    a. Take only 3 meals per day to decrease GI distress.

    b. Assess sedation prior to driving a vehicle.

    c. This drug will not interfere with your attempts to become pregnant.

    d. Take a "drug holiday" at lease once a week.

NURSING MANAGEMENT: EVERY GOOD NURSE SHOULD . . .

Multiple Choice

Circle the option that best answers the question or completes the statement.

1. Roy Gilger is receiving oral prednisone after a kidney transplant. To minimize adverse effects of the prednisone, the nurse should
   a. administer the drug on an empty stomach.
   b. administer the drug with milk or food.
   c. decrease the dose in times of physical stress.
   d. decrease the dose if proton pump inhibitors are prescribed.

2. Stella Rogers receives prednisone because of adrenal insufficiency. She is take one dose every day. To most closely mimic normal physiologic action of glucocorticoids, the nurse should instruct Ms. Rogers to take the drug
   a. early in the morning.
   b. late in the evening.
   c. in the middle of the day.
   d. at anytime of day.

3. Tom Fowler receives fludrocortisone (Florinef), a mineralocorticoid, for his Addison disease. The nurse would evaluate the drug therapy as being effective if
   a. hypertension develops.
   b. hypokalemia occurs.
   c. weight increases.
   d. all of the above
   e. none of the above

4. Linda Tyler is to begin therapy with fludrocortisone (Florinef) for Addison disease. Teaching about fludrocortisone drug therapy should include which of the following?
   a. Decrease potassium intake.
   b. Increase sodium intake.
   c. Stop drug therapy during periods of illness.
   d. Wear or carry a Medics Alert bracelet or card.

5. Oscar Haynes is to begin aminoglutethimide (Cytadren) therapy for Cushing syndrome. The nurse should monitor which of the following while Mr. Haynes receives aminoglutethimide?
   a. thyroid function
   b. blood pressure
   c. adrenal insufficiency
   d. all of the above
   e. none of the above

CASE STUDY

Beula Sommers is 65 years old and has chronic asthma. She receives a limited income from her social security pension. She is given a prescription to start beclomethasone, an inhaled glucocorticoid. The drug is administered through a metered-dose inhaler. She is to take one puff twice a day.

1) Why was a glucocorticoid ordered for Ms. Sommers?

2) What teaching is indicated for the beclomethasone therapy? (Need help? See Chapter 36, Drugs Affecting the Lower Respiratory System)

CRITICAL THINKING CHALLENGE

Beula Sommers receives inhaled beclomethasone for 2 years and then is started on oral prednisone. She has been taking the oral prednisone for 1 year when she is brought to the emergency room with severe hypotension. Her lab work shows her sodium levels to be low and her potassium levels to be elevated. She appears somewhat dehydrated, and her temperature is 100 degrees although her white count is not elevated.

1) What is your assessment of these findings?

2) What explanations might account for the presence of these findings?

CHAPTER 41

Drugs Affecting Blood Glucose Levels

TOP TEN THINGS TO KNOW ABOUT DRUGS AFFECTING BLOOD GLUCOSE LEVELS

1. All insulins manage hyperglycemia by promoting cellular glucose uptake and metabolism. Insulins vary by peak, onset, and duration of action. The standard source of insulins is now recombinant DNA, or human. Pork sources are still available but are used only if specifically ordered. Insulins are used in type 1 diabetes and sometimes in type 2 diabetes.

2. Excessive insulin produces hypoglycemia. Insufficient insulin produces hyperglycemia.

3. Regular insulin is rapid acting and short lasting. It may be used alone or in combinations with longer-acting insulins such as NPH.

4. All insulins are given subcutaneously. Only regular insulin may also be given intravenously.

5. Patient teaching about insulin should include how to administer accurately, diet modifications, exercise, testing for blood glucose, storage of insulin, and disposal of used needles and syringes.

6. Glyburide is an oral, sulfonylureas hypoglycemic agent. It stimulates insulin release and reduces glucagon levels. It is used in type 2 diabetes. It should not be used in a patient allergic to sulfa drugs. Gastrointestinal upset is a common adverse effect.

7. Metformin is an oral biguanide hypoglycemic agent used in type 2 diabetes. It suppresses hepatic glucose production, enhances insulin sensitivity in the muscle, and promotes glucose uptake. It requires some pancreatic insulin to work. Hypoglycemia may occur if used concurrently with sulfonylureas hypoglycemic agents, such as glyburide.

8. Acarbose is an oral alpha-glucosidase inhibitor hypoglycemic agent used in type 2 diabetes. It delays the digestion of carbohydrates, resulting in a smaller postprandial rise of blood glucose. Use oral glucose tablets if hypoglycemia occurs because cane sugar found in candy and orange juice will not be absorbed due to the drug.

9. Rosiglitazone is a thiazolidinedione oral hypoglycemic agent used in type 2 diabetes where insulin use is needed but glucose control has not been achieved. It lowers the blood glucose levels by improving the cellular response to insulin (makes insulin have more effect on cell). It can also be used in type 1 in addition to insulin. Monitor liver enzyme function before therapy and closely throughout the first year of therapy because hepatotoxicity is possible.

10. Glucagon, a naturally occurring substance, is given as a drug therapy to restore consciousness in extreme hypoglycemia. It stimulates glycogenolysis in the peripheral tissues.

KEY TERMS

Crossword puzzle

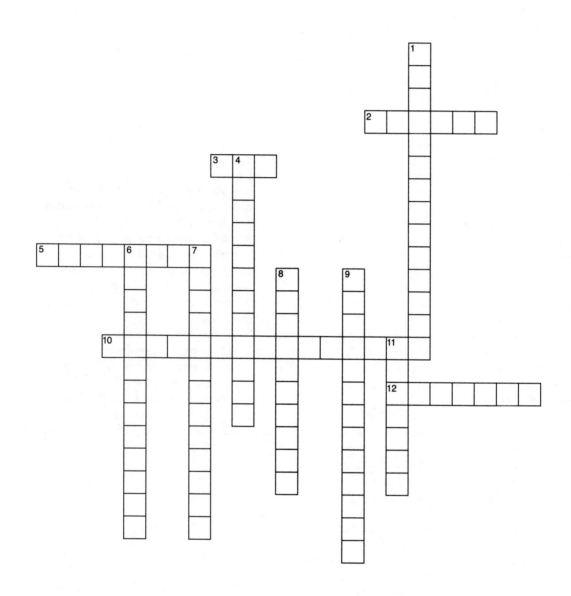

Across

2. Type of acidosis caused by accumulation of lactic acid due to tissue hypoxia, drug reaction, or unknown etiology
3. Abbreviation for hyperosmolar hyperglycemic state
5. Form of diabetes characterized by an alteration in carbohydrate utilization
10. Formation of glucose from non-carbohydrates, such as proteins or fats
12. Rebound phenomenon of reactive hyperglycemia

Down

1. Hydrolysis of glycogen to glucose
4. Deficit of glucose in the bloodstream
6. State of absolute insulin deficiency
7. Class of oral hypoglycemic agents
8. Islets of _____
9. Excess of glucose in the bloodstream
11. Hormone that promotes glucose utilization, protein synthesis, and the formation and storage of neutral lipids

PHYSIOLOGY AND PATHOPHYSIOLOGY: THE BODY HUMAN

Essay

1. Which two hormones have the most influence on the regulation of blood glucose?

2. Identify the cells in the islets of Langerhans and the hormones they produce.

3. What are the functions of insulin?

4. What is the single most important factor influencing the rate of insulin synthesis and release?

5. Other than insulin, what other factors influence blood glucose levels?

CORE DRUG KNOWLEDGE: JUST THE FACTS

Multiple choice

Circle the option that best answers the question or completes the statement.

1. The onset of NPH is approximately
   a. 30 to 60 minutes.
   b. 1 to 1.5 hours.
   c. 1 to 2.5 hours.
   d. 4 to 8 hours.

2. Regular insulin is effective for approximately
   a. 3 to 4 hours.
   b. 8 to 12 hours.
   c. 24 hours.
   d. more than 36 hours.

3. The peak effect of long-acting insulin occurs approximately _____ after administration.
   a. 10 to 30 hours
   b. 7 to 15 hours
   c. 4 to 12 hours
   d. 2 to 4 hours

4. Which of the following types of insulin can be given intravenously?
   a. regular
   b. intermediate acting
   c. long acting
   d. any of the above

5. To decrease the potential for lipodystrophy, the patient should
   a. monitor glucose levels.
   b. dip urine for ketones daily.
   c. rotate injection sites.
   d. trim toenails evenly.

6. Ingestion of alcohol with insulin therapy may result in
   a. hyperglycemia.
   b. hypoglycemia.
   c. both a and b.
   d. neither a or b.

7. Which of the following insulin preparations is used in the insulin pump delivery system?
   a. NPH
   b. Lente
   c. Lispro
   d. Ultralente

8. Maximal effects of glyburide (DiaBeta) occur within
   a. 40 to 60 minutes.
   b. 10 to 25 minutes.
   c. 2 hours
   d. 3 to 4 hours.

9. Sulfonylurea drugs are contraindicated for use in patients with an allergy to
   a. insulin.
   b. sulfonamides.
   c. aminoglycosides.
   d. penicillin.

10. Which of the following drugs should be used for type 2 diabetes during pregnancy?
    a. glyburide (DiaBeta)
    b. glucagon
    c. insulin
    d. rosiglitazone (Avandia)

11. Which of the following statements is correct concerning repaglinide (Prandin)?
    a. It is unsuitable for use with elderly patients.
    b. It is contraindicated for patients with renal insufficiency.
    c. It has an extremely long half-life and duration of action.
    d. It can be omitted when the patient skips a meal.

12. The effects of metformin (Glucophage) include
    a. suppression of hepatic glucose production.
    b. lowers triglyceride levels.
    c. enhances insulin sensitivity.
    d. all of the above.

13. Metformin (Glucophage) should be administered
    a. with meals.
    b. 1 hour before meals.
    c. 2 hours after meals.
    d. at bedtime.

14. Which of the following adverse effects is SPECIFIC to metformin (Glucophage) therapy?
    a. hypoglycemia
    b. GI distress
    c. lactic acidosis
    d. diarrhea

15. Acarbose (Precose) works by
    a. sensitizing insulin receptors.
    b. decreasing carbohydrate absorption from the small intestine.
    c. increasing insulin secretion from the pancreas.
    d. decreasing hepatic production of glucose.

16. Acarbose is contraindicated for use in patients with
    a. diverticulitis.
    b. hepatic insufficiency.
    c. anemia.
    d. chronic obstructive pulmonary disease (COPD).

17. Thiazolidinedione antiglycemics such as rosiglitazone (Avandia) work by
    a. enhancing insulin production.
    b. sensitizing insulin receptors.
    c. decreasing hepatic production of glucose.
    d. inhibiting carbohydrate absorption from the small intestine.

18. Rosiglitazone (Avandia) may be given concurrently with
    a. metformin (Glucophage).
    b. glyburide (DiaBeta).
    c. acarbose (Precose).
    d. all of the above.

19. The duration of action of glucagon is approximately
    a. 24 hours.
    b. 5 to 10 minutes.
    c. 1 to 2 hours.
    d. 6 to 12 hours.

Matching

Match the following types of insulin with the correct duration of action.

1. _____ isophane (NPH)
2. _____ regular (Humulin R)
3. _____ lispro (Humalog)
4. _____ insulin glargine (Lantus)
5. _____ insulin zinc (Lente)
6. _____ regular (Iletin II)
7. _____ zinc suspension (Ultralente)
8. _____ insulin aspart (NovoLog)
9. _____ regular (Novolin R)
a. Ultra-fast acting
b. Fast acting
c. Intermediate acting
d. Long acting

Matching

Match the following oral agents with their appropriate class

1. _____ metformin (Glucophage)
2. _____ rosiglitazone (Avandia)
3. _____ nateglinide (Starlix)
4. _____ glipizide (Glucotrol)
5. _____ tolbutamide (Orinase)
6. _____ pioglitazone (Actos)
7. _____ glyburide (DiaBeta)
8. _____ repaglinide (Prandin)
9. _____ acarbose (Precose)
10. _____ miglitol (Glyset)
a. Sulfonylureas
b. Biguanides
c. Alpha-glucosidase inhibitors
d. Thiazolidinediones
e. Meglitinides

CORE PATIENT VARIABLES: PATIENTS, PLEASE

Multiple choice

Circle the option that best answers the question or completes the statement.

1. James Lewis, age 38, has type 1 diabetes and takes regular insulin. He is hospitalized for pneumonia. As you enter Mr. Lewis' room, you note that he is trembling and tachycardic. He complains of a headache and of feeling nervous. You suspect that Mr. Lewis is experiencing

   a. hyperglycemia.

   b. hypoglycemia.

   c. hyperosmolar hypergylcemic states.

   d. none of the above.

2. Harry Turner has type 1 diabetes. He is switching his regimen to include lispro (Humalog) insulin. What instructions should be given to Mr. Turner regarding the administration of this medication? Administer the medication

   a. 1 hour before meals.

   b. 1 hour after meals.

   c. 10 to 15 minutes before a meal.

   d. only at bedtime.

3. Diane Pestolesi, age 22, takes NPH insulin twice a day. NPH was administered to Mrs. Pestolesi at 0730. At what time is Mrs. Pestolesi MOST likely to experience a hypoglycemic episode?

   a. 0830 to 0900

   b. 0930 to 1130

   c. 1130 to 1930

   d. 1030 to 1200

4. Tamara Smith has just been diagnosed with type 1 diabetes. She is prescribed a combination of regular and intermediate-acting insulin. When preparing this combination, Mrs. Smith should be taught to draw up which medication first?

   a. regular insulin

   b. intermediate-acting insulin

   c. it does not matter

5. Ken Harris, age 54, is admitted to the hospital after a fall down his stairs. Mr. Harris also has type 2 diabetes and COPD. He takes glyburide QD and albuterol (Proventil) prn. Mr. Harris also has a history of alcoholism and has been clean and sober for 5 years. He admits to "falling off the wagon" when he fell down the stairs. Mr. Harris rings the call light and tells you he has chest pain, shortness of breath, blurred vision and feels faint. You suspect

   a. hypoglycemia.

   b. hyperglycemia.

   c. disulfiramlike reaction.

   d. hyperosmolar hypergylcemic states.

6. Janice Hobbs, age 43, has type 2 diabetes. She has taken glyburide (DiaBeta) but experiences hypoglycemia frequently. Which of the following drugs would be helpful in treating Ms. Hobbs' diabetes?

   a. metformin (Glucophage)

   b. regular insulin

   c. repaglinide (Prandin)

   d. tolbutamide (Tolinase)

7. Vicky Torres takes metformin (Glucophage) for her diabetes. Which of the following interventions would be necessary throughout therapy?

   a. serial CBC

   b. electrocardiogram (ECG)

   c. periodic hepatic and renal function studies

   d. baseline arterial blood gas

8. Julianna Page is hospitalized for complications of a tubal ligation. She has a history of type 2 diabetes and takes acarbose (Precose). Mrs. Page is experiencing a hypoglycemia episode. Which of the following interventions would be appropriate?

   a. orange juice

   b. hard candy

   c. milk and crackers

   d. oral glucose tablet

9. Gerry DeJesus has been hospitalized for brittle type 1 diabetes. Upon entering Mr. DeJesus' room, you find him unconscious with a glucometer reading of 32. Which of the following drugs would be most appropriate to treat Mr. DeJesus?

   a. IV glucose

   b. glucagon IM

   c. diazoxide

   d. dissolved glucose tablets

10. Kiera Aloi calls the clinic and tells you her mother had an insulin reaction and was found unconscious. Kiera states she gave her mother a glucagon injection 20 minutes ago and she woke up but is still groggy and does not make sense. Which of the following instructions would you give?

   a. "Let her wake up on her own, then give her something to eat."

   b. "Place a couple of hard candies in her mouth."

   c. "Just let her sleep. She needs the rest."

   d. "Give her another injection and call the paramedics."

NURSING MANAGEMENT: EVERY GOOD NURSE SHOULD . . .

Use this information to complete the decision tree on page 233.

Your patient is a type 1 diabetic and is hospitalized for cellulitis of the left foot. His medication orders include the following:

NPH insulin 20 units SC Q AM before breakfast
Sliding scale with regular insulin SC, before meals and at bedtime:

   If blood glucose is 70–160 give zero units
   If blood glucose is 161–200 give 2 units
   If blood glucose is 201–240 give 4 units
   If blood glucose is 241–280 give 6 units
   If blood glucose is 281–310 give 8 units
   If blood glucose is < 70 or > 310 contact physician

CASE STUDY

Susan Parsons is a 60-year-old African American. She is 30 pounds over her ideal weight. She has been diagnosed with type 2 diabetes. She has a history of allergy to penicillin and sulfa drugs. She is to start on metformin (Glucophage), an oral antihyperglycemic drug.

1. Why was Ms. Parsons not started on insulin?

2. Why was Ms. Parsons not started on a sulfonylurea such as glyburide?

3. What teaching is necessary for Ms. Parsons?

CRITICAL THINKING CHALLENGE

Ms. Parsons is on metformin for 1 year. Her blood glucose levels have been stabilized at 120. At this time, she cuts her right foot and develops an infection. She is hospitalized. Her blood glucose level now is 297. Would you expect to see any changes made in Ms. Parson's drug therapy to control her diabetes? Why or why not?

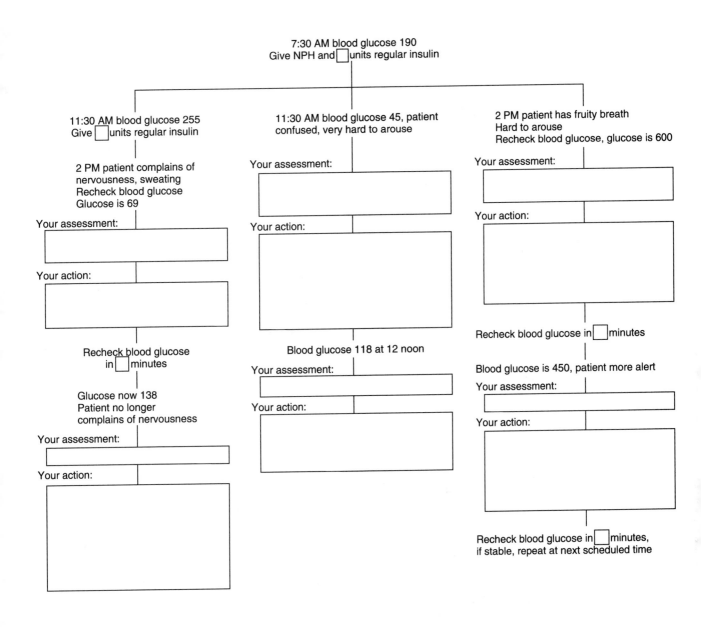

7:30 AM blood glucose 190
Give NPH and ☐ units regular insulin

11:30 AM blood glucose 255
Give ☐ units regular insulin

2 PM patient complains of
nervousness, sweating
Recheck blood glucose
Glucose is 69

Your assessment:

Your action:

Recheck blood glucose
in ☐ minutes

Glucose now 138
Patient no longer
complains of nervousness

Your assessment:

Your action:

11:30 AM blood glucose 45, patient
confused, very hard to arouse

Your assessment:

Your action:

Blood glucose 118 at 12 noon

Your assessment:

Your action:

2 PM patient has fruity breath
Hard to arouse
Recheck blood glucose, glucose is 600

Your assessment:

Your action:

Recheck blood glucose in ☐ minutes

Blood glucose is 450, patient more alert

Your assessment:

Your action:

Recheck blood glucose in ☐ minutes,
if stable, repeat at next scheduled time

CHAPTER 42

Drugs Affecting Men's Health And Sexuality

TOP TEN THINGS TO KNOW ABOUT DRUGS AFFECTING MEN'S HEALTH AND SEXUALITY

1. Testosterone is the primary male sex hormone. Adequate levels of sex hormones are needed to develop the sexual and reproductive organs, create and maintain the secondary sexual characteristics, and induce and stop the growth spurt of adolescence. Testosterone also causes retention of sodium, potassium, and phosphorus and decreased urinary excretion of calcium.

2. Testosterone is used as a replacement therapy for males with low or absent endogenous testosterone. In postmenopausal women, testosterone may be used in advanced, inoperable metastatic breast cancer.

3. Most adverse effects of testosterone are related to high doses of the drug. The most common male adverse effects are gynecomastia, excessive frequency and duration of penile erections, decreased ejaculatory volumes, and oligospermia (low sperm counts). Females will experience masculinization if they receive testosterone.

4. Other adverse effects of testosterone are related to the actions of testosterone on fluid and electrolytes. They include hypernatremia, hypercalcemia, hyperchloremia, hyperkalemia, hyperphosphatemia, fluid overload, edema, and hypercholesterolemia.

5. Sildenafil is used in the treatment of erectile dysfunction. It is administered orally, usually 1 hour before sexual activity. Sildenafil is effective only with accompanying sexual stimulation. Sildenafil promotes vasodilation and increases blood flow to the penis; this helps to achieve and maintain an erection.

6. Sildenafil should not be used if nitrates are also used. Adverse effects are usually mild and transient.

7. Finasteride is used to treat benign prostatic hyperplasia (BPH) and male pattern baldness; the dose for male hair loss is much smaller than for BPH. Two separate trade names are used to differentiate these preparations.

8. Finasteride prevents testosterone from being converted to dihydrotestosterone (DHT; the hormone responsible for prostate growth). This decreases the circulating DHT levels and also boosts testosterone levels. These changes improve BPH-related symptoms, increase maximum urinary flow rates, and decrease prostate size.

9. With male pattern hair loss, DHT is found in increased amounts in the scalp. Finasteride decreases scalp and serum DHT concentrations in these men.

10. Topical minoxidil is used to treat male pattern baldness. It can also be used in women with diffuse hair loss or thinning in the frontal parietal areas. Exact cause of action is unknown. At least 4 months of twice-daily applications are needed for hair growth. Therapy will be effective in more than half of patients but must be continued to maintain the new hair.

KEY TERMS

True/false

Mark true or false for each of the following statements. If the statement is false, replace the underlined words with the correct words that will make the statement correct.

1. _____ <u>Luteinizing hormones</u> are naturally occurring or synthetic steroidal compounds that produce the masculinization and tissue building properties of testosterone.
2. _____ During puberty, the pituitary gland secretes large volumes of <u>FSH</u> and <u>LH</u>.
3. _____ <u>Benign prostatic hypertrophy</u> is the inability to achieve or maintain an erection in at least every three of four attempts at intercourse.
4. _____ Prostatic enlargement that is not caused by cancer is called <u>erectile dysfunction.</u>
5. _____ <u>Male pattern baldness</u> is also known as androgenetic alopecia.

PHYSIOLOGY AND PATHOPHYSIOLOGY: THE BODY HUMAN

Essay

1. What is the primary male sex hormone(s)?

2. In addition to maintaining male secondary sexual characteristics, what effect does testosterone have on the body?

3. How does the body achieve an erection?

CORE DRUG KNOWLEDGE: JUST THE FACTS

Multiple choice

Circle the option that best answers the question or completes the statement.

1. Which of the following disorders IN WOMEN may be treated with testosterone?
   a. delayed puberty
   b. breast cancer
   c. hair loss
   d. decreased libido

2. Testosterone may be contraindicated for use in patients with cardiovascular disorders because of the potential for
   a. arrhythmias.
   b. tachycardia.
   c. bradycardia.
   d. congestive heart failure (CHF).

3. Adverse effects of testosterone therapy in females include
   a. breast enlargement.
   b. loss of voice.
   c. menstrual irregularities.
   d. hair loss.

4. Patients using testosterone (Testaderm TTS) should replace the patch
   a. weekly.
   b. daily.
   c. monthly.
   d. every other day.

5. In contrast to patients using testosterone (Testaderm TTS), patients using Androderm transdermal patches should replace the patch
   a. weekly.
   b. daily.
   c. monthly.
   d. every other day.

6. Appropriate pharmacotherapy with anabolic steroids includes all of the following EXCEPT
   a. improvement of athletic performance.
   b. controlling metastatic breast cancer in women.
   c. hereditary angioedema.
   d. specific anemias.

7. Adverse effects of anabolic steroids include damage to the
   a. heart.
   b. kidneys.
   c. liver.
   d. eyes.

8. Erectile dysfunction is currently treated with
   a. testosterone.
   b. minoxidil (Rogaine).
   c. finasteride (Proscar).
   d. sildenafil (Viagra).

9. Sildenafil (Viagra) is contraindicated for patients with serious _____ problems.
   a. hematopoietic
   b. respiratory
   c. urinary
   d. cardiovascular

10. Benign prostatic hypertrophy is currently treated with
    a. testosterone.
    b. minoxidil (Rogaine).
    c. finasteride (Proscar).
    d. sildenafil (Viagra).

11. In addition to BPH, finasteride may be used in the treatment of
    a. erectile dysfunction.
    b. adrenal suppression.
    c. migraine headache.
    d. male pattern baldness.

12. Minoxidil (Rogaine) should be applied to
    a. wet hair and scalp after shampooing.
    b. wet hair and scalp 2 times a day.
    c. dry hair and scalp after shampooing and drying.
    d. dry hair and scalp 2 times a day.

CORE PATIENT VARIABLES: PATIENTS, PLEASE

Multiple choice

Circle the option that best answers the question or completes the statement.

1. Harrison Kennedy, age 12, takes testosterone due to a family history of delayed puberty. Harrison should be monitored for which of the following adverse effects?
    a. altered bone maturation
    b. excessive hair growth
    c. testicular atrophy
    d. tachycardia

2. During testosterone therapy, Harrison should have which of the following lab tests monitored?
    a. CBC
    b. electrolytes
    c. renal and hepatic function
    d. all of the above

3. Henry Velker, age 14, is taking testosterone. Patient education for Henry should include the potential for
    a. headaches.
    b. impotence.
    c. gynecomastia.
    d. testicular hypoplasia.

4. Appropriate follow-up care for prepubescent boys receiving testosterone treatment includes
    a. weekly testosterone levels.
    b. radiographs every 6 months.
    c. monthly CBC and creatinine.
    d. daily testosterone levels for the first 2 weeks.

5. Benny Oldman, age 42, is receiving testosterone for adrenal insufficiency. Which of the following lab tests should be monitored during therapy?
    a. cholesterol, liver function tests, and a CBC
    b. chest x-ray, CBC, and urinalysis
    c. cholesterol and urinalysis
    d. liver function and chest x-ray

6. Oliver Bradshaw has just been diagnosed with erectile dysfunction. He is being started on sildenafil (Viagra). Appropriate patient teaching should include instructions to take the medication
    a. 6 to 10 hours before sexual activity.
    b. with a high-fat meal to increase its absorption.
    c. approximately 1 hour before sexual activity.
    d. 3 to 4 hours before sexual activity.

7. Your patient presented to the clinic with a request for sildenafil (Viagra). While taking his medical history, you note that he has a history of hypertension, diabetes mellitus, and depression. In his social history, you note that he is a pack-a-day smoker. What advice would you give this patient?
    a. "This must be used cautiously with you due to your medical history and current smoking status."
    b. "This drug is contraindicated for you, but, if you use it only weekly, you should be OK."
    c. "You can use this drug without any problems."
    d. "You can use this drug, but be sure not to take any other medications for at least 2 hours before you take it."

8. Mary Ellison comes to the clinic for advice about her hair loss. She states that her husband takes finasteride (Propecia) and his hair growth is "great." She wants to know if she may also have a prescription for finasteride. What is your best response?
    a. "Why don't you try some of your husband's pills to see if it works for you."
    b. "That should be no problem."
    c. "Finasteride is actually contraindicated for women because it causes birth defects."
    d. "I can get you a few samples to try."

9. Jack Frost is taking finasteride (Proscar) for BPH. He complains of erectile dysfunction, decreased libido, and decreased volume of ejaculate. With your knowledge of this drug, what would you tell Mr. Frost?

   a. "If I were you, I would stop this drug today."

   b. "These are expected adverse effects to the drug. Sometimes they go away on their own."

   c. "These are expected adverse effects to the drug. You have to choose if you want to be able to urinate or have sexual activity."

   d. "Sounds like you have an allergy to the drug."

10. Leonard Gilbert has male pattern baldness and is starting minoxidil (Rogaine) therapy. He asks, "Just when will I see a difference in my hair?" What is your best response?

    a. 1 week

    b. 1 month

    c. 4 months

    d. 6 months

NURSING MANAGEMENT: EVERY GOOD NURSE SHOULD...

Multiple choice

Circle the option that best answers the question or completes the statement.

1. Jake Phillips, 11 years old, has been diagnosed with hypogonadism. He is to start on testosterone (short acting) as replacement therapy. The nurse should do which of the following to minimize adverse effects from the drug therapy?

   a. administer the drug intravenously

   b. verify that x-rays are taken every 6 months

   c. assess BUN and creatinine levels regularly

   d. all of the above

   e. none of the above

2. Gordon Miller, 28 years old, is to be started on Testoderm TTS, a transdermal system of testosterone administration, for treatment of his secondary hypogonadotropic hypogonadism. Which of the following should the nurse include in teaching for Gordon?

   a. Apply the patch to skin that is dry and irritated.

   b. Replace the patch every 2 hours.

   c. Apply the patch to skin on the arm, back, or upper buttocks.

   d. Secure the patch to the skin using an Ace wrap.

3. Frank Capristi, 58 years old, is to start on sildenafil for erection dysfunction. He has a family history of cardiovascular disease and currently is being treated for elevated blood cholesterol levels with lovastatin. He takes no other medications. Patient education for Frank should include

   a. sexual stimulation is needed for sildenafil to be effective.

   b. take the drug about 1 hour before sexual intercourse.

   c. if symptoms of chest pain, shortness of breath, or nausea occur during intercourse, stop sexual activity.

   d. all of the above.

   e. none of the above.

4. Robert Bryan, 73 years old, lives with his daughter, 30 years old, and her family. Robert has BPH and is to be started on finasteride, an androgen inhibitor. He has trouble swallowing pills. His daughter tells you that she frequently crushes medication for him to help him swallow it. To minimize adverse effects, the nurse should

   a. insist Robert swallow the pills whole.

   b. show Robert how to insert the pill through the urethra.

   c. instruct the daughter not to handle or to get any crushed or broken drug on her skin.

   d. teach the daughter to administer the drug just before her father urinates.

5. Mike Timmons, 32 years old, is in the clinic for a routine visit. During that time, he tells the nurse of his plan to buy minoxidil to treat his thinning hair line. He says, "I'll give it a try for a little while and see if it helps." Patient education regarding this drug therapy should include

   a. this drug is only available by prescription.

   b. fine, soft colorless hair may grow first.

   c. this drug may increase your blood pressure.

   d. hair growth should be seen within 2 weeks.

CASE STUDY

Eduardo Feliz, 52 years old, has been a diabetic for 35 years and has coronary artery disease, which is nonsymptomatic at this time. He is to be started on testosterone topical patches because it was found that his endogenous testosterone levels are greatly below normal levels.

What lab values should be monitored when Eduardo returns for a follow-up visit, 6 weeks after starting drug therapy?

CRITICAL THINKING CHALLENGE

When Eduardo returns for a second follow-up visit, 12 weeks after starting drug therapy, he complains of being short of breath, and that his wedding ring is tight. On examination, you auscultate rales and crackles in his lungs and you see that he has +2 edema in his hands and feet.

What is a possible cause of these symptoms?

CHAPTER 43

Drugs Affecting Women's Health and Sexuality

TOP TEN THINGS TO KNOW ABOUT DRUGS AFFECTING WOMEN'S HEALTH AND SEXUALITY

1. Estrogens and progestin are the primary female sex hormones. Adequate levels of sex hormones are needed to develop the sexual and reproductive organs, create and maintain the secondary sexual characteristics, induce and stop the growth spurt of adolescence, create a normal menstrual cycle, and achieve and maintain a pregnancy.

2. Estrogen also affects the cardiovascular system (positively and negatively depending on dose, route, and whether the woman is menopausal), increases bone density, maintains tone and elasticity of urogenital structures, and may have a role in maintaining memory function. Other actions of estrogen include increased fluid retention, protein anabolism, and conservation of calcium and phosphorus.

3. Conjugated estrogen is used as hormone replacement therapy (HRT) when endogenous levels of estrogen are low or absent, as treatment of abnormal uterine bleeding, and as treatment for moderate to severe vasomotor response (hot flashes) during menopause. Additional uses for postmenopausal women include prevention of osteoporosis and cardiovascular disease. In males, it is used as palliative therapy in prostatic and breast cancers.

4. Estrogen replacement therapy (especially if combined with progestin) in postmenopausal women may slightly increase the risk of breast cancer. This is still being researched. Women with significant risk for breast cancer (strong family history, previous breast cancer, history of benign breast tumors, early menarche, late-in-life first pregnancy, no children) may not be candidates for hormone replacement therapy.

5. Adverse effects of estrogen are related to estrogen's effects on the body and may be dose related. Common adverse effects include menstrual changes (breakthrough bleeding, changes in menstrual flow, dysmenorrhea, premenstrual-like syndrome), nausea, headache, bloating, photosensitivity, and breast tenderness.

6. Progestins are composed of progesterone and its derivatives. They regulate, through stimulation or inhibition, the secretion of pituitary gonadotropins, thus regulating development of ovarian follicle. Progestins also inhibit spontaneous uterine contractions.

7. Progestins are used to treat amenorrhea and dysfunctional uterine bleeding. Progestins are given with estrogen as HRT; the combination helps prevent endometrial cancer but may increase the risk of breast cancer.

8. Oral contraceptives are combinations of estrogen and progestins. Formulations with high doses of estrogen may cause serious adverse effects (thromboembolism, stroke, myocardial infarction). Therefore, the lowest effective dose of estrogen should be used.

9. Alendronate inhibits normal and abnormal bone resorption. It is used to treat and prevent osteoporosis in postmenopausal women, and to treat Paget disease.

10. Gastrointestinal (GI) complaints are common adverse effects from alendronate. Very specific administration techniques help to minimize or prevent these problems. Teach the patient to take alendronate at least 30 minutes before eating, drinking any beverage other than plain water, or taking any other medication. The patient should also not lie down after taking alendronate.

KEY TERMS

True/false

Mark true or false for each of the following statements. If the statement is false, replace the underlined words with the words that will make the statement correct.

1. _____ The female body produces six different <u>progestins.</u>
2. _____ <u>Estrogen</u> is the primary endogenous progestational substance.
3. _____ <u>Estrogen,</u> which is secreted by the hypothalamus and then perfused throughout the anterior pituitary, stimulates the release of <u>gonadotropin-releasing hormone</u> and <u>progestins.</u>
4. _____ The ending of monthly menstrual cycles is known as <u>menopause.</u>
5. _____ <u>Paget disease,</u> characterized by low bone mineral density, is a loss in bone mass sufficient to compromise normal function.
6. _____ During the <u>proliferative phase,</u> the follicle is transformed into the corpus luteum, which secretes much progesterone and estrogen.
7. _____ During the <u>secretory phase,</u> estrogen increases the vascularity of the uterine lining, preparing it for implantation of a fertilized egg.
8. _____ The female sex <u>hormones</u> are responsible for the production of female sexual characteristics.
9. _____ <u>Osteoporosis</u> is an idiopathic bone disease characterized by chronic, focal areas of bone destruction.

PHYSIOLOGY AND PATHOPHYSIOLOGY: THE BODY HUMAN

Essay

1. What is the primary female sex hormone(s)?

2. Which of the estrogen hormones is the most potent?

3. In addition to maintaining female secondary sexual characteristics, what effect does estrogen have on the body?

4. Describe the hormonal control of the menstrual cycle.

CORE DRUG KNOWLEDGE: JUST THE FACTS

Multiple choice

Circle the option that best answers the question or completes the statement.

1. Which of the following disorders is an INAPPROPRIATE use of conjugated estrogen?
    a. HRT in female hypogonadism
    b. male castration
    c. primary ovarian failure
    d. abnormal uterine bleeding

2. Long-term use of conjugated estrogen as monotherapy may increase the risk for
    a. brain tumors.
    b. pancreatic cancer.
    c. uterine cancer.
    d. lung cancer.

3. Conjugated estrogens may be given safely to patients with
    a. non-estrogen-dependent neoplastic diseases.
    b. undiagnosed abnormal genital bleeding.
    c. active thrombophlebitis or thromboembolic disorders.
    d. history of cerebrovascular accident (CVA).

4. Conjugated estrogens are considered a pregnancy category _____ drug.
    a. A
    b. B
    c. D
    d. X

5. Common adverse effects to the use of conjugated estrogens include all of the following EXCEPT:
    a. breakthrough bleeding.
    b. shortness of breath.
    c. nausea and vomiting.
    d. bloating and abdominal cramps.

6. Which of the following drugs are used in the treatment of ovulatory failure?
    a. clomiphene (Clomid)
    b. conjugated estrogens
    c. progestins
    d. all of the above

7. Use of ovulatory stimulants may result in
   a. menorrhagia.
   b. multiple births.
   c. amenorrhea.
   d. metrorrhagia.

8. Danazol (Danocrine) is used in the management of
   a. primary ovarian failure.
   b. endometriosis.
   c. birth control.
   d. amenorrhea.

9. Progesterone would be INEFFECTIVE for which of the following?
   a. secondary amenorrhea
   b. dysfunctional bleeding
   c. birth control
   d. pituitary tumor

10. Adverse effects to progesterone birth control pills are
    a. less serious than those with estrogen.
    b. more serious than those with estrogen.
    c. similar to those experienced with estrogen.
    d. more frequent than those with estrogen.

11. Megestrol acetate (Megace), a progestinlike progesterone, is used in the treatment of
    a. AIDS
    b. CVA.
    c. pregnancy complications.
    d. COPD.

12. What is the route of administration for Norplant?
    a. subdermal
    b. subcutaneous
    c. intrathecal
    d. intramuscular

13. Which of the following drugs may be taken while breast-feeding?
    a. progesterone
    b. estrogen-progesterone birth control pills
    c. estrogen
    d. None of the above

14. Mifepristone (Mifeprex) is used to
    a. stop conception.
    b. treat ovarian failure.
    c. abort an early pregnancy.
    d. treat adrenal insufficiency.

15. Alendronate (Fosamax) is used in the management of
    a. unwanted pregnancy.
    b. primary ovarian failure.
    c. hair loss.
    d. osteoporosis.

CORE PATIENT VARIABLES: PATIENTS, PLEASE

Multiple choice

Circle the option that best answers the question or completes the statement.

1. Georgia Hanes, age 54, came to the clinic due to a lack of menstruation in the past 12 months. Laboratory tests confirm Mrs. Hanes is postmenopausal. Mrs. Hanes states she is confused about the use of estrogen after menopause. Which of the following facts is correct about estrogen use after menopause?
   a. There is a decreased risk for breast cancer in women with a family history of breast cancer.
   b. There is an increased risk for cardiac events in women without a history of coronary heart disease.
   c. Postmenopausal women on estrogen have an increase in bone density.
   d. It decreases the risk for uterine cancer.

2. Hillary Adams, age 62, has been prescribed both estrogen and progestin for her postmenopausal symptoms. Ms. Adams states, "My friends all just take estrogen. Why do I have to take both pills?" Your best response would be
   a. "This is the regimen that your health care provider prefers."
   b. "Because you still have your uterus, you may get endometriosis if the estrogen is given unopposed by progesterone."
   c. "It is important for you to bleed each month so we know that you are not pregnant."
   d. "This combination is better than single-agent therapy."

3. Eleanor Noble, age 66, comes to the clinic for a checkup after a CVA. She is actively involved in rehabilitation and uses a cane to ambulate. Mrs. Noble tells you she is concerned that she might "break something" if she should fall and wishes to take estrogen and progesterone to reduce her osteoporosis risk. Which of the following statements would be most appropriate?

   a. "You are really doing your homework. It sounds like a good idea."

   b. "You should really finish your rehab before we consider any new drugs."

   c. "With your history of stroke, these medications are not suggested for use."

   d. "I think you should only take progesterone because you had a stroke."

4. Beverly Willis, age 14, comes to the clinic after a therapeutic abortion. Beverly states she still plans to have intercourse, and can't always remember to take her contraception. For this patient, what would be an appropriate form of birth control?

   a. intrauterine devide (IUD).

   b. condoms and foam.

   c. Depo-Provera

   d. cyclic birth control pills.

5. Melissa Taylor, age 19, comes to the clinic for a routine checkup. She states she had an intrauterine progesterone insert placed approximately 4 months ago. Melissa is concerned that her normal 2-day flow has been increased to 5 days. Which of the following statements would be most appropriate?

   a. "It sounds like the device may have perforated the uterus."

   b. "This is an expected change with use of the insert."

   c. "This may be the beginning of endometriosis."

   d. "You probably have a pelvic infection."

6. Gilda Benson, age 42, comes to the clinic requesting birth control pills. Gilda states she has been divorced for 2 years and is now ready "to do some serious dating." Which of the following statements from Gilda's health status history would contraindicate the use of birth control pills?

   a. first pregnancy at age 16

   b. smoked 1 pack per day until 2 years ago

   c. COPD

   d. deep vein thrombosis

7. Valerie Newis, age 16, has been prescribed triphasic birth control pills. Valerie calls the clinic and states that she has forgotten to take her pill for 2 days. Which of the following statements is most appropriate?

   a. "Take all three pills today and continue your pack."

   b. Take 2 pills today and 2 pills tomorrow and continue your pack."

   c. "Stop taking the pack and start a new pack in 4 days."

   d. "Take one pill a day and don't forget any more."

8. Mary Fox has just had a progesterone IUD placed for birth control. Patient education should include

   a. "This needs to be replaced in one year."

   b. "This does not need to be replaced for 5 years."

   c. "Should you become pregnant, this will just fall out."

   d. "This should stop your monthly menstrual cycle."

9. Your patient took mifepristone (Mifeprex) 3 weeks ago. She comes to the clinic with a complaint of continued vaginal bleeding. With your knowledge of this drug, which of the following is appropriate?

   a. Tell the patient this is normal and to return if bleeding continues more than 2 weeks.

   b. Obtain orthostatic vital signs. If normal, send her home.

   c. Obtain a CBC and have her evaluated by the health care provider.

   d. Call for paramedics.

10. Your patient is taking alendronate (Fosamax) for the prevention of osteoporosis. Patient education should include

   a. "Take it first thing in the morning with a glass of orange juice."

   b. "Take it at bedtime with a glass of milk."

   c. "Take it first thing in the morning, with water, before you eat or drink anything else."

   d. "Lie down after taking the medication for 30 minutes."

NURSING MANAGEMENT: EVERY GOOD NURSE SHOULD . . .

Multiple choice

Circle the option that best answers the question or completes the statement.

1. You are the nurse working in the GYN department of an outpatient center. Patients frequently ask you what you think about estrogen use and if they are candidates to take estrogen. Which of these patients may be appropriate candidates for estrogen use?

   a. Maria, 20 years old, diagnosed with primary ovarian failure

   b. Kay, 30 years old, post bilateral salpingo-oophorectomy (removal of fallopian tubes and ovaries) secondary to multiple bouts of pelvic inflammatory disease

   c. Olga, 55 years old, complaining of hot flashes and vaginal dryness

   d. all of the above

   e. none of the above

2. Sylvia Parker, 57 years old, has been prescribed estrogen hormone replacement therapy after menopause. Teaching for Ms. Parker should include

   a. "Take the drug for 3 weeks, then stay off the drug for 1 week."

   b. "Sun exposure will promote the effectiveness of the estrogen."

   c. "X-rays will need to be taken every 6 months."

   d. "Sudden, severe headaches may occur and are not serious."

3. Darla Stevens, 19 years old, is to receive progesterone for treatment of primary amenorrhea. To maximize the therapeutic effect and to minimize the adverse effects from drug therapy, the nurse should

   a. assess Darla for thrombophlebitis before and during therapy.

   b. verify that Darla is not pregnant before beginning drug therapy.

   c. administer the progesterone daily for 6 to 8 days per order.

   d. do all of the above.

   e. do none of the above.

4. You are teaching a class on birth control to women who are 6 weeks postpartum. Which of the following statements should be included?

   a. Levonorgestrel implants prevent pregnancy for up to 2 years.

   b. Intrauterine progesterone inserts have no serious adverse effects.

   c. Estrogen-progestin combination oral contraceptives are the best choice for women over 35 years who smoke cigarettes.

   d. All of the above.

   e. None of the above.

5. You are the nurse practitioner working in a practice with OB-GYN physicians in the United States. Shari Nelson, 22 years old, is a patient who has come to see you because she is concerned that she became pregnant after a rape that occurred 4 weeks ago. You confirm that she is pregnant, and because she wishes to terminate this pregnancy you prescribe mifepristone. Patient education for Shari must include

   a. a discussion of the facts contained in the FDA Medication Guide, after she has obtained a copy and read it.

   b. verification that she can return to the office for two follow-up appointments.

   c. instruction that she will need to take 3 tablets in the presence of the nurse practitioner.

   d. all of the above.

   e. none of the above.

CASE STUDY

Lorinda Wyatt, 20 years old, is 6 weeks postpartum after vaginal delivery. She has come for her checkup. She questions you about resuming birth control. Her record indicates that she was on Ortho-Norvum 7/7/7, a triphasic oral contraceptive before becoming pregnant. She has been breast-feeding but is planning to stop when she returns to work in the next week. She has not yet had a menstrual period since she delivered. Consider Lorinda's core patient variables. What advice would you give her regarding resuming birth control?

CRITICAL THINKING CHALLENGE

Lorinda asks if there is a better form of birth control than the Ortho-Novum 7/7/7 oral contraceptives. She says, "I got pregnant while I was using those pills. I really wasn't planning on becoming pregnant right now. I definitely want to wait awhile before I get pregnant again."

What questions might you want to ask Lorinda to more completely assess her?

CHAPTER 44

Drugs Affecting Uterine Motility

TOP TEN THINGS TO KNOW ABOUT DRUGS AFFECTING UTERINE MOTILITY

1. Drug therapy may be used to induce labor, augment (improve) labor, or stop labor that begins preterm.

2. Oxytocin, a synthetic form of an endogenous hormone, is given by intravenous (IV) infusion to initiate or augment labor when clinically indicated. Oxytocin is also used intramuscularly (IM) to control postpartum bleeding, and through a nasal spray to initiate milk letdown before pumping or breast-feeding.

3. There is a three-phase response to oxytocin therapy: incremental phase, stable phase, and hyperstimulation.

4. Adverse effects of oxytocin are dose related. Most common maternal adverse effects are nausea, vomiting, uterine hypertonicity, and cardiac tonicity. Water intoxification is uncommon but can be fatal. The most common fetal adverse effect is bradycardia.

5. Monitor maternal vital signs, length of contractions, time between contractions, fetal heart rate, fetal movement, and maternal fluid status when giving oxytocin. Always administer with IV pump and piggyback the diluted drug onto main IV line.

6. Tocolytic drugs are given to stop preterm labor long enough (24 to 48 hours) to give the mother corticosteroids, which assist in preparing the baby's lungs for delivery, and allow the mother to be transported to another facility if needed (e.g., to a facility with a neonatal intensive care).

7. Ritodrine, a beta agonist, has relatively selective preference for uterine receptors. It is used to control preterm labor after 20 weeks' gestation but is used infrequently due to adverse effects.

8. Adverse effects of ritodrine are dose related and secondary to beta stimulation. Maternal and fetal tachycardia and increases in maternal blood pressure occur in nearly all patients. Antidote for overdose is a beta blocker.

9. Terbutaline, another beta agonist, is also used to stop preterm labor, but this is an unlabeled and controversial use. It has no advantages over ritodrine for controlling preterm labor. Terbutaline is primarily used as a bronchodilator.

10. Magnesium sulfate is the drug of choice to treat or prevent seizures associated with preeclampsia, eclampsia, and pregnancy-induced hypertension. It has some effect on controlling preterm labor, but this is an unlabeled use. Monitor blood levels carefully to prevent overdose. Administer by IV pump.

KEY TERMS

Anagrams

Using the following definitions, unscramble each of the following sets of letters to form a word. Write your response in the spaces provided.

1. pregnancy before labor starts

   T N A P M U T E R A
   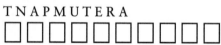

2. uterine relaxants used to stop labor

   T O O T C Y L S I C
   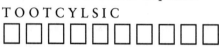

3. after delivery of the fetus

   P T M U S O T P R A
   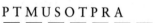
   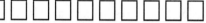

4. fibrillation and prolonged contraction of the uterus

   R U E N E I T Y A T E T N
   ☐☐☐☐☐☐☐☐☐☐☐☐☐

5. uterine stimulants used to initiate or augment contraction

   Y I C X O T S I O
   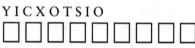

6. onset of labor

   M P R A N I T R U A T
   ☐☐☐☐☐☐☐☐☐☐☐☐

PHYSIOLOGY AND PATHOPHYSIOLOGY: THE BODY HUMAN

Essay

1. In the uncomplicated pregnancy, when should labor begin?

2. In addition to stimulation of the uterus, what are the actions of endogenous oxytocin?

3. What are the regulatory processes involved in the control of uterine motility?

4. In the intrapartal period, what adaptations are required by the cardiovascular system?

5. In the intrapartal period, what changes occur in the respiratory system?

6. In the intrapartal period, what major change occurs in the hemopoietic system?

7. In the intrapartal period, what are the expected changes in the renal system?

8. In the intrapartal period, what occurs in the gastrointestinal (GI) system?

CORE DRUG KNOWLEDGE: JUST THE FACTS

Multiple choice

Circle the option that best answers the question or completes the statement.

1. What methods of administration are appropriate for inducing labor with oxytocin (Pitocin)?
   a. oral
   b. intramuscular
   c. intravenous
   d. all of the above

2. What is the initial dose of oxytocin (Pitocin) to stimulate labor?
   a. 0.5 to 1 mU/minute
   b. 5 to 10 mU/minute
   c. 2 to 3 mU/minute
   d. 4 to 8 mU/minute

3. Maximum effect from oxytocin (Pitocin) administration occurs within
   a. 1 minute.
   b. 40 minutes.
   c. 2 hours.
   d. 4 hours.

4. Before oxytocin (Pitocin) therapy is initiated, which of the following should occur?
   a. 10 hours of nonprogressing labor
   b. fetal distress
   c. assessment of pelvic adequacy
   d. uterine tetany

5. The primary pharmacotherapeutics for ergonovine maleate (Ergotrate) and methylergonovine maleate (Methergine) is
   a. suppression of uterine motility.
   b. induction of labor.
   c. prevention of postpartum hemorrhage.
   d. all of the above.

6. Which of the following drugs may be used to induce an abortion?
   a. carboprost (Hemabate)
   b. dinoprostone (Prepidil)
   c. ergonovine maleate (Ergotrate)
   d. both a and b

7. Ritodrine (Yutopar) works by
   a. stimulation of alpha receptor sites in the uterine smooth muscle.
   b. inhibition of alpha receptor sites in the uterine smooth muscle.
   c. stimulation of beta receptor sites in the uterine smooth muscle.
   d. inhibition of beta receptor sites in the uterine smooth muscle.

8. Ritodrine (Yutopar) is contraindicated for use in patients taking
   a. beta agonists and corticosteroids.
   b. inhaled anticholinergic agents.
   c. H2 antagonists.
   d. antibiotics.

9. Patients receiving ritodrine (Yutopar) should be positioned on their
   a. back.
   b. right side.
   c. left side.
   d. any of the above.

10. To maximize therapeutic benefits from magnesium sulfate, the serum level should be
    a. 1.5 to 3 mEq/L.
    b. 16 to 25 mEq/L.
    c. 7 to 10 mEq/L.
    d. 4 to 7 mEq/L.

CORE PATIENT VARIABLES: PATIENTS, PLEASE

Multiple choice

Circle the option that best answers the question or completes the statement.

1. Allison Mays, age 26, is receiving IV oxytocin (Pitocin) to enhance labor. She complains of dry mouth and requests ice water. Allison should be monitored for which of the following?
   a. dehydration
   b. water intoxication
   c. urinary frequency
   d. bradycardia

2. Doris Perez has been in labor for 6 hours. Favorable induction with oxytocin (Pitocin) is most likely to occur if Mrs. Perez has a Bishop's score of
   a. 1 to 2.
   b. 0 to 1.
   c. 3 to 4.
   d. greater than 5.

3. Barbara Harris is receiving oxytocin (Pitocin) to stimulate delivery. Barbara is experiencing contractions lasting 90 seconds with resting pressure of 18 mmHg. Which of the following interventions would be most appropriate?
   a. continue the infusion at the current rate
   b. increase the infusion rate
   c. stop the infusion and call the health care provider
   d. continue the infusion and call the health care provider

4. Your patient is receiving IV oxytocin (Pitocin) to stimulate labor. To safely administer this medication, the nurse should
   a. give the drug by rapid IVP.
   b. piggyback the drug into the primary IV line.
   c. give the drug IVP over 5 to 6 minutes.
   d. not give IV; give SC only.

5. Nancy Fox is receiving ritodrine (Yutopar) for preterm labor. Which of the following occurrences would necessitate cessation of the drug?
   a. fetal tachycardia
   b. maternal hypertension
   c. persistent maternal tachycardia above 140
   d. maternal headache

6. Mrs. Fox (as above) has been receiving ritodrine (Yutopar) for 3 days. Which of the following interventions should be done?

   a. Monitor vital signs.

   b. Monitor glucose.

   c. Monitor for fetal distress.

   d. all of the above

7. Erika Wilson is 35 weeks pregnant and has preterm contractions. Mrs. Wilson has been prescribed ritodrine (Yutopar). She asks, "It's so close to my due date, why can't I just deliver?" Which of the following is the best response?

   a. "Infants born this early have difficulty breathing."

   b. "Delaying delivery gives your baby an opportunity to fully develop and avoid complications."

   c. "Maternal hemorrhaging may occur with delivery at this time."

   d. "Your baby might have brain damage if it is born this early."

8. Alda Babusek has preeclampsia and is brought to the hospital. For prevention of seizures due to preeclampsia, you would anticipate treatment for Mrs. Babusek with which of the following drugs?

   a. magnesium sulfate

   b. oxytocin (Pitocin)

   c. ritodrine (Yutopar)

   d. terbutaline (Brethine)

9. Alexis Cahill has just delivered a baby boy. She has been receiving magnesium sulfate for eclampsia for the past 24 hours. Baby Cahill should be monitored for which of the following?

   a. tachycardia

   b. hypertension

   c. respiratory depression

   d. all of the above

NURSING MANAGEMENT: EVERY GOOD NURSE SHOULD . . .

Multiple choice

Circle the option that best answers the question or completes the statement.

1. Before beginning therapy with oxytocin, the nurse should

   a. verify that there is a contraindication to vaginal delivery is contraindicated.

   b. confirm significant cephalopelvic disproportion.

   c. assess that cervical ripening is favorable through Bishop's scoring.

   d. determine if fetal distress is present but delivery is not imminent.

2. Which of the following solutions is appropriate to use to dilute oxytocin for IV administration?

   a. 5% dextrose in lactated Ringer's

   b. 20% dextrose in water

   c. 0.2% sodium chloride

   d. none of the above; oxytocin should not be diluted

3. Your patient is receiving oxytocin for induction of labor. Her contractions begin to occur every 1 minute 50 seconds, and last 1 minute 40 seconds. The nurse should

   a. increase the oxytocin rate.

   b. increase the concentration of the oxytocin.

   c. shut off the oxytocin.

   d. decrease the rate of the mainline fluids.

4. Which of the following solutions would be appropriate to dilute ritodrine for IV infusion?

   a. 0.9% normal saline

   b. 5% dextrose and lactated Ringer's

   c. 5% dextrose and 0.9% normal saline

   d. 5% dextrose and water

5. To minimize adverse effects during ritodrine infusion, the nurse should

   a. use an IV pump.

   b. position patient on her right side.

   c. encourage high fluid intake.

   d. do all of the above.

   e. do none of the above.

CASE STUDY

Jenny Sampson is pregnant with a gestation of 40 weeks. She has been in labor for 6 hours but has not progressed in the labor. Bishop's scale indicates a score of 7. Her vital signs are: pulse 84, respirations 18, and blood pressure 110/70. She is started on oxytocin IV infusion 1 mU/minute. The order states to increase the rate every 60 minutes by 1 mU/minute until effective contractions occur.

1. Are these orders appropriate for Jenny? Why or why not?

2. What actions of the nurse are indicated to maximize therapeutic effect and minimize adverse effects of the oxytocin?

CRITICAL THINKING CHALLENGE

Jenny continues on the oxytocin infusion for 4 hours, with the rate being increased each hour per order. Jenny now has contractions every 2 minutes 30 seconds, which last 90 seconds. She is 10 cm dilated. She says she feels like she has to have a bowel movement.

1. What is your assessment of Jenny's condition?

2. What actions should the nurse take now?

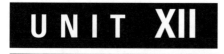

UNIT XII

Antineoplastic Drugs

CHAPTER 45

Drugs for Treating Neoplastic Disorders: Cell Cycle-Specific Drugs

TOP TEN THINGS TO KNOW ABOUT DRUGS FOR TREATING NEOPLASTIC DISORDERS: CELL CYCLE-SPECIFIC DRUGS

1. Cell cycle-specific drugs are toxic to the cell at a particular phase of the cell cycle and cause no significant harm during the other phases. The major toxicities of antineoplastic drugs are seen on rapidly dividing cells, such as the bone marrow, gastrointestinal (GI) mucosa, hair follicles, and gonadal cells. Avoid use in pregnancy.

2. 5-Fluorouracil (5-FU), an antimetabolite, works in the S phase of cell division and interferes with the synthesis of DNA and RNA by acting as a false antimetabolite causing thymine deficiency (thymine is needed for DNA and RNA cell division and growth). 5-FU, like other antimetabolites, are most effective against tumors with a high growth fraction. It is used to treat various solid tumors, especially malignant GI tumors.

3. Myelosuppression (anemia, leukopenia, and thrombocytopenia) is the dose-limiting adverse effect of 5-FU. Monitor WBC closely at nadir. GI effects (stomatitis, esophagopharyngitis, intractable vomiting, diarrhea, GI ulceration, and bleeding) are also serious adverse effects.

4. Vincristine, a vinca alkaloid, works in the M (mitotic) phase of cell division by preventing cell division in the metaphase stage of mitosis. It is used in treating acute lymphoblastic leukemia and some other cancers. Dose-limiting adverse effects are neurologic (motor, sensory, and autonomic neuropathy). Severity of neurotoxicity is related to cumulative dose. Vincristine is only given intravenously (IV). It is a vesicant. Use extravasation precautions.

5. Etoposide, a podophyllotoxin, works in the G_2 and S phases of the cell cycle preventing cells from entering mitosis and prophase by inhibiting DNA synthesis. Etoposide is used in combination therapy for refractory testicular tumors and small-cell lung cancer.

6. Myelosuppression (granulocytopenia) is etoposide's dose-limiting adverse effect. Monitor white blood cell (WBC) count closely at nadir. Etoposide may be given by mouth (PO) or IV. It causes nausea and vomiting when given PO; it is an irritant when given IV.

7. Paclitaxel (a taxane) inhibits the normal dynamic reorganization of the microtubular network during interphase and mitosis. Paclitaxel also prevents transition from the G_0 and G_1 phase into the S phase by blocking cellular response to protein growth factors. Paclitaxel is used in treating ovarian and breast cancers. Myelosuppression and neurotoxicity are dose-limiting adverse effects of paclitaxel.

8. Hypersensitivity reactions occur in about 10% of patients who receive paclitaxel during the first 10 minutes of the infusion. Premedicate with corticosteroids (Decadron), diphenhydramine (Benadryl), and H2 antagonist (Cimetidine) to prevent severe reactions.

9. Topotecan HCl, a semisynthetic derivative of camptothecin, inhibits the enzyme needed for maintaining DNA structure during replication, transcription, and translation of genetic materials (S phase). This inhibition leads to breakage of DNA strands and cell death. Topotecan is used to treat patients with metastatic ovarian cancer after failure of initial or subsequent chemotherapy. It is also effective in treating small-cell lung cancer. The dose-limiting toxicity of topotecan is myelosuppression, especially neutropenia. Assess adequacy of bone marrow reserve before starting therapy and reassess WBC at nadir. Hematopoietic growth factors may be needed.

10. Hydroxyurea, a miscellaneous antineoplastic agent, is used in managing hematologic cancers. It is an inhibitor of the enzyme ribonucleotide reductase, causing inhibition of DNA, without inhibiting RNA or protein synthesis. It is S phase specific and may hold other cells in the G_1 phase of the cell cycle. Myelosuppression (especially leukopenia) is the major toxicity and is dose related.

KEY TERMS

Crossword puzzle

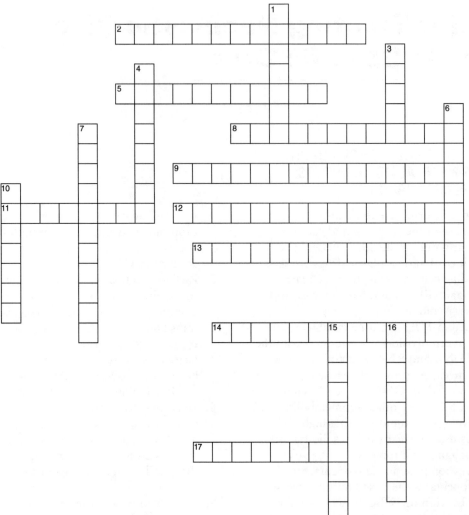

Across

2. Type of therapy given after induction therapy has achieved a complete remission
5. This therapy involves the use of adjuvant chemotherapeutic drugs during the preoperative or perioperative periods
8. Term that describes the use of cytotoxic agents to destroy cancer cells
9. Ability of the body to react to radiation treatment after it is completed
11. Any agent causing irritation
12. After complete remission is achieved, the same agents used for induction therapy are given at higher doses
13. Fraction of the cell population that is in any phase of the cell cycle
14. Chemotherapeutic drugs that are most effective during a particular phase of the cycle are known as cell _____
17. This therapy is administered after radiation or surgery to destroy residual tumor cells

Down

1. This therapy is given to a patient whose symptoms have recurred or whose treatment by another regimen has failed
3. Time at which the maximum cytotoxic effect is exerted on the bone marrow
4. Extremely acidic drugs that may cause significant and undesired tissue damage
6. Drugs that act independently of a specific cell cycle are called cell _____
7. This therapy involves using single or combination, low-dose cytotoxic drugs on a long-term basis
10. Process of reproduction of cells, resulting in the formation of two daughter cells
15. This therapy is done to control symptoms, provide comfort, and improve patient's quality of life if a cure is not achievable
16. This term commonly describes treatment of hematologic concerns

PHYSIOLOGY AND PATHOPHYSIOLOGY: THE BODY HUMAN

Matching

Match the following phases of the reproductive cell cycle.

1. _____ mitotic spindles constructed and RNA synthesized

2. _____ waiting for reproductive stimulus

3. _____ cell division

4. _____ DNA and RNA assembled

5. _____ resting phase

a. G_0

b. G_1

c. S

d. G_2

e. M

Essay

1. What are the four phases of mitosis?

2. What is cytokinesis?

3. Describe generation time.

4. What differentiates the cancer cell from the normal cell?

5. Define first-order kinetics.

CORE DRUG KNOWLEDGE: JUST THE FACTS

Multiple choice

Circle the option that best answers the question or completes the statement.

1. Antimetabolites such as 5-fluorouracil (5-FU) inhibit tumor growth by
   a. interfering with the metaphase of mitosis.
   b. inhibiting DNA synthesis in the S and G_2 phases.
   c. inhibiting the normal dynamic reorganization of the microtubular network during interphase and mitosis.
   d. inducing thiamine deficiency, which deprives the cells of DNA and RNA.

2. Which of the following would necessitate close monitoring of a patient receiving 5-FU therapy?
   a. poor nutritional status
   b. depressed bone marrow function
   c. concurrent serious infection
   d. all of the above

3. 5-FU therapy is particularly effective in the treatment of
   a. central nervous system (CNS) lesions.
   b. malignant GI tumors.
   c. lymphoma.
   d. leukemia.

4. Which of the following adverse effects would necessitate cessation of therapy with 5-FU?
   a. WBC >3500
   b. constipation
   c. stomatitis
   d. hypertension

5. Which of the following chemotherapeutic agents is most useful in the treatment of lymphoblastic leukemia?
   a. floxuridine (FUDR)
   b. etoposide (VePesid)
   c. vincristine (Oncovin)
   d. docetaxel (Taxotere)

6. Patients receiving vincristine (Oncovin) should be closely monitored for
   a. fever spike.
   b. extravasation.
   c. diarrhea.
   d. hypertension.

7. Which of the following drugs may be used in combination therapy because of its minimal effect on myelosuppression?
   a. vincristine (Oncovin)
   b. teniposide (Vumon)
   c. 5-FU
   d. hydroxyurea (Hydrea)

8. Administration of etoposide (VePesid) should be
   a. IVP within 3 minutes.
   b. IVPB over 30 to 60 minutes.
   c. IVP over 10 minutes.
   d. IVPB over 1 to 2 hours.

9. An adverse effect associated with etoposide (VePesid) therapy is
   a. bronchospasm and cough.
   b. CNS depression and tachycardia.
   c. increased intraocular pressure and visual disturbances.
   d. radiation recall and alopecia.

10. Paclitaxel (Taxol) therapy has been very successful in patients with
    a. brain and uterine cancer.
    b. uterine and breast cancer.
    c. GI and uterine cancer.
    d. brain and pancreatic cancer.

11. Patients receiving paclitaxel (Taxol) may experience which of the following adverse effects?
    a. hypersensitivity reaction
    b. neurotoxicity
    c. myelosuppression
    d. all of the above

12. A unique adverse effect associated with docetaxel (Taxotere) therapy is
    a. fluid retention syndrome.
    b. increased appetite.
    c. increased thickness of hair.
    d. decreased intraocular pressure.

13. Topotecan HCl (Hycamtin) works by
    a. inhibiting the activity of an enzyme involved in gene transcription and DNA replication.
    b. inhibiting DNA synthesis in the S and G_2 phases
    c. inhibiting the normal dynamic reorganization of the microtubular network during interphase and mitosis.
    d. inducing thiamine deficiency, which deprives the cells of DNA and RNA.

14. Which of the following statements concerning drug–drug interactions of topotecan HCl (Hycamtin) is accurate?
    a. There are no known drug–drug interactions.
    b. There are a few drug–drug interactions, but they are minor.
    c. There are a few drug–drug interactions, and they are serious.
    d. There are many drug–drug interactions, and they are serious.

15. Hydroxyurea (Hydrea) is used in the management of
    a. breast cancer.
    b. prostate cancer.
    c. pulmonary cancer.
    d. hematologic cancers.

16. Patients receiving hydroxyurea (Hydrea) should be cautioned about the potential for
    a. photosensitivity.
    b. sedation.
    c. constipation.
    d. fluid overload.

17. Generally speaking, the chemotherapeutic agents are pregnancy category _____ drugs.
    a. A or B
    b. B or C
    c. D or X
    d. C or D

18. Generally speaking, the most important lab test to monitor for patients receiving chemotherapy is the
    a. liver function.
    b. renal function.
    c. platelet count.
    d. CBC with differential.

CORE PATIENT VARIABLES: PATIENTS, PLEASE

Multiple choice

Circle the option that best answers the question or completes the statement.

1. Justine George is prescribed 5-fluorouracil (5-FU) drug therapy. Which of the following adverse effects would limit the use of this drug therapy?
   a. hepatotoxicity
   b. neurotoxicity
   c. myelosuppression
   d. pulmonary toxicity

2. Before initiating 5-FU therapy, which of the following should be documented?
   a. pulmonary function results
   b. condition of skin, nails, and hair
   c. visual acuity
   d. blood pressure

3. Eleanor Parker is receiving 5-FU therapy. She is scheduled to receive her third cycle. Before initiating this infusion, the nurse should evaluate Mrs. Parker's

    a. WBC and differential count.

    b. urinalysis.

    c. BUN and creatinine.

    d. hepatic enzymes.

4. Jeffrey Reiser is prescribed vincristine (Oncovin) therapy. Jeffrey develops a loss of deep tendon reflexes and weakness. He also complains of constipation. You suspect

    a. hepatotoxicity.

    b. neurotoxicity.

    c. pulmonary toxicity.

    d. cardiotoxicity.

5. During an infusion of etoposide (VePesid), Harry Farmer develops facial flushing, bronchospasm, and tachycardia. This might be due to

    a. pulmonary toxicity.

    b. infusing medication too long.

    c. rapid infusion.

    d. cardiotoxicity.

6. Nancy Blevins is receiving combination therapy with paclitaxel (Taxol) and cisplatin (Platenol). Which of the drugs should be administered first?

    a. paclitaxel

    b. cisplatin

    c. It does not matter.

    d. They should never be used in combination.

7. Which of the following interventions are necessary when Ms. Blevins receives paclitaxel (Taxol)?

    a. Shield medication from light.

    b. Assess vital signs frequently during first 15 minutes of infusion.

    c. Monitor urine output for discoloration.

    d. Assess level of consciousness during first 15 minutes of infusion.

8. To minimize the potential for fluid retention syndrome with docetaxel (Taxotere) therapy, which of the following premedications may be administered?

    a. corticosteroids

    b. histamine antagonists

    c. diuretics

    d. all of the above

9. Carole Falk is receiving topotecan HCl (Hycamtin). She asks, "How many times do I need to get this drug?" What is your best response?

    a. "This is the only time."

    b. "You will need only five doses."

    c. "You will need one dose for 5 consecutive days and need to repeat that series three more times."

    d. "You need to get it one time every 21 days for four courses."

10. Marilyn Greenburg is receiving hydroxyurea (Hydrea) for leukemia. Which of the following should be closely monitored with Mrs. Greenburg?

    a. hepatic function

    b. pulmonary function

    c. CBC

    d. ECG

11. When calculating the correct dose of hydroxyurea (Hydrea) for Mrs. Greenburg, which of the following is correct?

    a. Use actual weight.

    b. Use maximum weight in the past 6 months.

    c. Use ideal weight.

    d. Use actual or ideal weight, whichever is lower.

12. Gretchen Hall is receiving chemotherapeutic drugs for breast cancer. She asks, "What does that word 'nadir' mean?" You would respond

    a. that is the length of time it takes for the drug to clear your body.

    b. that is the length of time before your hair starts to fall out.

    c. that is the period that the drug can cause the most damage to your white cells.

    d. that is the period that the drug works the hardest.

NURSING MANAGEMENT: EVERY GOOD NURSE SHOULD . . .

Multiple choice

Circle the option that best answers the question or completes the statement.

1. Rob Fisher, 51 years old, is receiving 5-FU for stomach cancer. He has been on 5-FU for 5 days when he develops mouth sores. What teaching is appropriate regarding management and treatment of these mouth sores?

    a. Drink hot tea with honey and lemon.

    b. Rinse the mouth after every meal with a commercial mouthwash.

    c. Eat more gelatin and pudding.

    d. Use aspirin to control the discomfort.

2. Lois Wilder is to begin receiving vincristine as treatment for her lymphoblastic leukemia. Which of the following would be most important for the nurse to emphasize in patient education?

    a. Brush hair vigorously.

    b. Eat a bland, low-residue diet.

    c. Report immediately if heart rate seems slow.

    d. Report immediately if IV site is burning or looks red.

3. Lois receives several doses of vincristine. This time while checking the IV site during drug infusion, the nurse notices some swelling at the insertion site. An appropriate nursing action would be to

    a. turn off the infusion.

    b. administer isotonic sodium thiosulfate.

    c. apply iced compresses.

    d. do all of the above.

    e. do none of the above.

4. To minimize the risk of a hypersensitivity reaction to etoposide, a podophyllotoxin, the nurse should

    a. administer the drug by IV push.

    b. administer the drug slowly over at least 30 to 60 minutes.

    c. make sure the patient has a call light handy.

    d. make sure the patient's family stays with the patient.

5. Julia Jordan, 30 years old, is to receive paclitaxel for treatment of breast cancer, because other treatment has not been effective. She is concerned that she will lose her hair and asks whether this is likely with paclitaxel treatment. The best response of the nurse would be

    a. "No, hair loss does not occur with paclitaxel."

    b. "Yes, hair loss may occur and may be severe."

    c. "Yes, hair loss may occur, but it is usually mild and unnoticeable."

    d. "You shouldn't worry about possible hair loss; other adverse effects are more important."

6. Nick Willis is to receive hydroxyurea and then radiation for treatment of acute blastic leukemia. To minimize adverse effects from the drug therapy, the nurse should

    a. monitor the CBC before and during therapy.

    b. begin drug therapy 1 week before radiation therapy.

    c. monitor for elevated BUN and creatinine levels.

    d. do all of the above.

    e. do none of the above.

7. Which of the following should the nurse do to prevent accidental personal exposure to hazardous drugs such as antineoplastics?

    a. Use caution when purging IV lines with an antineoplastic.

    b. Discard syringes that held antineoplastics in the trash can at the patient's bedside.

    c. Use a gauze pad around the IV tubing when disconnecting it from the angiocath after drug administration.

    d. Wash your hands during drug preparation if you are eating while preparing the drug.

CASE STUDY

Gordon Meyers is 63 years old and has colorectal cancer. He is to receive 5-FU 450 mg/m^2 IV on days 1 through 5, and day 28 of drug therapy, then weekly thereafter. Additionally, he is to receive levamisole 50 mg PO every 8 hours for days 1 through 3 of therapy, then every 2 weeks for 1 year.

1. Why is Mr. Meyers receiving these two drug therapies? (Hint: Need help? See Chapter 33.)

2. Discuss the monitoring that should be done for Mr. Meyers while he receives these drug therapies.

CRITICAL THINKING CHALLENGE

Mr. Meyers complains that he is having diarrhea and that the stools are black.

1. What is your assessment of these findings?

2. What actions should you take when Mr. Meyers reports these findings to you?

CHAPTER 46

Drugs for Treating Neoplastic Disorders: Cell Cycle-Nonspecific Drugs

TOP TEN THINGS TO KNOW ABOUT DRUGS FOR TREATING NEOPLASTIC DISORDERS: CELL CYCLE-NONSPECIFIC DRUGS

1. Cell cycle-nonspecific drugs kill cells regardless of their phase in the cell cycle. This nonspecificity is why these drugs are considered more toxic than cell cycle-specific drugs. They should be avoided in pregnancy.

2. Cyclophosphamide is an alkylating agent that is derived from nitrogen mustard. When the liver metabolizes cyclophosphamide, it becomes a cytotoxic agent. The active metabolite has broad-spectrum antitumor effects. Cyclophosphamide is used in the treatment of hematologic cancers as well as solid tumors.

3. The dose-limiting adverse effect of cyclophosphamide is leukopenia. Long-term lower dose therapy can cause secondary cancers later in the patient's life. High-dose therapy can cause hemorrhagic cystitis; to prevent this, give the uroprotectant drug, mesna, and hydrate the patient well, before, during, and after therapy.

4. Carmustine, a nitrosoureas drug, is used in the palliative therapy of several disorders. It works by alkylating DNA and RNA and, thus, blocking synthesis and repair.

5. Adverse effects of carmustine include nausea and vomiting, delayed bone marrow suppression (thrombocytopenia and leukopenia 6 weeks after drug administration), and pulmonary toxicity (associated with prolonged therapy and higher cumulative doses). To minimize adverse effects, give antiemetics within 2 hours of treatment, monitor WBC, and prevent infection.

6. Doxorubicin, an antitumor antibiotic, has wide clinical activity, particularly against hematologic cancers and solid tumors. Doxorubicin blocks the synthesis of RNA and DNA. Doxorubicin also binds to nucleic acids, causing destruction and prolonged tissue damage.

7. Adverse effects of doxorubicin are acute (nausea, vomiting, bone marrow suppression, mucositis, alopecia, and other cutaneous reactions), chronic (cardiotoxicity, the dose-limiting toxicity; cumulative dose influences cardiotoxicity; children and older adults are more susceptible), and local (extravasation injury and radiation recall). To minimize adverse effects, give cardioprotective drugs, like dexrazoxane, with treatment, and prevent extravasation (good IV technique, use large veins, monitor closely during infusion).

8. Tamoxifen, an antiestrogen, is used to treat advanced breast cancer in postmenopausal women. It competes with estrogen for binding sites in tissues and, thus, deprives estrogen-sensitive tumors of estrogen.

9. Most patients do not have adverse effects from short-term use of tamoxifen. The infrequent adverse effects of tamoxifen are related to loss of estrogen's effects (hot flashes, vaginal bleeding or discharge, menstrual irregularities, fluid retention). Possible serious effects are liver abnormalities, which may be fatal, and endometrial cancer (with long-term use). Increased bone and tumor pain (disease flare) are signs of positive tumor response.

10. Combination chemotherapy uses two or more drugs against a tumor. Combination therapy maximizes cell kill, has a broader range of kill, increases duration of remission, and minimizes emergence of cancer cells resistant to chemotherapy. Dosage of each drug can be kept to a minimum, thus decreasing serious toxicities from each drug.

KEY TERMS

Fill in the blanks

Read each statement carefully and, using the chapter's key terms, write your answer in the space provided.

1. Drugs that mimic the actions of radiation therapy on cells are named _____.

2. The _____ and _____ are a diverse group of drugs that are beneficial in treating neoplasms that originate from tissues whose growth is hormonally mediated.

3. To limit the potential toxicities of chemotherapeutic drugs, _____ may be used.

4. Cytoxin, a type of _____ drug, has a broad spectrum of antitumor activity.

5. _____ are a subcategory of the alkylating drugs, which are highly lipid soluble.

6. *Streptomyces* bacteria broths are the etiology of most _____.

7. A positive tumor response to drug therapy may be indicated by a local _____.

8. Antineoplastic drugs that are not limited to a specific phase in the cell's life cycle are called _____.

9. The most commonly used _____ is doxorubicin.

10. _____ occurs within 24 hours of receiving chemotherapy.

11. Vomiting 5 days after chemotherapy is referred to as _____.

12. The _____ is the number of cells that make up the tumor.

13. Drugs that have a high potential for causing severe nausea and vomiting are called _____.

CORE DRUG KNOWLEDGE: JUST THE FACTS

Multiple choice

Circle the option that best answers the question or completes the statement.

1. Pharmacotherapeutics for cyclophosphamide (Cytoxan) include all of the following EXCEPT
   a. uterine cancer.
   b. hematologic cancers.
   c. stem cell transplantation.
   d. pancreatic cancer.

2. In addition to hematopoietic abnormalities, adverse effects associated with high-dose cyclophosphamide (Cytoxan) therapy include
   a. sterile hemorrhagic cystitis and diabetes insipidus.
   b. nephrotoxicity and diabetes insipidus.
   c. ototoxicity and CNS sedation.
   d. syndrome of inappropriate antidiuretic hormone (SIADH) and hemorrhagic cystitis.

3. Patients receiving cyclophosphamide (Cytoxan) should be informed for the potential development of
   a. secondary malignancies.
   b. excessive hair growth.
   c. gray-colored skin.
   d. gout.

4. Patients receiving PO cyclophosphamide (Cytoxan) should be advised to
   a. limit fluids to 4 glasses per day.
   b. increase ingestion of green leafy vegetables.
   c. increase fluid consumption to 10 to 12 glasses per day.
   d. decrease intake of sodium.

5. Cisplatin (*cis*-platinum) is well known for its ability to cause
   a. hair loss.
   b. nausea and vomiting.
   c. hyperkalemia.
   d. sedation.

6. Pharmacotherapeutics for carmustine (BCNU) include
   a. uterine cancer.
   b. brain tumors.
   c. pancreatic cancer.
   d. breast cancer.

7. Doxorubicin given in a liposome formulation change the _____ of the drug.
   a. pharmacotherapeutics
   b. pharmacokinetics
   c. pharmacodynamics
   d. contraindications

8. Patients receiving doxorubicin (Adriamycin) should be monitored frequently for
   a. CNS depression.
   b. respiratory depression.
   c. thrombophlebitis.
   d. extravasation.

9. The major limiting factor of doxorubicin (Adriamycin) therapy is
   a. hepatotoxicity.
   b. nephrotoxicity.
   c. neurotoxicity.
   d. cardiotoxicity.

10. The major limiting factor of bleomycin (Blenoxane) therapy is
    a. pulmonary toxicity.
    b. cardiotoxicity.
    c. nephrotoxicity.
    d. hepatotoxicity.

11. First-line therapy for advanced breast cancer in postmenopausal women is
    a. bleomycin (Blenoxane).
    b. tamoxifen (Nolvadex).
    c. streptozocin (Zanosar).
    d. cisplatin (Platinol).

12. In the treatment of breast cancer, tamoxifen (Nolvadex) works by
    a. increasing estrogen reception at receptor sites.
    b. decreasing androgen reception at receptor sites.
    c. inhibiting DNA synthesis in tumor cells.
    d. depriving estrogen-sensitive tumors of estrogen.

13. Which of the following statements concerning adverse effects of tamoxifen (Nolvadex) therapy is correct?
    a. There are many adverse effects, and most are very significant.
    b. There are few adverse effects, but all are very significant.
    c. There are few adverse effects, and they are modest.
    d. There are many adverse effects, and most are life threatening.

14. Although each cycle cell nonspecific drug has different dose-limiting factors, they all have a potential common adverse effect that requires frequent monitoring of
    a. CBC.
    b. liver enzymes.
    c. pulmonary function tests.
    d. renal function.

CORE PATIENT VARIABLES: PATIENTS, PLEASE

Multiple choice

Circle the option that best answers the question or completes the statement.

1. Kenny Tijion, age 27, is prescribed cyclophosphamide (Cytoxan). Mr. Tijion states, "What type of reaction will I probably have to this drug?" Which of the following is the best response?
   a. "Your hair will probably fall out, almost right away."
   b. "You will probably experience nausea and vomiting."
   c. "This drug causes severe constipation."
   d. "Probably none."

2. Mr. Tijion is receiving cyclophosphamide (Cytoxan). He complains of dizziness, nasal stuffiness, and rhinorrhea. What is your best action?
   a. stop the infusion immediately
   b. give diphenhydramine (Benadryl) IVP
   c. slow the infusion rate
   d. a and b

3. Your patient is to receive cyclophosphamide (Cytoxan). To administer this drug safely, the nurse should
   a. prehydrate the patient orally and intravenously with at least 1 to 2 L of normal saline solution with potassium and magnesium additives.
   b. keep the patient NPO until the solution is infused.
   c. prehydrate the patient with tap water.
   d. decrease fluid ingestion 24 hours before administration of cyclophosphamide.

4. Which of the following patients has an increased risk for adverse effects if given carmustine (BCNU) therapy? Patients with
   a. cardiovascular disorders
   b. pulmonary disorders
   c. integumentary disorders
   d. CNS disorders

5. Benny Falk is receiving carmustine (BCNU). He complains of an intense burning sensation at his IV site. What should you do?
   a. Increase the rate of infusion and bring an ice compress.
   b. Increase the rate of infusion and bring a warm compress.
   c. Decrease the rate of infusion and bring a warm compress.
   d. Decrease the rate of infusion and bring an ice compress.

6. Susan Bevins had chemotherapy and radiation therapy 6 months ago. Today, she comes to the clinic with a complaint of blisters, swelling, and skin loss at the site of her cancer. After reviewing her chart, you note that she received doxorubicin (Adriamycin). With your knowledge of this drug, you suspect Mrs. Bevins is experiencing
   a. a delayed hypersensitivity.
   b. chemotherapy extravasation.
   c. radiation recall.
   d. a routine sunburn.

7. Mary Redler, age 66, is receiving doxorubicin (Adriamycin) therapy. To minimize the potential for cardiotoxicity, Mrs. Redler has been prescribed dexrazoxane (Zinecard). The nurse should administer dexrazoxane
   a. 3 hours after completion of doxorubicin infusion.
   b. 24 hours before initiation of doxorubicin infusion.
   c. 30 minutes before initiation of doxorubicin infusion.
   d. 1 hour after completion of doxorubicin infusion.

8. Which of the following instructions should be given to Mrs. Redler concerning doxorubicin (Adriamycin) therapy?
   a. "You may feel very sleepy after therapy."
   b. "This drug may turn your urine a reddish color."
   c. "Many patients have intractable hiccups after therapy."
   d. "Some patients may experience a floating sensation during therapy."

9. Michael Linde comes to the clinic for a follow-up visit after carmustine (BCNU) therapy 3 weeks ago. Mr. Linde states he feels "OK" but now feels better knowing that his CBC is not abnormal. Which of the following statements is most appropriate?
   a. "We need to continue to check your lab values because this drug can cause bone marrow suppression weeks after administration."
   b. "You can see your regular doctor in 6 months now."
   c. "You are one of the lucky ones, but it's best to get rechecked in a few months."
   d. "This drug doesn't usually affect the results of your CBC."

10. Allison Bennet takes digoxin (Lanoxin) for atrial fibrillation. Ms. Bennet has lymphoma and is prescribed carmustine (BCNU). During therapy, Ms. Bennet's digoxin dose may need to be
    a. increased.
    b. decreased.
    c. unchanged.

NURSING MANAGEMENT: EVERY GOOD NURSE SHOULD . . .

Multiple choice

Circle the option that best answers the question or completes the statement.

1. Louis Breckstein, 68 years old, has small-cell lung cancer and is receiving cyclophosphamide, an alkylating agent, as treatment. To minimize adverse effects from the cyclophosphamide, the nurse should
   a. administer diuretics to increase urinary output.
   b. prehydrate with 1 to 2 L of normal saline with potassium and magnesium.
   c. administer an aminoglycoside antibiotic.
   d. limit dietary potassium and magnesium.

2. Herminie Nunez, 43 years old, is to receive long-term cyclophosphamide therapy to treat her chronic leukemia. Which of the following should be included in her teaching?

   a. She may experience amenorrhea.

   b. Nausea, vomiting, and anorexia are possible adverse effects.

   c. A secondary malignancy is possible later in life.

   d. all of the above

   e. none of the above

3. Lee Ann is 8 years old and receiving doxorubicin to treat leukemia. To minimize adverse effects, the nurse should

   a. use a small, peripheral vein to administer doxorubicin.

   b. offer aspirin to relieve discomforts from drug administration.

   c. monitor for rales and dyspnea.

   d. monitor for reddish-colored urine.

4. Hilary Rosemblum is 58 years old and has right breast cancer. She is receiving tamoxifen. She complains of bone pain and pain in her right breast. The most appropriate action of the nurse is to

   a. hold the next dose of tamoxifen.

   b. decrease the next dose of tamoxifen.

   c. administer the next dose of tamoxifen as ordered.

   d. contact the physician immediately.

5. Glynda Thomas is receiving carmustine, a nitrosoureas, as treatment for a brain tumor. She returns in 6 weeks for a second treatment. Before administering the next dose, the nurse should check Glynda's

   a. weight.

   b. blood pressure.

   c. platelets.

   d. BUN.

6. You are to administer IV doxorubicin. Before starting the infusion, you should

   a. verify patency of IV site.

   b. apply ice to the arm.

   c. apply a tourniquet above the IV insertion site.

   d. massage the vein.

CASE STUDY

Selma Goldberg, 47 years old, has been diagnosed with ovarian cancer. She is to receive the following chemotherapy:

Doxorubicin 60 mg/m^2 IV every 21 days
Cyclophosphamide 300 mg/m^2 IV on day 1 every 4 weeks

1. What is the rationale for two different antineoplastic drugs being ordered?

2. Describe the adverse effects that Selma is most likely to experience while on these two drugs.

CRITICAL THINKING CHALLENGE

When Selma returns to restart the drug cycle, she has diagnostic tests done before the next doses of doxorubicin and cyclophosphamide. The findings include

BUN	20
Creatinine	1.2
Platelets	101,000
WBC	4,200
SGOT	33
SGPT	33
ECG	normal sinus rhythm

1. What is your evaluation of the combined chemotherapy up to this date?

2. Should you administer the next doses of cyclophosphamide and doxorubicin?

Antimicrobial Drugs

CHAPTER 47

Principles of Antimicrobial Therapy

TOP TEN THINGS TO KNOW ABOUT THE PRINCIPLES OF ANTIMICROBIAL THERAPY

1. Antimicrobial drugs are classified by their susceptible organism or by their mechanism of action.
2. Antimicrobials work in six ways. They inhibit: bacterial cell wall synthesis, protein synthesis, nucleic acid synthesis, metabolic pathways, and viral enzymes. Lastly, they disrupt cell membrane permeability.
3. Selective toxicity is the ability of a drug to suppress or kill an infecting microbe without harming the patient's cells.
4. Microbes develop resistance to antimicrobial therapy due to production of drug-inactivating enzymes, changes in receptor structure, changes in drug permeation and transport, development of alternative metabolic pathways, emergence of drug-resistant microbes, and antimicrobial usage that facilitates the development of resistance.
5. Resistance is more likely to occur from the use of broad-spectrum drugs. Resistance is facilitated if the drug dose is too low, the time between doses is too long, therapy stops too soon, or the drug is used prophylactically.
6. Four important antibiotic-resistant microbes are methicillin-resistant *Staphylococcus aureus* (MRSA), penicillin-resistant *Streptococcus pneumoniae*, vancomycin-resistant *Enterococci* (VRE), and multiple drug-resistant *Mycobacterium tuberculosis*.

7. Drug selection to treat an infection is based on identification of the pathogen, drug susceptibility, drug spectrum, drug dose, duration of therapy, site of infection, and patient assessment.
8. Gram staining and culturing determine the organism, whereas a sensitivity test determines which antimicrobials are effective in killing the organism. Culture and sensitivity tests should be done before administration of any antimicrobial drug.
9. Empiric therapy or broad-spectrum drugs may be used before an organism has been identified. Combination drug therapy is often used initially for severe infections, or for mixed infections. There are advantages and disadvantages to combination therapy.
10. The patient's response to drug therapy (positive and negative) should be assessed carefully. For drug therapy that may cause serious adverse effects, monitor serum drug levels, peak and trough levels, and other relevant lab values. Individualize monitoring based on the patient, the drug therapy, and the infecting microbe.

CHAPTER 48

Antibiotics Affecting the Bacterial Cell Wall

TOP TEN THINGS TO KNOW ABOUT ANTIBIOTICS AFFECTING THE BACTERIAL CELL WALL

1. Drugs that affect the bacterial cell wall permeate the cell wall and bind to molecular targets on the cytoplasmic membrane in the cell. They then disrupt the strength of the cell wall. This permits the high oncotic pressure inside the cell to draw fluid into the cell. Fluid is drawn in until the cell bursts. The patient's immune system cleans up the debris and fights any remaining infection.

2. Penicillins were the first antibiotics used clinically. Penicillins are also called beta-lactam antibiotics because their chemical structure contains a beta-lactam ring, which is needed for antibacterial action. Some penicillins also have an additional side chain in their chemical structure, which gives different properties to the drug.

3. Penicillins may be narrow spectrum, broad spectrum, or extended spectrum; they may also be penicillinase resistant.

4. Penicillin G, the prototype penicillin, is a narrow-spectrum, bactericidal drug that is effective against mostly gram-positive organisms. It is most commonly given intravenously (IV). The most serious adverse effect is allergic reactions. Most common adverse effects are gastrointestinal (GI). For optimum effectiveness, administer doses around the clock. Assess patients carefully, especially during first dose, for allergic reactions.

5. Patients allergic to one penicillin should be considered allergic to all penicillins. Carbapenems also have a beta-lactam ring structure and may create a cross-sensitivity in patients allergic to a penicillin. Monobactam antibiotics have a significantly different chemical structure from other beta-lactams and are safe to give to penicillin-allergic patients.

6. Cephalosporins are similar to penicillins in structure and activity. Four generations of cephalosporins have been introduced, each with a different spectrum of activity. Cephalosporins are the most commonly prescribed antibiotics; this is leading to cephalosporin-resistant bacteria.

7. Cefazolin, the prototype cephalosporin, is a first-generation drug. Patients allergic to penicillin may have cross-sensitivity to cefazolin. Most frequent adverse effects are hypersensitivity and GI; nephrotoxicity is possible and is more likely if the patient also receives aminoglycoside antibiotics. Acute alcohol intolerance (disulfiramlike reaction) may occur as an interaction of cefazolin and alcohol.

8. If penicillins or cephalosporins are given intramuscularly (IM), use a deep muscle, and verify anatomic landmarks carefully to avoid accidental intravessel administration.

9. Vancomycin, a tricyclic glycopeptide antibiotic, is the only drug in its class. In addition to altering the bacterial cell wall, it also inhibits the synthesis of RNA. Because of serious toxicity, vancomycin is used only in serious infections when other antibiotics have failed. Vancomycin-resistant *Enterococcus* (VRE) is becoming a common problem.

10. Vancomycin has adverse effects of nephrotoxicity, ototoxicity, and significant histamine release (resulting in anaphylactoid reactions and "red-man" or "red-neck" syndrome). Administer drug slowly IV (at least over 60 minutes), and avoid extravasation. Monitor peak and trough levels and hepatic and renal function. Assess for change in balance and hearing loss.

KEY TERMS

Matching

Match the following key terms with their definitions:

1. _____ bacterial cell envelope

2. _____ beta-lactam

3. _____ beta-lactamases

4. _____ cephalosporinases

5. _____ penicillinases

6. _____ penicillin-binding proteins

a. Composed of a thick cell wall and cytoplasmic membrane

b. Enzymes that inactivate penicillin

c. Located inside the bacterial cell wall

d. Active chemical structure of many antibiotics

e. Enzymes that inactivate cephalosporins

f. Enzymes that disrupt the beta-lactam ring

CORE DRUG KNOWLEDGE: JUST THE FACTS

Multiple choice

Circle the option that best answers the question or completes the statement.

1. Which of the following classes of antibiotics is MOST likely to induce an allergic reaction?
   a. aminoglycosides
   b. macrolides
   c. penicillins
   d. cephalosporins

2. Generally speaking, penicillin G is INEFFECTIVE in the management of
   a. most gram-negative bacteria infections.
   b. gram-positive anaerobic infections.
   c. gram-positive spirochete infections.
   d. endocarditis prophylaxis.

3. Which of the following routes is INAPPROPRIATE for administration of penicillin?
   a. PO
   b. SC
   c. IM
   d. IV

4. Before the administration of penicillin, it is important to
   a. check the CBC results.
   b. determine if any previous reactions to antibiotics have occurred.
   c. ask the patient to void.
   d. check the patient's pregnancy status.

5. Repository forms of penicillin G include
   a. penicillin VK.
   b. penicillin G potassium.
   c. penicillin G sodium.
   d. procaine penicillin G.

6. Penicillin has a cross sensitivity to which of the following drug classes?
   a. aminoglycosides
   b. cephalosporins
   c. erythromycins
   d. tetracyclines

7. In contrast to narrow-spectrum penicillins, aminopenicillins such as amoxicillin (Amoxil) have increased effectiveness against
   a. gram-negative bacteria infections.
   b. gram-positive anaerobic infections.
   c. gram-positive spirochete infections.
   d. endocarditis prophylaxis.

8. Extended-spectrum penicillins are extremely effective against
   a. gonorrhea.
   b. *Streptococcus*.
   c. *Pseudomonas*.
   d. *Staphylococcus*.

9. Beta-lactamase inhibitors are given in conjunction with penicillin to
   a. change the protein binding sites.
   b. increase the spectrum of activity.
   c. target the enzyme that may destroy penicillin.
   d. decrease the potential for adverse effects.

10. A benefit of aztreonam (Azactam) therapy is that it
    a. has increased spectrum of activity.
    b. may be used in penicillin-allergic patients.
    c. has decreased potential for adverse effects.
    d. has decreased potential for drug–drug interactions.

11. What is the difference between imipenem (Primaxin) and meropenem (Merrem)?

    a. Meropenem has a narrow spectrum of activity, and imipenem does not.

    b. Imipenem has a narrow spectrum of activity, and meropenem does not.

    c. Meropenem is easily inactivated and must be administered with cilastatin.

    d. Imipenem is easily inactivated and must be administered with cilastatin.

12. What is the major difference between the different "generations" of cephalosporin agents?

    a. pharmacodynamics

    b. spectrum of activity

    c. emergence of drug resistance

    d. ability to induce allergic responses

13. Generally speaking, cephalosporin antibiotics should be taken for

    a. 7 to 10 days.

    b. 2 to 3 days.

    c. 1 to 5 days.

    d. 10 to 21 days.

14. Hypersensitivity to cephalosporins frequently presents with

    a. shortness of breath.

    b. hives.

    c. nausea and vomiting.

    d. maculopapular rash.

15. Vancomycin is used in the management of

    a. sexually transmitted diseases.

    b. urinary tract infection.

    c. serious systemic bacterial infections.

    d. cellulitis.

16. The most serious adverse effects to vancomycin are

    a. sinus tachycardia and hypotension.

    b. ototoxicity and nephrotoxicity.

    c. hepatotoxicity and neurotoxicity.

    d. histamine release and phlebitis.

CORE PATIENT VARIABLES, PATIENTS, PLEASE

Multiple choice

Circle the option that best answers the question or completes the statement.

1. Chelsea Lincoln is prescribed penicillin V for a dental infection. Which of the following instructions would you give?

    a. "Take the medication with food for best results."

    b. "Although it is ordered QID, you can double the dose and take it BID."

    c. "You can take it every other day if you experience GI distress."

    d. "Take the medication 1 hour before or 2 hours after a meal."

2. Yancy Jones, age 86, has pneumonia and is prescribed penicillin. Mr. Jones has a history of renal insufficiency. Which of the following lab tests should be done before initiating therapy?

    a. pulmonary function tests

    b. BUN and creatinine

    c. ALT and AST

    d. urinalysis

3. Quincy Redler is hospitalized with bacteremia. He is prescribed IV penicillin G and gentamicin. How would you administer these drugs?

    a. Wait at least 2 hours between administration of these drugs.

    b. Wait 30 minutes between administration of these drugs.

    c. Administer each drug on an alternate day.

    d. Administer the first drug, flush the tubing, then administer the second drug.

4. Jack Palmer comes to the clinic and is diagnosed with an infection. When asked about allergies, Mr. Palmer stated, "I have an allergy to penicillin, but I can take ampicillin." With your knowledge about these drugs, you know that

    a. this is a possibility because they are two different types of penicillins.

    b. Mr. Palmer should not take any form of drug with "cillin" in its name if he has an allergy to penicillin.

    c. as long as they are not taken together, it is all right for Mr. Palmer to take either drug.

    d. none of the above.

5. Danny Gillespie has just received an injection of IM procaine penicillin. Within 30 seconds, he became confused and agitated and ran from the exam room. You suspect
   a. Mr. Gillespie has been taking some type of illicit drugs.
   b. an allergy to penicillin.
   c. a toxic response of penicillin.
   d. a procaine reaction.

6. Hannah Clark is being treated with cefazolin and gentamicin. Because of this combination, Mrs. Clark has an increased risk for
   a. cardiotoxicity.
   b. hepatotoxicity.
   c. ototoxicity.
   d. nephrotoxicity.

7. Jim Verlan takes warfarin for deep vein thrombosis (DVT) prophylaxis. He has recurrent cellulitis in his leg and is prescribed cefixime (Suprax). You would anticipate Mr. Verlan's warfarin dose to be
   a. increased.
   b. decreased.
   c. unchanged.

8. Geoffrey Baines has an order for IV cefazolin (Kefzol). As you take the medication out of the refrigerator, you note that the solution was reconstituted yesterday. You should
   a. allow the solution to warm for 15 minutes, then administer.
   b. give the infusion now.
   c. call the pharmacy and have a replacement sent.
   d. warm the solution in the microwave, then administer.

9. Frieda Williams has been receiving IV cefazolin for the past 24 hours, and the next dose is now due. You note that the culture and sensitivity test has returned and reports that her infection is resistant to cephalosporins. You should
   a. hang the cefazolin, and write a note in the progress notes.
   b. hang the cefazolin.
   c. hold the cefazolin, contact the health care provider, and get an order for a new antibiotic.
   d. Hold the cefazolin, and tell the next shift to discuss the test results with the doctor when he or she makes rounds in the evening.

10. Nelson Olson is receiving vancomycin therapy. To minimize adverse effects, the health care provider has ordered peak-and-trough blood levels. When is the optimal time for you to obtain the peak blood level?
    a. 30 minutes before the next infusion
    b. 20 minutes after the onset of the infusion
    c. 1 hour before the next infusion
    d. 1 hour after the completion of the infusion

11. Michael Richards is scheduled to receive IV vancomycin. To safely administer this medication, the nurse should infuse it
    a. over 20 minutes.
    b. over 60 minutes.
    c. over 2 to 3 hours.
    d. within 10 minutes.

12. Lillian Fields is ordered to have vancomycin PO. Mrs. Fields states, "My friend had this drug, but she got it in her veins. Isn't that a better way to get it?" What is your response?
    a. "Since your problem is in your GI system, giving the drug this way will have a localized action on the gut."
    b. "Why don't you ask the doctor that question."
    c. "I'm sure your friend received a different drug."
    d. "I have no idea."

NURSING MANAGEMENT: EVERY GOOD NURSE SHOULD . . .

Multiple choice

Circle the option that best answers the question or completes the statement.

1. Which of the following will maximize the therapeutic effect of penicillin G?
   a. administer with milk
   b. administer the doses only during normal waking hours
   c. administer IV forms directly out of the refrigerator
   d. administer the drug for at least 2 days after patient feels better

2. Joe Scott is to be discharged on cefazolin, a cephalosporin. The nurse should teach Mr. Scott to avoid which of the following while on drug therapy?

   a. wine

   b. potassium chloride elixirs (such as Kay Ciel)

   c. cough medicine

   d. all of the above

   e. none of the above

3. Armand Perez, 23 years old, is receiving vancomycin as treatment of endocarditis. To minimize adverse effects from the drug therapy, the nurse should administer the drug by

   a. IV push.

   b. slow IV infusion.

   c. subcutaneous injection.

   d. oral route.

4. You are to administer the first IV dose of penicillin G to Rosalie Abramson, 64 years old, to treat her pneumonia. To minimize adverse effects, you should

   a. determine if a sputum culture and sensitivity has been obtained.

   b. ask her if she has any drug allergies.

   c. monitor her closely during drug administration.

   d. do all of the above.

   e. do none of the above.

5. You are to administer procaine penicillin to a patient in the outpatient department who has syphilis. To maximize therapeutic effects and minimize adverse effects, you should

   a. administer into the deltoid muscle.

   b. keep in the refrigerator until time of administration.

   c. locate anatomic landmarks to determine the injection site.

   d. do all of the above.

   e. do none of the above.

6. Gloria Trotter, 33 years old, has a mixed infection and is receiving cefazolin, a cephalosporin, and gentamicin, an aminoglycoside antibiotic. To minimize adverse effects, the nurse should most closely monitor which lab value?

   a. hematocrit

   b. aPTT

   c. BUN

   d. cefazolin blood levels

CASE STUDY

Marion Maraglia, 42 years old, is receiving vancomycin 1 g IV every 6 hours for osteomyelitis. This morning, she fell while going to the bathroom. She is not injured. As you help her back to bed, she laughs a little and says to you, "I don't know what came over me. I'm acting like I'm tipsy." Later, you hear her complain to the housekeeper that there must be crickets in her room, because she keeps hearing little noises. The housekeeper checks the room carefully and assures her there are no crickets in the room.

1. What assessment do you make of these incidents?

2. Are there any additional data you would like to help confirm your assessment?

CRITICAL THINKING CHALLENGE

After obtaining an order, you have a peak-and-trough level drawn around the next scheduled dose of vancomycin. The results are trough = 12 μg/mL; peak = 65 μg/mL.

1. What is your assessment of these lab findings?

2. What action would you take based on your assessment?

CHAPTER 49

Drugs Affecting Protein Synthesis

TOP TEN THINGS TO KNOW ABOUT DRUGS AFFECTING PROTEIN SYNTHESIS

1. Drugs that affect protein synthesis in the bacteria may be either bactericidal or bacteriostatic. These drugs are usually reserved for serious infections. Superinfections may occur with the use of these drugs.

2. Gentamicin, an aminoglycoside, works by entering the bacterial cell and binding to ribosomes; this causes the cell to produce amino acids that do not link correctly, thus preventing bacterial reproduction, weakening the cell wall, leading to cell wall rupture and death. Many bacteria can resist all aminoglycosides from entering their cells; to overcome this, gentamicin is often given with other antibiotics to increase their effectiveness or alter the cell wall, allowing the gentamicin to enter.

3. Gentamicin is reserved for serious infections due to severe adverse effects of nephrotoxicity, ototoxicity, neurotoxicity, and others. Monitor drug peak and trough levels to dose appropriately and prevent adverse effects.

4. Clindamycin, a lincosamide, is used to treat serious to life-threatening infections. It works by entering the bacterial cell, binding to bacterial ribosomes, suppressing protein synthesis, and causing cell death. Most common adverse effects are gastrointestinal (GI); serious adverse effects are pseudomembranous colitis and blood abnormalities.

5. Erythromycin, a macrolide, inhibits RNA-dependent protein synthesis at the chain elongation step. This either prevents the cell from dividing or causes cell death. It is the drug of choice for penicillin-allergic patients. Absorption is diminished by food, dairy products, and antacids. Causes frequent GI distress even if given intravenously (IV). IV infusions are very irritating to the veins, so administer very slowly.

6. Linezolid, an oxazolidinone, was developed to treat methicillin-resistant *Staphylococcus aureus* (MRSA) infections; it is also used to treat vancomycin-resistant *Enterococcus* (VRE) infections. Approval may be required from the infectious disease department or committee before the drug is administered to a patient. Linezolid blocks the early stages of protein synthesis, unlike other antibiotics;

this may prevent the development of resistance and cross resistance. Linezolid also is a monoamine oxidase (MAO) inhibitor. Drug–food interactions can be serious; avoid foods with tyramine, caffeine, and alcohol. Most common adverse effects are GI.

7. Quinupristin/dalfopristin are the only streptogramins and are marketed as a combination drug. Quinupristin/dalfopristin are used to treat life-threatening VRE infections ("superbugs"). Approval may be required from the infectious disease department or committee before the drug is administered to a patient. Quinupristin/dalfopristin irreversibly blocks ribosome functioning, thus inhibiting protein synthesis. Quinupristin/dalfopristin is a potent inhibitor of P450, so many drug interactions are possible. Administer by IV infusion, preferably through a central line. Flush lines with 5% dextrose and water only.

8. Tetracycline, one of the tetracyclines, retards bacterial growth by inhibiting protein synthesis and preventing cell division and replication. It is used to treat a variety of serious infections (e.g., Rocky Mountain spotted fever) when penicillin cannot be used, and to treat acne vulgaris, and chlamydia. Overuse is leading to resistance. Dairy products and antacids interfere with the absorption of tetracycline.

9. Adverse effects of tetracycline include GI (most common), photosensitivity (advise patients to stay out of direct sunlight), and mottling and discoloration of developing teeth (avoid use in pregnancy and in children younger than 8 years old).

10. Chloramphenicol has a broad range of activity but is reserved for serious infections where other antibiotics have been ineffective. Chloramphenicol inhibits protein synthesis in both bacterial and human cells. Life-threatening adverse effects include "gray-baby syndrome" (newborns get progressive blue-gray skin and vasomotor collapse), blood dyscrasias, and reversible or nonreversible bone marrow depression (dose-related or non–dose-related). Serious adverse effects are optic neuritis (blindness) and peripheral neuritis. Monitor drug levels.

KEY TERMS

Matching

Match the following key terms with their definitions:

1. _____ azotemia
2. _____ cylindruria
3. _____ hyposthenuria
4. _____ nephrotoxicity
5. _____ ototoxicity
6. _____ peak and trough
7. _____ proteinuria
8. _____ pyuria
9. _____ xeroderma
10. _____ xerophthalmia

a. Pus in the urine
b. Adverse effect affecting the kidneys
c. Determines if drug levels remain therapeutic
d. Casts in the urine
e. Dryness of the skin
f. Excessive urea levels in the blood
g. Dryness of the conjunctiva
h. Loss of the ability to concentrate urine
i. Adverse effect affecting hearing
j. Protein in the urine

CORE DRUG KNOWLEDGE: JUST THE FACTS

Multiple choice

Circle the option that best answers the question or completes the statement.

1. Patients with aminoglycoside therapy should be monitored for
   a. cardiotoxicity and nephrotoxicity.
   b. ototoxicity and nephrotoxicity.
   c. peripheral neuropathy and cardiotoxicity.
   d. hepatotoxicity and ototoxicity.

2. What is the correct time to obtain a trough level of gentamicin?
   a. 30 minutes after IM administration
   b. 60 minutes after IV administration
   c. 2 hours before the next dose
   d. 30 minutes before the next dose

3. Which of the following statements concerning drug–drug interactions with gentamicin is correct? There are:
   a. many interactions, and most are very significant.
   b. many interactions, and most are insignificant.
   c. very few interactions, and most are significant.
   d. very few interactions, and most are insignificant.

4. The appropriate route of administration for neomycin is
   a. oral.
   b. subcutaneous.
   c. intramuscular.
   d. intravenous.

5. Clindamycin is reserved for the management of
   a. severe systemic gram-positive bacteria.
   b. severe systemic gram-negative bacteria.
   c. infections by bacteria with known sensitivity.
   d. anaerobes only.

6. Although clindamycin is reserved for serious infections, topical clindamycin is useful in the treatment of
   a. hives.
   b. Stevens-Johnson syndrome.
   c. acne vulgaris.
   d. pruritus.

7. Clindamycin is associated with the development of
   a. hearing loss.
   b. pseudomembranous colitis.
   c. azotemia.
   d. migraine headaches.

8. The antibiotic class of choice for penicillin-allergic patients is
   a. cephalosporins.
   b. macrolides.
   c. fluoroquinolones.
   d. aminoglycosides.

9. The most common adverse effects of erythromycin affect the _____ system.
   a. central nervous
   b. respiratory
   c. hematopoietic
   d. GI

10. A benefit of clarithromycin therapy is
    a. BID dosing.
    b. less expensive than erythromycin.
    c. alternate-day dosing.
    d. all of the above.

11. Linezolid (Zyvox) is indicated for use in the management of
    a. pseudomembranous colitis.
    b. bacterial meningitis.
    c. methicillin-resistant *Staphylococcus aureus*.
    d. all of the above.

12. The pharmacokinetics of linezolid (Zyvox) is unusual in that
    a. the oral formulation has a duration twice as long as the IV formulation.
    b. the oral formulation has 100% bioavailability.
    c. the IV formulation has 98% bioavailability.
    d. the IV onset is longer than the PO onset.

13. The most common adverse effects associated with the use of linezolid (Zyvox) include
    a. pseudomembranous colitis.
    b. rebound hypertension.
    c. diarrhea, headache, nausea, and vomiting.
    d. constipation.

14. Quinupristin/dalfopristin (Synercid) is indicated for the management of
    a. brain abscesses.
    b. pseudomembranous colitis.
    c. trichomoniasis.
    d. vancomycin-resistant *Enterococcus*.

15. Potential serious adverse effects to quinupristin/dalfopristin (Synercid) include all of the following EXCEPT
    a. pseudomembranous colitis.
    b. superinfection.
    c. vancomycin-resistant *Enterococcus*.
    d. hepatotoxicity.

16. During quinupristin/dalfopristin (Synercid) therapy, the nurse should arrange for which of the following lab tests?
    a. hepatic function and bilirubin
    b. complete blood count (CBC) and renal function
    c. hepatic and renal function
    d. hepatic function and CBC

17. To maximize the absorption of tetracycline, the patient should avoid concurrent administration of
    a. antacids containing calcium.
    b. fluids.
    c. corticosteroids.
    d. all of the above.

18. Adverse reactions to tetracycline include
    a. increased ocular pressure.
    b. photosensitivity.
    c. cardiac arrhythmias.
    d. kidney stones.

19. Use of outdated tetracycline may induce
    a. bronchospasm.
    b. CNS sedation.
    c. exfoliative rash.
    d. renal failure.

20. Chloramphenicol is the drug of choice in the treatment of
    a. methicillin-resistant *Staphylococcus aureus*.
    b. serious systemic fungal infections.
    c. brain abscesses.
    d. urinary tract infections.

21. A serious adverse effect associated with chloramphenicol therapy in newborn infants is
    a. gray-baby syndrome.
    b. red-neck syndrome.
    c. pseudomembranous colitis.
    d. hypotension.

22. In an adult, a frequent serious adverse effect associated with chloramphenicol therapy is
    a. hepatic insufficiency.
    b. diverticulitis.
    c. CNS depression.
    d. aplastic anemia.

CORE PATIENT VARIABLES: PATIENTS, PLEASE

Multiple choice

Circle the option that best answers the question or completes the statement.

1. Justine Black is receiving IV gentamicin (Garamycin) therapy. After the blood tech draws a specimen, Ms. Black asks, "Why are they taking so much blood?" Which of the following is the best response?

   a. "They want to be sure that this is the right drug for you."

   b. "It is important to keep gentamicin level within a certain range to avoid adverse effects."

   c. "The lab frequently makes mistakes and has to redraw the specimen."

   d. "They are really only taking a little bit each time."

2. Your patient has been receiving IV gentamicin (Garamycin) for the past 2 days. She is scheduled for surgery today. To ensure the patient's safety, the nurse should

   a. be sure to tape a note to the front of the chart documenting the administration of gentamicin.

   b. refrain from giving any benzodiazepine as a preoperative medication.

   c. refrain from giving any anticholinergic before surgery.

   d. ask the anesthesiologist for an increased dose of premedication.

3. Your patient is to start PO clindamycin. To maximize the therapeutic effects of the drug, the nurse should administer the first dose

   a. on an empty stomach.

   b. with a high-fat meal.

   c. with small, frequent meals.

   d. with grapefruit juice.

4. Your patient is using clindamycin lotion on her skin. She complains that the skin is extremely dry. You would suggest

   a. hydration.

   b. moisturizing cream.

   c. hydration and moisturizing cream.

   d. soaking in a bathtub.

5. Leslie Reynolds, age 66, is hospitalized with serious infection and is receiving IV clindamycin. Mrs. Reynolds should be monitored for which of the following symptoms?

   a. rash

   b. facial rigidity

   c. respiratory depression

   d. blood-tinged diarrhea

6. Barbara Venture, age 55, has had type 1 diabetes since age 12. She experiences diabetic gastroparesis. Which of the following drugs may be helpful in this disorder?

   a. cefixime

   b. neomycin

   c. erythromycin

   d. lincomycin

7. Zachary Miller has asthma and takes theophylline. He has an acute exacerbation of bronchitis and is prescribed erythromycin. Zachary should be monitored for

   a. treatment failure of erythromycin.

   b. treatment failure of theophylline.

   c. toxicity of erythromycin.

   d. all of the above.

8. Your patient has an order for IV erythromycin. To safely administer this medication, the nurse should

   a. dilute with sterile water and administer refrigerated solutions within 8 hours.

   b. dilute with normal saline and administer nonrefrigerated solutions within 24 hours.

   c. dilute with sterile water and administer refrigerated solutions within 24 hours.

   d. dilute with normal saline and administer nonrefrigerated solutions within 8 hours.

9. During linezolid (Zyvox) therapy, the nurse should assist the patient to choose a diet that limits the intake of

   a. potassium.

   b. sugar.

   c. salt.

   d. tyramine.

10. Henry Talbot is receiving linezolid (Zyvox) therapy. Despite the attempts by the staff to educate Mr. Talbot to his dietary restrictions, he insists on having food brought in by his wife and family. The nurse should monitor Mr. Talbot's

    a. weight.

    b. lung sounds.

    c. blood pressure.

    d. intake and output.

11. Your patient is scheduled to receive IV quinupristin/dalfopristin (Synercid). To safely administer this medication, the nurse should flush the line with

    a. D_5W.

    b. saline.

    c. heparin.

    d. saline or heparin.

12. The optimal infusion time for IV quinupristin/dalfopristin (Synercid) is

    a. 20 minutes.

    b. 1 hour.

    c. 10 minutes.

    d. 1 minute.

13. Helen Noon has been diagnosed with acne vulgaris and placed on tetracycline therapy. What assessment should be done before initiating therapy?

    a. pregnancy status

    b. blood pressure

    c. skin turgor

    d. temperature

14. Kimberly Payne, age 16, comes to the prenatal clinic crying and states her boyfriend has been diagnosed with chlamydia. His doctor gave him a prescription for doxycycline for both himself and Kimberly. Which of the following statements would be most appropriate?

    a. "Take the medication. Let's gets this resolved before it causes you any discomfort."

    b. "You can take the medication, but be sure you take your prenatal vitamins at least 2 hours after the doxycycline."

    c. "It's best you do not take this medication because it may cause problems with the baby's teeth and bones."

    d. "I would advise against it, but you can do what you wish."

15. Marshall Kelly has recently completed a 10-day series of chemotherapy. He is now diagnosed with bacterial meningitis and is prescribed chloramphenicol. Mr. Kelly should be closely monitored for

    a. bone marrow suppression.

    b. renal toxicity.

    c. ototoxicity.

    d. superinfection.

NURSING MANAGEMENT: EVERY GOOD NURSE SHOULD . . .

Multiple choice

Circle the option that best answers the question or completes the statement.

1. Sam Gerber, 65 years old, is receiving gentamicin, an aminoglycoside, for peritonitis. To minimize adverse effects, the nurse should

    a. monitor intake and output closely.

    b. assess for tinnitus.

    c. assess for loss of balance.

    d. do all of the above.

    e. do none of the above.

2. You are administering IV erythromycin, a macrolide, to your patient to treat bacterial endocarditis. The patient complains of burning during the infusion. The most appropriate initial action of the nurse is to

    a. document that the patient is allergic to erythromycin.

    b. apply a warm compress to the vein.

    c. slow down the rate of the infusion.

    d. remove the IV from the patient.

3. Anna Hoffman, 24 years old, is receiving clindamycin for treatment of pelvic inflammatory disease. She begins to have diarrhea, with loose stools five or six times a day. The nurse should

    a. obtain order for an antidiarrheal.

    b. obtain order for laboratory examination of the stool specimen.

    c. obtain order for a high-roughage diet.

    d. do all of the above.

    e. do none of the above.

4. Olanda Morris, 20 years old, with a 2-year-old child at home, is to be discharged on tetracycline as treatment for a chlamydia infection. Patient education should emphasize which of the following?

   a. Take the drug with milk.

   b. Stop taking the drug when symptoms are gone.

   c. Exposure to sunlight will increase effectiveness of drug.

   d. Keep this drug secured and out of reach of children.

5. Marshall Burns is receiving chloramphenicol for meningitis. For which of the following adverse effects should the nurse withhold administration of the drug and contact the physician?

   a. excessive bruising

   b. elevation of hepatic enzymes

   c. fatigue

   d. all of the above

   e. none of the above

6. You are to administer a dose of quinupristin/dalfopristin to David Hudson for a severe VRE infection. David is NPO and has a peripherally inserted central catheter (PICC) line in his left arm. He also receives diazepam for seizures. The most appropriate nursing action would be to

   a. administer the drug orally.

   b. flush the PICC line before and after the drug is given with D_5W solution.

   c. flush the PICC line after the drug is given with heparin flush solution.

   d. notify the physician that you cannot safely administer this drug.

7. Which of the following foods should a patient who is receiving linezolid avoid?

   a. blue cheese

   b. strawberries

   c. graham crackers

   d. carrots

CASE STUDY

Larry Pearson, 54 years old, has type 1 diabetes. He is known to have diminished renal function. He has developed osteomyelitis after he cut his foot on a piece of glass and it didn't heal. After a culture and sensitivity is done on his foot, it is learned that the infecting organism is resistant to many antibiotics. It is susceptible to gentamicin, and Mr. Pearson is started on this drug therapy. The order reads: Start gentamicin 60 mg Q 8 hours. Peak and trough level after third dose. Pharmacist to follow and adjust dose based on lab work.

1. Consider Mr. Pearson's core patient variables. What core patient variables place Mr. Pearson at additional risk for adverse effects from the gentamicin?

2. Why are peak and trough levels ordered? When should the nurse collect them? Are there any special concerns with collecting peak and trough samples?

CRITICAL THINKING CHALLENGE

You are the nurse administering the first two doses of gentamicin to Mr. Pearson. You know that a peak and trough are ordered around the next dose.

1. What implications does this have on your administration of gentamicin?

2. In addition to administering the drug therapy and monitoring for its effectiveness and adverse effects, are there any other actions you feel are appropriate when caring for Mr. Pearson?

CHAPTER 50

Miscellaneous Antibiotics

TOP TEN THINGS TO KNOW ABOUT MISCELLANEOUS ANTIBIOTICS

1. Miscellaneous antibiotics have a mechanism of action other than disrupting the cell wall or protein synthesis of bacteria.
2. Miscellaneous antibiotics include the fluoroquinolones, rifampin, metronidazole, and polymyxin B.
3. Ciprofloxacin, a fluoroquinolone, is bactericidal and works by inhibiting DNA gyrase, an enzyme needed for bacterial DNA replication. Human DNA is not affected.
4. Ciprofloxacin is most effective against aerobic gram-negative organisms. It has previously been used extensively for serious gram-negative infections, but some types of bacteria have developed resistance to ciprofloxacin.
5. Ciprofloxacin has a prolonged postantibiotic effect. This means that organisms will not resume growing for 2 to 6 hours after exposure to the drug, even when the drug blood level is too low to be detected.
6. The most common adverse effects of ciprofloxacin are gastrointestinal (GI); arthropathy (joint disease) is possible and is the most serious adverse effect. Children under 18 are more at risk of arthropathy.
7. Give ciprofloxacin through a large vein and infuse slowly over 60 minutes to reduce risk of venous irritation.
8. If the patient has GI adverse effects from oral ciprofloxacin, small, frequent meals should be given.
9. Polymyxin B is an older antibiotic used to treat most gram-negative bacteria.
10. Polymyxin B is administered by topical, ophthalmic, and otic routes, and is frequently mixed with other drugs.

KEY TERMS

Fill in the blanks

Read each statement carefully and, using the chapter's key terms, write your answer in the space provided.

1. The _____ agents are a relatively new, synthetic, broad-spectrum class of antibiotics.

2. Despite undetectable drug levels, organisms may not resume growing for 2 to 3 hours after exposure to ciprofloxacin. This is called a _____.

3. The most significant adverse effect to the use of ciprofloxacin is _____.

CORE DRUG KNOWLEDGE: JUST THE FACTS

Multiple choice

Circle the option that best answers the question or completes the statement.

1. How do fluoroquinolone antibiotics work? They
   a. interrupt cell wall synthesis.
   b. inhibit DNA replication.
   c. block the action of folic acid.
   d. interrupt protein synthesis.

2. Ciprofloxacin (Cipro) is available in all of the following dosage forms EXCEPT
   a. oral.
   b. parenteral.
   c. topical.
   d. inhalation.

3. Fluoroquinolones such as ciprofloxacin (Cipro) are INEFFECTIVE in the management of
   a. gram-negative organisms.
   b. aerobic gram-positive organisms.
   c. anaerobic organisms.
   d. sexually transmitted diseases.

4. The most frequent adverse effects to ciprofloxacin (Cipro) therapy affect the _____ system.
   a. GI
   b. central nervous
   c. hematopoietic
   d. respiratory

5. Unlike ciprofloxacin (Cipro), enoxacin (Penetrex) is approved for the management of
   a. genitourinary infections only.
   b. anaerobic infections.
   c. meningitis.
   d. acne only.

6. Gatifloxacin (Tequin) is unique in that it
   a. needs to be taken every 4 hours.
   b. has bioequivalent oral and parenteral formulations.
   c. has no photosensitivity activity.
   d. has no drug–drug interactions.

7. Levofloxacin (Levaquin) should be administered
   a. QD.
   b. QOD.
   c. QID.
   d. BID.

8. When administered for systemic circulation, polymyxin B may induce
   a. cardiotoxicity.
   b. immunotoxicity.
   c. hepatotoxicity.
   d. nephrotoxicity.

CORE PATIENT VARIABLES: PATIENTS, PLEASE

Multiple choice

Circle the option that best answers the question or completes the statement.

1. Donna Hill brought her 5-year-old son to the clinic today. He was diagnosed with an eye infection and placed on ophthalmic ciprofloxacin (Cipro). Mrs. Hill asks, "My pediatrician says that this drug is not OK for kids. Why did this doctor order it?" What is your best response?
   a. "Just because one doctor does not want to use it doesn't mean all of them feel the same way."
   b. "This is something you should ask the doctor."
   c. "Your pediatrician is right. Oral preparations of this drug should not be given to children, but the topical drops are approved."
   d. "No, I think you are wrong."

2. Mary Ellis, age 25, has been prescribed ciprofloxacin (Cipro) for a respiratory infection. Patient teaching should include which of the following instructions?

   a. If taking birth control pills, use a backup method while taking the drug.

   b. Do not use any bronchodilator inhalers while taking this drug.

   c. Wear high-top shoes to avoid tendon rupture.

   d. Stop the medication as soon as you feel better.

3. Murray Talbert has just been prescribed ciprofloxacin (Cipro) for a skin infection. After reviewing Mr. Talbert's medical record, you note that he has a history of gastroesophageal reflux disease (GERD). Patient teaching for Mr. Talbert should include which of the following instructions?

   a. Do not take any medication for your stomach while taking this drug.

   b. Take any antacids at least 1 hour before or 2 hours after the Cipro.

   c. Be sure to take the Cipro at the same time you take your vitamins.

   d. Take Cipro with a full glass of cranberry juice.

4. Alice Waters has an order for IV ciprofloxacin (Cipro). To administer this medication safely, the nurse should

   a. dilute in 5 mL NS and infuse IVP over 1 to 2 minutes.

   b. dilute in 10 mL sterile water and infuse IVP in 30 seconds.

   c. infuse IVPB over 15 to 20 minutes.

   d. infuse IVPB over 1 hour.

5. Ginger Wells has just completed a 7-day course of ciprofloxacin (Cipro). Ginger calls the clinic today and complains of a thick white vaginal discharge. You suspect a

   a. hypersensitivity reaction.

   b. toxic reaction.

   c. suprainfection.

   d. sexually transmitted disease.

NURSING MANAGEMENT: EVERY GOOD NURSE SHOULD . . .

Multiple choice

Circle the option that best answers the question or completes the statement.

1. To minimize adverse effects from ciprofloxacin, the nurse should teach the patient to

   a. use a sunscreen.

   b. limit fluid intake.

   c. take a double dose if one is missed.

   d. eat three large meals.

2. Greta Hampstead, 55 years old, takes theophylline for her chronic obstructive pulmonary disease (COPD). She is started on ciprofloxacin to treat peritonitis. To minimize adverse effects, the nurse should

   a. encourage aerobic exercise.

   b. monitor for tachycardia and insomnia.

   c. place the patient's bed in front of a sunny window.

   d. administer the theophylline in the morning and the ciprofloxacin in the evening.

3. Jean Fox has been taking oral ciprofloxacin at home to treat pneumonia from *Klebsiella pneumoniae*. She calls the advice line for her HMO and complains to you, the advice nurse, that she must be allergic to ciprofloxacin because she has terrible nausea and abdominal pain since she started the drug. You should advise her to

   a. stop taking the drug because she is allergic to it.

   b. crush the drug and mix in a small amount of yogurt.

   c. take the drug after meals.

   d. eat small, frequent meals, but continue the drug.

CASE STUDY

Judy Lancaster, 28 years old, has been prescribed ciprofloxacin to treat a severe urinary tract infection. She will be taking the drug orally at home, 500 mg twice a day.
Describe the patient education that Judy needs about ciprofloxacin.

CRITICAL THINKING CHALLENGE

Three days later, Judy Lancaster returns to the
outpatient center complaining that her symptoms have
not improved much. She tells you that she has taken
the drug twice a day for the last 3 days as prescribed.
Her lab report from 3 days ago indicates that the
bacteria are susceptible to ciprofloxacin.
What other questions might you ask to determine why
she is still having symptoms of a urinary tract
infection?

CHAPTER 51

Drugs for Treating Urinary Tract Infections

TOP TEN THINGS TO KNOW ABOUT DRUGS FOR TREATING URINARY TRACT INFECTIONS

1. Sulfamethoxazole-trimethoprim is a combination of a sulfonamide and another antibiotic. The name is abbreviated as SMZ-TMP. Some sources list it as trimethoprim-sulfamethoxazole or TMP-SMZ.

2. SMZ-TMP interferes with the synthesis of folic acid (folate) needed for biosynthesis of RNA, DNA, and proteins. This prevents the formation of new bacteria, so SMZ-TMP is bacteriostatic. Avoid giving to patients with folate deficiency disorders.

3. SMZ-TMP is used to treat a variety of organisms and illnesses, including urinary tract infections (UTI), respiratory infections (such as *Pneumocystis carinii* pneumonia [PCP] seen in HIV and AIDS), gastrointestinal (GI) infections, and sexually transmitted diseases.

4. Immunocompromised patients are more likely to have adverse effects from SMZ-TMP.

5. Nausea, vomiting, and diarrhea are the most common adverse effects of SMZ-TMP. Serious adverse effects are crystalluria (resulting in renal damage), allergic reactions (such as urticaria, pruritus, photosensitivity, and Stevens-Johnson syndrome), and hematologic effects (such as anemia and agranulocytosis).

6. To minimize adverse effects from SMZ-TMP, give with food, and increase fluid intake to at least 1.5 L/day, unless contraindicated by the physical condition of the patient.

7. Other antibiotic classes are also used to manage UTI. These include cephalosporins, fluoroquinolones, penicillins, and tetracycline.

8. Urinary tract antiseptics work by a local action in the urinary tract. They do not achieve high serum levels and so have few systemic effects. There is no prototype.

9. Urinary tract antiseptics include methenamine (avoid giving to patients with upper UTI or indwelling urinary catheters because these don't allow sufficient time for drug to work), nitrofurantoin, nalidixic, and cinoxacin.

10. Phenazopyridine is a urinary analgesic. It does not have antibacterial activity, but it relieves pain, burning, frequency, and urgency due to irritation of the urinary tract from the UTI. Phenazopyridine will make the urine look orange or red.

KEY TERMS

Anagrams

Using the following definitions, unscramble each of the following sets of letters to form a word. Write your response in the spaces provided.

1. A recurrent UTI caused by a different organism from the initial infection

   N R O E I I N T F C E

   □□□□□□□□□□□

2. Infection of the bladder

   S C I Y T S I T   □□□□□□□□

3. Another term for acute urethral syndrome

   S U I R T E I T R H

   □□□□□□□□□□

4. Infection of the kidneys

   S P I Y T E I L R O H N P E

   □□□□□□□□□□□□□□

5. A recurrent UTI caused by the same organism from the initial infection

   E R S E P L A   □□□□□□□

6. Symptoms of a UTI after the initial infection resolved

   T R N E E C R U R

   □□□□□□□□□

7. Infection caused by microbes invading the prostate

   S P I R T O I S T T A

   □□□□□□□□□□□

8. Potential adverse effect to the use of sulfonamides

   A C I R R Y U S L T L A

   □□□□□□□□□□□□

9. First-line drugs in the management of UTI

   S S E U D L I F M O A N

   □□□□□□□□□□□□

10. Necessary for the biosynthesis of RNA, DNA and proteins

    A B A P   □□□□

PHYSIOLOGY AND PATHOPHYSIOLOGY: THE HUMAN BODY

Essay

1. Name the components of the urinary system.

2. Identify the host defenses that protect an individual from a UTI.

3. Why are women more prone to UTIs than men?

CORE DRUG KNOWLEDGE: JUST THE FACTS

Multiple choice

Circle the option that best answers the question or completes the statement.

1. Pharmacotherapeutics of SMZ-TMP include all of the following EXCEPT
   a. *Pneumocystis carinii* pneumonia.
   b. Legionnaire's disease.
   c. histoplasmosis.
   d. urinary tract infections.

2. Sulfonamides work by
   a. inhibiting protein synthesis.
   b. interfering with folic acid synthesis.
   c. disrupting cell wall matrix.
   d. inhibiting replication of DNA.

3. During therapy with sulfamethoxazole-trimethoprim (SMZ-TMP), the patient should be advised to
   a. avoid sunlight.
   b. avoid cranberry juice or foods that acidify urine.
   c. increase fluid intake.
   d. do all of the above.

4. A potential adverse effect associated with the administration of sulfamethoxazole-trimethoprim (SMZ-TMP) is
   a. crystalluria.
   b. congestive heart failure.
   c. iron deficiency anemia.
   d. migraine headache.

5. A potential adverse effect to the infant who receives sulfamethoxazole-trimethoprim (SMZ-TMP) from breast-feeding is
   a. kernicterus.
   b. hepatitis.
   c. pancreatitis.
   d. aplastic anemia.

6. A benefit of fosfomycin (Monurol) therapy is
   a. one-time-a-day dosing.
   b. 3-day duration of therapy.
   c. one-time-only dosing.
   d. one-time-a-week dosing.

7. Which of the following statements concerning urinary tract antiseptics is accurate?
   a. They reach low systemic levels.
   b. They have many adverse effects due to their toxicity.
   c. They have many drug–drug interactions.
   d. They are the drug of choice for acute UTI.

8. Nitrofurantoin (Macrodantin) is associated with adverse effects in the
   a. CNS.
   b. cardiovascular system.
   c. pulmonary system.
   d. urinary system.

9. Treatment with which of the following drugs will result in bright orange-red urine?
   a. phenazopyridine (Pyridium)
   b. sulfisoxazole (Novosoxazole)
   c. nitrofurantoin (Macrodantin)
   d. spectinomycin

10. Although phenazopyridine (Pyridium) is frequently used in the management of UTI, it
    a. has more adverse effects than benefits.
    b. has no antibacterial activity.
    c. is more frequently used in the management of viral illness.
    d. is not FDA approved.

CORE PATIENT VARIABLES: PATIENTS, PLEASE

Multiple choice

Circle the option that best answers the question or completes the statement.

1. Malcolm Jeffreys, age 66, is a homeless alcoholic who comes to the clinic with a complaint of dysuria and hematuria. Mr. Jeffreys is diagnosed with pyelonephritis and started on a course of SMZ-TMP. Due to Mr. Jeffreys' health status history, which of the following lab tests would be appropriate before initiating therapy?
   a. renal function and arterial blood gas
   b. folate level and complete blood count (CBC)
   c. hepatic enzymes and folate level
   d. arterial blood gas and hepatic enzymes

2. To maximize the effects of SMZ-TMP, Mr. Jeffreys should be advised to take the medication
   a. on an empty stomach.
   b. with a glass of cranberry juice.
   c. with a high-fat meal.
   d. at bedtime.

3. Vincent Hayes is taking sulfamethoxazole-trimethoprim (SMZ-TMP) for PCP prophylaxis. What instructions should be given to Mr. Hayes?
   a. Limit your intake of water.
   b. Drink at least 4 glasses of cranberry juice per day.
   c. Increase your fluids to at least 1 liter per day.
   d. Increase your intake of dairy products.

4. Because Mr. Hayes (#3 above) will be taking sulfamethoxazole-trimethoprim (SMZ-TMP) for a long period of time, the nurse should arrange for periodic laboratory testing to include
   a. uric acid levels and liver function.
   b. pulmonary function tests and CBC.
   c. ophthalmic examinations and renal function tests.
   d. CBC, liver function, and renal function tests.

5. Jeffrey Taylor is taking sulfamethoxazole-trimethoprim (SMZ-TMP) for PCP prophylaxis. Jeffrey comes to the clinic today with a complaint of fatigue, sore throat, and easy bruising. What do you suspect may be the problem?

   a. viral pharyngitis

   b. anemia

   c. strep throat

   d. mononucleosis

6. Ginny Archangelo has been prescribed fosfomycin (Monurol) for her acute UTI. Patient education should include instructions to

   a. drink the medication immediately after dissolving the powder.

   b. crush the capsules and mix in apple sauce.

   c. inhale the metered-dose inhaler as needed.

   d. let the dissolved powder sit for 1 hour before consuming.

7. Viola Gibbs, age 81, has a urinary tract infection. Mrs. Gibbs has an indwelling catheter. Which of the following medications would be INAPPROPRIATE for the treatment of Mrs. Gibbs' UTI?

   a. sulfamethoxazole-trimethoprim (SMZ-TMP)

   b. sulfisoxazole (Novosoxazole)

   c. methenamine (Hiprex)

   d. nitrofurantoin (Furadantin)

8. Barbara Thompson has pyelonephritis. She complains of a constant burning sensation in her lower abdomen and frank pain with voiding. Which of the following drugs would be helpful in alleviating the discomfort Ms. Thompson is experiencing?

   a. phenazopyridine (Pyridium)

   b. nitrofurantoin (Macrodantin)

   c. methenamine (Hiprex)

   d. sulfasalazine (Azulfidine)

NURSING MANAGEMENT: EVERY GOOD NURSE SHOULD . . .

Multiple choice

Circle the option that best answers the question or completes the statement.

1. Greg Upton, 50 years old, is being given a prescription for sulfamethoxazole-trimethoprim to treat a urinary tract infection. Teaching for Mr. Upton should emphasize which of the following?

   a. Take the drug with food if GI upset occurs.

   b. Drink at least 1,500 mL per day.

   c. Use sunscreen and protective clothing outside.

   d. all of the above

   e. none of the above

2. Karen Coombs is 74 years old and is uroseptic. She is started on IV sulfamethoxazole-trimethoprim. To minimize the risk of adverse effects, the nurse should closely monitor Ms. Coombs'

   a. CBC.

   b. fasting blood glucose/sugar (FBG or FBS).

   c. daily weight.

   d. distance vision.

3. Thomas Catalini, 24 years old, has AIDS and has received SMZ-TMP therapy for several months to prevent *Pneumocystis carinii* infections. As part of ongoing assessment and evaluation of therapy, the nurse should

   a. determine intake and output levels.

   b. assess for urine pH below 5.5.

   c. assess urine for crystals.

   d. do all of the above.

   e. do none of the above.

4. You are to administer SMZ-TMP via IV infusion to Harry Karman for a severe urinary tract infection. To minimize adverse effects you should

   a. administer as an IV bolus.

   b. refrigerate diluted solutions before administration.

   c. avoid flushing IV lines used to administer SMZ-TMP.

   d. all of the above

   e. none of the above

CASE STUDY

Anthony Ramirez, 44 years old, is to be started on oral SMZ-TMP for a urinary tract infection. As the nurse about to administer the first dose, you ask if he is allergic to sulfa drugs used as antibiotics. He tells you, no, the only drug allergy he has is to hydrochlorothiazide, which he took for his blood pressure. The next day, he tells you that the soap in the bed linen must be bothering him because he is very itchy. On examination, you see reddened areas, some of them raised, over his chest and back.
What is your assessment?

CRITICAL THINKING CHALLENGE

What piece of data did the nurse overlook that contributed to Mr. Ramirez' rash and itchiness?

CHAPTER 52

Drugs for Treating Mycobacterial Infections

TOP TEN THINGS TO KNOW ABOUT DRUGS FOR TREATING MYCOBACTERIAL INFECTIONS

1. Drug therapy to treat tuberculosis (TB) frequently includes three or four drugs because multi-drug resistance TB has developed. Unless the organism is resistant to isoniazid (INH), isoniazid is always included in the treatment for TB.

2. Isoniazid can be used as prophylaxis or as treatment of TB. INH is bactericidal or bacteriostatic; it works by disrupting the synthesis of the tuberculin bacterial cell wall. Isoniazid may also possibly inhibit plasma monoamine oxidase (MAO) inhibitor.

3. Common adverse effects of isoniazid include hepatitis and peripheral neuropathy.

4. To minimize the adverse effect of hepatitis, avoid giving INH to patients who already have hepatitis or who have a history of INH-induced hepatitis, monitor liver enzymes carefully, and teach patients to avoid alcohol.

5. To minimize and prevent peripheral neuropathy, give vitamin B_6 (pyridoxine) and complete routine eye examinations. To prevent drug–food interactions, avoid excessive tyramine-rich food and histamine-rich food.

6. Other drugs used to treat TB are rifampin, ethambutol, pyrazinamide (PZA), and streptomycin.

7. Main adverse effects from other TB drugs include optic neuritis (ethambutol), hepatotoxicities, arthralgias, gastrointestinal (GI), and photosensitivity (pyrazinamide), nephrotoxicity, and ototoxicity (streptomycin).

8. Rifampin is used to treat TB and leprosy. It inhibits bacterial and mycobacterial RNA synthesis. Adverse effects are similar to INH, especially hepatic injury. Rifampin will also discolor body fluids (urine, saliva, tears, sputum) and can permanently stain soft contact lenses. Rifampin has many drug interactions because it is a potent inducer of the P450 hepatic enzyme system.

9. Patients with TB may also have HIV or AIDS. Determine other drug therapy because many HIV and AIDS drugs are contraindicated with rifampin.

10. Teach patients about the risk of multidrug-resistant TB and the importance of completing entire course of drug therapy to treat TB.

KEY TERMS

True/false

Mark true or false for each of the following statements. If the statement is false, replace the underlined words with the words that will make the statement correct.

_____ 1. <u>Mycobacteria</u> are slow-growing microbes that cause disease in humans.

_____ 2. <u>Mycobacterium leprae</u> is spread by inhalation of spores into the lungs.

_____ 3. The combination of the primary lung lesion and lymph node granulomas is referred to as <u>leprosy.</u>

_____ 4. <u>Multiple-drug therapy</u> is used for patients with a positive skin test but a negative chest x-ray.

_____ 5. <u>Hansen's disease</u> and leprosy are the same disease.

_____ 6. <u>M leprae</u> frequently causes disease in patients who are HIV positive.

_____ 7. <u>Mycobacterium avium</u> complex is a disease that mainly affects the skin.

_____ 8. High fevers, chills, diarrhea, and weight loss are symptoms of <u>leprosy.</u>

_____ 9. <u>M avium</u> causes leprosy.

CORE DRUG KNOWLEDGE: JUST THE FACTS

Multiple choice

Circle the option that best answers the question or completes the statement.

1. Isoniazid is the drug of choice in the management of
   a. Hansen disease.
   b. *Mycobacterium avium* complex.
   c. tuberculosis.
   d. a and c.

2. Isoniazid (INH) works by
   a. inhibiting protein synthesis.
   b. inhibiting synthesis of the bacterial cell wall.
   c. disrupting the change of RNA to DNA.
   d. interfering with folic acid synthesis.

3. The most frequent adverse effects associated with the use of INH are
   a. renal failure and increased seizure activity.
   b. CNS depression and peripheral neuropathy.
   c. memory impairment and renal failure.
   d. hepatitis and peripheral neuropathy.

4. Which of the following statements concerning INH is correct?
   a. INH has very few drug–drug interactions, but the few are very significant.
   b. INH has very few drug–drug interactions, and they are very insignificant.
   c. INH has many drug–drug interactions, and most are very significant.
   d. INH has many drug–drug interactions, but they are very insignificant.

5. To minimize the potential for peripheral neuropathy, INH may be given in combination with
   a. rifampin (Rifadin).
   b. pyridoxine (B$_6$).
   c. spectinomycin.
   d. ethambutol (Myambutol).

6. A serious adverse effect associated with the administration of ethambutol (Myambutol) is
   a. optic neuritis.
   b. hepatitis.
   c. pancreatitis.
   d. CNS depression.

7. Pyrazinamide (PZA) therapy may exacerbate
   a. congestive heart failure.
   b. diabetes.
   c. gout.
   d. asthma.

8. Rifampin (Rifadin) works by
   a. inhibiting protein synthesis.
   b. inhibiting synthesis of the bacterial cell wall.
   c. disrupting RNA synthesis.
   d. interfering with folic acid synthesis.

9. Like INH, rifampin (Rifadin) may cause injury to the
   a. kidneys.
   b. liver.
   c. heart.
   d. lungs.

10. Which of the following statements concerning drug–drug interactions with rifampin (Rifadin) is accurate?

    a. Rifampin has very few drug–drug interactions, but the few are lethal.

    b. Rifampin has very few drug–drug interactions, and they are very insignificant.

    c. Rifampin has many drug–drug interactions, and most are very significant.

    d. Rifampin has many drug–drug interactions, but they are very insignificant.

11. Which of the following drugs would be INAPPROPRIATE for use in the treatment of leprosy?

    a. dapsone (Avlosulfan)

    b. clofazimine (Lamprene)

    c. spectinomycin

    d. rifapentine (Priftin)

12. The most serious adverse effect to dapsone (Avlosulfan) therapy affects the _____ system.

    a. hematopoietic

    b. cardiovascular

    c. respiratory

    d. integumentary

CORE PATIENT VARIABLES: PATIENTS, PLEASE

Multiple choice

Circle the option that best answers the question or completes the statement.

1. Elliott Reynolds, age 51, has recently been exposed to TB. Mr. Reynolds had a negative TB skin test 6 months ago; however, the current test is positive. Which of the following interventions should be done while Mr. Reynolds receives INH prophylaxis?

    a. baseline CBC and repeat CBC every 6 months

    b. baseline renal function tests and repeat test every 3 months

    c. baseline hepatic function test and repeat test every month

    d. baseline pyridoxine level and repeat test every 6 months

2. Noel Easton is receiving INH for TB prophylaxis. Mr. Easton comes to the clinic today with a complaint of fatigue, anorexia, nausea, and vomiting. You suspect Mr. Easton is experiencing

    a. hepatitis.

    b. peripheral neuropathy.

    c. tyramine reaction.

    d. all of the above.

3. Hillary Welker has been taking triple antimicrobial therapy for active TB for the past 3 months. Ms. Welker comes to the clinic today and complains that her contact lenses have turned red. Which of the following medications may have caused this problem?

    a. INH

    b. rifampin (Rifadin)

    c. ethambutol (Myambutol)

    d. spectinomycin

4. Jennifer Consle has been diagnosed with active TB. Ms. Consle has multiple medical problems including HIV, steroid-dependent asthma, and type 2 diabetes. Which of the following drugs, given concurrently with her previously prescribed medications, would be the most problematic?

    a. spectinomycin

    b. ethambutol (Myambutol)

    c. pyrazinamide (PZA)

    d. rifampin (Rifadin)

5. Henry Thomas, age 33, is taking multidrug therapy for TB. Mr. Thomas has a history of hepatic dysfunction. Which combination of drugs would be contraindicated for Mr. Thomas?

    a. INH and rifampin

    b. INH and ethambutol

    c. rifampin and spectinomycin

    d. ethambutol and PZA

6. Colin Hayes, age 32, is taking triple antimicrobial therapy for TB. He takes isoniazid (INH), rifampin (Rifadin), and ethambutol (Myambutol). In addition to serial liver function tests, which of the following should be done for Mr. Hayes?

    a. chest x-ray

    b. ophthalmology exam

    c. ECG

    d. HbA_{1C}

7. Jenna Hayes, age 30, is also taking triple antimicrobial therapy for TB. She takes isoniazid (INH), rifampin (Rifadin), and ethambutol (Myambutol). In addition to serial liver function tests, which of the following should be done for Mrs. Hayes?

    a. chest x-ray

    b. ECG

    c. ophthalmology exam

    d. uric acid level

8. Mrs. James is to receive IV rifampin (Rifadin). To safely administer this medication, the nurse should

    a. premedicate the patient with IV diazepam (Valium).

    b. administer IVP over 30 seconds.

    c. infuse IVPB over 3 hours.

    d. administer IVP over 2 to 3 minutes.

NURSING MANAGEMENT: EVERY GOOD NURSE SHOULD . . .

Multiple choice

Circle the option that best answers the question or completes the statement.

1. Martin Ulmer, 35 years old, has been diagnosed with active TB. He is prescribed isoniazid, rifampin, and ethambutol. He protests at taking so many medicines. The best action of the nurse would be to

    a. rotate the drugs, offering one each day.

    b. only administer the isoniazid, and mark the others as "refused."

    c. force him to take all three drugs.

    d. explain the rationale for triple-drug therapy.

2. Patient education about INH should include limiting the intake of which of the following?

    a. avocados

    b. chocolate

    c. tuna fish

    d. all of the above

    e. none of the above

3. To minimize adverse effects from isoniazid, the nurse should monitor

    a. SGOT and SGPT levels.

    b. creatinine clearance.

    c. BUN.

    d. vital capacity.

4. You work in a large city as a nurse in the health department. Because the incidence rate of TB is very high in the city, with multidrug resistance becoming more of a problem, the deputy director of the health department has issued a directive that the health department will actively work with patients to confirm their adherence with prescribed drug therapy. You would, therefore, expect to do which of the following for the patients you visit who have active TB and have been prescribed drug therapy?

    a. Instruct the caregiver to encourage the patient to take the medication.

    b. Tell the patient that as long as one of the drugs prescribed is taken he or she will be cured.

    c. Give each patient the pills and watch him or her swallow them.

    d. Ask the patient if he or she is taking the medicine.

CASE STUDY

Jerry Bowen, 38 years old, is homeless. He is an alcoholic and has been diagnosed with TB. He comes to the clinic that provides health care for the homeless every day to get his medication (INH, rifampin, ethambutol, and pyrazinamide).

1. What adverse effects is he most at risk for?

2. What will you do to minimize these adverse effects?

CRITICAL THINKING CHALLENGE

To help keep Jerry Bowen from drinking alcohol, the doctor has also prescribed disulfiram (Antabuse). When he returns to the clinic the next time, the nurse notices that Mr. Bowen's mood is very changeable. He came into the visit acting very angry with the nurse and the other staff members, but, after a short while, he was cracking jokes and talking nonstop. He tells the nurse he hopes she won't punish him too much for being so abrupt.

1. What may have brought this on?

2. What action should you take?

CHAPTER 53

Drugs for Treating Viral and Fungal Diseases

TOP TEN THINGS TO KNOW ABOUT DRUGS FOR TREATING VIRAL AND FUNGAL DISEASES

1. Viral and fungal diseases range from mildly annoying to life-threatening infections.
2. There are few effective antiviral drugs, because eradicating the virus also may damage the host's cells.
3. Acyclovir, an antiviral drug, competes for a position in the DNA chain of the herpes virus and then terminates DNA synthesis. Uninfected cells allow for minimum uptake of acyclovir. It is used to treat herpes simplex (cold sores, genital sores), herpes zoster (shingles), Epstein-Barr virus, and cytomegalovirus (CMV). It has no effect on HIV.
4. Use acyclovir during periods of active lesions. Teach patient to wear gloves and wash hands when applying topically to prevent spread of infection. Generally well tolerated; nephrotoxicity from crystallization may occur. Encourage PO fluids.
5. Fungal infections are systemic, dermatophytic (skin), or in the mucous membranes.
6. Amphotericin B, a polyene antifungal, is fungicidal or fungistatic, and works by binding to membrane sterols in fungal cell membranes, resulting in increased cell permeability, cell leakage, and death. Damage to host cells can also occur. Amphotericin B is used in treating progressive and potentially fatal systemic infections due to severe adverse effects.
7. Adverse effects of amphotericin B include nephrotoxicity (in more than 80% of patients), infusion-related reactions, electrolyte abnormalities, anemia, leukopenia, thrombocytopenia, and others. Administer other drugs as ordered before infusion to decrease adverse effects, administer a test dose before full dose (central line preferred), use in-line filter and IV pump, keep patient well hydrated, and monitor electrolytes, complete blood count (CBC), renal and hepatic function throughout therapy. Educate patients as to likelihood of transfusion reaction and other adverse effects.

8. Nystatin, an antifungal related to amphotericin B, is not used for systemic infections. It is used to treat topical, vaginal, and oral fungal infections. Oral suspension of nystatin should be swished through the mouth and then swallowed or spit out, as directed by prescriber. Oral troches should be dissolved in mouth.
9. Fluconazole, an azole antifungal, is used to treat esophageal, oropharyngeal, and vulvovaginal candidiasis, and in systemic fungal infections where the patient cannot tolerate amphotericin B. It may be used prophylactically in immunocompromised patients with a CD4+ T cell count less than 200. Fluconazole works by altering the fungal cell membrane, resulting in increased cellular permeability and leakage of cell contents.
10. Most common adverse effects of fluconazole are gastrointestinal (GI), headache, and dizziness. Mild elevation in liver enzymes may occur, which usually return to pretreatment levels after drug therapy is over. The patient should be encouraged to avoid alcohol.

KEY TERMS

Crossword puzzle

Use the definitions in the list provided below to complete the crossword puzzle.

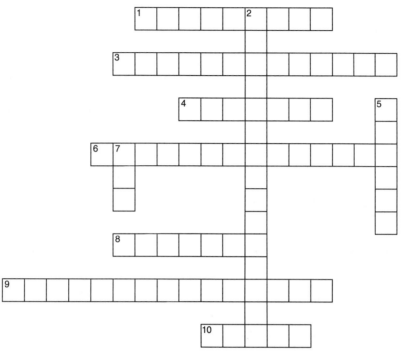

Across

1. Refers to the ability of a limited number of fungi that are capable of growing as yeasts at one temperature and as molds at another
3. Fungi that cannot grow at core body temperature
4. Virus that is spread by direct contact with fluid from active lesions
6. Most serious fungal infection that affects HIV-positive patients
8. Fungus that is almost always present on the skin
9. Type of herpes that is life threatening
10. Also known as ringworm

Down

2. Process needed to produce the activity of acyclovir
5. Type of herpes that is caused by the same virus that causes chickenpox
7. Common respiratory virus that affects children

PHYSIOLOGY AND PATHOPHYSIOLOGY: THE BODY HUMAN

Essay

1. What are the five steps of viral reproduction?

2. How do yeasts reproduce?

3. What are hyphae?

4. In the human host, where would you find an infection with a dermatophyte?

5. How is a systemic mycosis different than a dermatophyte?

CORE DRUG KNOWLEDGE: JUST THE FACTS

Multiple choice

Circle the option that best answers the question or completes the statement.

1. Which of the following viruses is unaffected by acyclovir (Zovirax)?
   a. herpes
   b. HIV
   c. cytomegalovirus (CMV)
   d. Epstein-Barr

2. What is the mechanism of action of acyclovir (Zovirax)?
   a. inhibition of viral cell wall
   b. disruption of protein synthesis
   c. termination of DNA synthesis
   d. increased permeability of viral cell wall

3. In the home environment, which of the following precautions should be taken with acyclovir (Zovirax)? Protect from
   a. air
   b. light
   c. heat
   d. all of the above

4. Which of the following drugs is INAPPROPRIATE in the treatment of CMV?
   a. penciclovir (Denavir)
   b. ganciclovir (Cytovene)
   c. cidofovir (Vistide)
   d. foscarnet (Foscavir)

5. In addition to influenza A, amantadine (Symmetrel) may be useful in the treatment of
   a. acetaminophen toxicity.
   b. diverticulitis.
   c. HIV disease.
   d. Parkinson's disease.

6. Which of the following statements concerning foscarnet (Foscavir) is correct?
   a. It is a highly efficient drug and has minimal adverse reactions or drug–drug interactions.
   b. It is a highly efficient drug and has few adverse effects but significant drug–drug interactions.
   c. It is a highly efficient drug and has a multitude of serious adverse effects and only a few insignificant drug–drug interactions.
   d. It is a highly efficient drug and has a multitude of serious adverse effects and significant drug–drug interactions.

7. Amphotericin B (Fungizone) is used to manage patients with a diagnosis of
   a. tinea.
   b. onychomycosis.
   c. a serious systemic mycotic disease.
   d. a serious systemic viral disease.

8. What is the mechanism of action of amphotericin B (Fungizone)?
   a. alters fungal cell membrane permeability
   b. inhibits protein synthesis
   c. disrupts fungal mitotic spindle structure
   d. interrupts DNA synthesis

9. Which of the following laboratory tests should be done before and throughout amphotericin B (Fungizone) therapy?
   a. CBC
   b. electrolytes
   c. renal function
   d. all of the above

10. Amphotericin B (Fungizone) is thought to have a suppressive effect on erythropoietin production. This may result in
    a. renal toxicity.
    b. hepatic toxicity.
    c. anemia.
    d. seizure activity.

11. Nystatin (Mycostatin), an antifungal drug nearly identical to amphotericin B (Fungizone), is indicated for the treatment of
    a. severe systemic mycoses.
    b. oral, cutaneous, mucocutaneous, or vaginal candidiasis.
    c. severe systemic viruses.
    d. HIV.

12. Flucytosine (5-FC) should be administered cautiously to patients receiving other medications that are known to induce
    a. hepatotoxicity.
    b. nephrotoxicity.
    c. hematologic toxicity.
    d. all of the above.

13. Which of the following drugs is used as primary fungal prophylaxis in immunocompromised patients?
    a. fluconazole (Diflucan)
    b. ketoconazole (Nizoral)
    c. butenafine (Mentax)
    d. amphotericin B (Fungizone)

14. The most common adverse effects to fluconazole (Diflucan) therapy affect the _____ system.
    a. neurologic
    b. gastrointestinal
    c. reproductive
    d. endocrine

15. Which of the following drugs is NOT indicated for use in the treatment of superficial mycoses?
    a. ciclopiroxolamine (Loprox)
    b. butenafine (Mentax)
    c. flucytosine (5-FC)
    d. tolnaftate (Tinactin)

16. Oseltamivir phosphate (Tamiflu) and zanamivir (Relenza) are used in the management of
    a. cytomegalovirus.
    b. herpes simplex.
    c. herpes zoster.
    d. influenza.

CORE PATIENT VARIABLES: PATIENTS, PLEASE

Multiple choice

Circle the option that best answers the question or completes the statement.

1. Henry Baker, age 36, is receiving IV acyclovir (Zovirax). Mr. Baker has additional medical problems including a seizure disorder, HIV, diabetes mellitus, and drug addiction. Which of Mr. Baker's medical problems requires cautious use of acyclovir?
   a. diabetes mellitus
   b. HIV
   c. seizures
   d. drug addiction

2. Janice King, age 34, is receiving IV acyclovir (Zovirax). To safely administer this drug, you should administer it
   a. over 20 minutes and keep the patient NPO.
   b. over 20 minutes and keep the patient well hydrated.
   c. over 60 minutes and keep the patient NPO.
   d. over 60 minutes and keep the patient well hydrated.

3. Your patient has received IV acyclovir (Zovirax). Because it was administered IV, you should monitor for adverse effects to the
   a. kidneys.
   b. liver.
   c. lungs.
   d. brain.

4. Jessica Vance, age 56, is receiving IV amphotericin B (Fungizone). Which of the following electrolyte imbalances may be induced by this therapy?
   a. hypokalemia
   b. hyponatremia
   c. hyperkalemia
   d. hypernatremia

5. Mrs. Vance (question #4) is at greatest risk for which of the following adverse effects?
   a. blurred vision
   b. arachnoiditis
   c. nephrotoxicity
   d. hypertension

6. Before initiation of amphotericin B (Fungizone) therapy, what information should be given to Mrs. Vance?

   a. "This infusion may make you feel tired. I'll leave the side rails down."

   b. "Many patients have a reaction to this medication. I will premedicate you to diminish this possible response."

   c. "This medication may cause a minor tingling at the IV site. Let me know if that occurs."

   d. "This infusion will last for about 30 minutes. I'll be back then to take it down."

7. Melanie Cane, age 28, is being treated with griseofulvin (Grisactin) for a fungal infection in her toenails. The nurse explains she may need to take the medication for 6 to 12 months. Which of the following instructions should also be given to Ms. Cane?

   a. "Keep this medication out of the light."

   b. "Take this medication with a fatty meal."

   c. "If you take birth control pills, use another method of contraception."

   d. "Stop taking the medication 1 week each month."

8. Beatrice Henson is receiving IV fluconazole (Diflucan). What is the appropriate rate of infusion for this medication?

   a. 200 mg over 20 minutes

   b. 200 mg per hour

   c. 200 mg over 3 to 4 hours

   d. 200 mg IV push over 2 minutes

9. Patrick Ying has HIV disease and is being prescribed fluconazole (Diflucan) for fungal prophylaxis. Mr. Ying also has type 2 diabetes and takes tolbutamide (Orinase). You would expect Mr. Ying's tolbutamide dose may need to be

   a. increased.

   b. decreased.

   c. unchanged.

10. Your neighbor comes over and states that she can feel a "herpes cold sore" coming. She asks, "Do you have anything I can take for it?" Your best response is

    a. "I'll see if I have any antibiotics."

    b. "I have some leftover penciclovir (Denavir). I'll get it for you."

    c. "There is a great OTC med called docosanol (Abreva) that you can get at the drug store."

    d. "I have some ganciclovir (Cytovene). Maybe that will help."

11. Your patient has the flu and is prescribed zanamivir (Relenza). Patient teaching should include how to

    a. use a metered-dose inhaler.

    b. use a diskhaler.

    c. give a SC injection.

    d. give an IM injection.

NURSING MANAGEMENT: EVERY GOOD NURSE SHOULD . . .

Multiple choice

Circle the option that best answers the question or completes the statement.

1. Jerry Mendelson is being treated for genital herpes with acyclovir. He calls the patient information hot line at his HMO and speaks to the nurse. He states that the lesions are now red and warm. What advice should the nurse give?

   a. Take aspirin and continue with the acyclovir.

   b. Stop taking the acyclovir.

   c. Come in to the health center to be examined.

   d. Take a warm bath.

2. Ashley Dougan is to receive amphotericin B for a systemic fungal infection. Before beginning the first dose, the nurse should

   a. administer a test dose.

   b. assess vital signs.

   c. administer antipyretic, such as ibuprofen.

   d. do all of the above.

   e. do none of the above.

3. During the infusion of amphotericin B, Ashley develops wheezing, nausea, and a drop in her blood pressure. The nurse should

   a. increase the rate of infusion.

   b. change the IV site to a peripheral line with a smaller vein.

   c. slow the IV rate.

   d. do all of the above.

   e. do none of the above.

4. Edgar Beck is receiving fluconazole prophylaxis against histoplasmosis due to his low CD4 and T cell counts. He develops diarrhea while on fluconazole. The nurse should

   a. discontinue the fluconazole.

   b. seek an order for an antidiarrheal.

   c. obtain stool cultures.

   d. do all of the above.

   e. do none of the above.

5. Elise Anderson has been treated with several antibiotics for a surgical infection after repair of a fractured hip. She now has oral candidiasis and is to receive nystatin suspension. To increase the effectiveness of the drug, the nurse should

   a. shake the suspension and apply to the surgical wound.

   b. mix the suspension in water and have the patient drink it.

   c. have the patient swish the suspension in her mouth before swallowing it.

   d. avoid shaking, draw up in a syringe, and administer to the back of the patient's throat.

CASE STUDY

Steve March, 38 years old, has a history of congestive heart failure. He takes digoxin, hydrochlorothiazide, and captopril for this. He was recently treated with prednisone, an oral steroid, for a severe asthmatic attack. Unfortunately, he has now developed a serious *Aspergillus* infection. The organism is resistant to the usually effective antibiotics, except for amphotericin B. He has orders to begin amphotericin B.

1. Consider the patient-related variables. Are there any that place him at increased risk of adverse effects from the amphotericin? If yes, what are they?

2. What can the nurse do to minimize possible adverse effects?

CRITICAL THINKING CHALLENGE

1. What factors do you think contributed to Mr. March developing a serious *Aspergillus* infection?

2. Should you give the amphotericin B?

CHAPTER 54

Drugs for Treating HIV and AIDS

TOP TEN THINGS TO KNOW ABOUT DRUGS FOR TREATING HIV AND AIDS

1. HIV infection and AIDS are chronic diseases that have a poor prognosis. HIV infection and effectiveness of drug therapy is monitored by CD4+ T cell counts and HIV RNA counts (viral load).

2. Pharmacotherapy may be used for symptomatic or asymptomatic patients. There are benefits and risks of treatment. Exact protocols and treatment strategies for HIV and AIDS are evolving constantly, as new drugs are being developed and more is learned about these infections.

3. Pharmacotherapy for HIV and AIDS is complex and requires lifestyle changes and accommodations by the patient. The timing of doses is very important. Some of the drugs need to be taken on an empty stomach and some with food. A great number of pills/capsules must be taken daily. All anti-HIV drugs have adverse effects that may decrease the quality of the patient's life. Drug therapy can be very expensive. These factors make it difficult for a patient to comply with drug therapy effectively.

4. Resistance can develop in all types of anti-HIV agents when the therapeutic regimen is not followed. Missing even one dose may affect a patient's response to therapy.

5. Zidovudine (AZT) is an antiretroviral (specifically, a nucleoside reverse transcriptase inhibitor) used to treat HIV infection; it was the first FDA-approved drug for treating HIV. It works by incorporating itself into the DNA of the virus. This stops the building process and prevents the creation of a new virus. It is the only antiretroviral used to reduce the risk of perinatal transmission of HIV. Fatty meals decrease absorption.

6. Common adverse effects of zidovudine are gastrointestinal (GI) intolerance, headache, rash, and fever. Serious adverse effects are blood dyscrasias (bone marrow depression, anemia, granulocytopenia, thrombocytopenia), and these occur fairly frequently. Monitor blood work for adverse effects and response to therapy.

7. Saquinavir is a protease inhibitor. Protease is responsible for packaging infected polyproteins so that the new virus carries the disease. Protease inhibitors block this step so that the new virus is noninfectious. Protease inhibitors also block reverse transcriptase (decrease viral replication) and inhibit replication of HIV in the macrophages (major reservoirs of HIV). It is used in combination therapy with reverse transcriptase inhibitors. Combination therapy enhances suppression of viral replication and limits the emergence of viral resistance.

8. Bioavailability of saquinavir is increased with high-fat, high-protein meals. It has many drug–drug interactions, so always check compatibility before coadministering. Common adverse effects are GI and central nervous system (CNS). Therapeutic adherence for every dose is crucial to prevent increases in viral load and drug resistance.

9. Nevirapine, a nonnucleoside reverse transcriptase inhibitor, is given as combination therapy with nucleoside reverse transcriptase inhibitors. Resistant viruses emerge rapidly if used alone. It works by binding directly with the reverse transcriptase, blocking RNA and DNA-dependent DNA polymerase activities. It is not given with protease inhibitors. Common adverse effects are rash (occasionally may become severe and life threatening), elevated hepatic enzymes, fever, headache, nausea, and vomiting. Escalate dose per recommended regimen to minimize adverse effects.

10. Patients with HIV infections are at high risk of developing opportunistic infections. Some of these infections occur so commonly that drug therapy for prophylaxis is routinely prescribed. Prophylaxis therapy is often used for *Pneumocystis carinii* pneumonia (sulfamethoxazole-trimethoprim), TB (isoniazid), and *Toxoplasma gondi* (sulfamethoxazole-trimethoprim), among others.

KEY TERMS

True/false

Mark true or false for each of the following statements. If the statement is false, replace the underlined words with the words that will make the statement correct.

_____ 1. A <u>provirus</u> is the virus before it exits the cell.

_____ 2. The <u>polymerase chain reaction test</u> and <u>viral load</u> test detect antibodies produced in response to HIV infection.

_____ 3. Viral load indicates the <u>current immunologic status of the patient.</u>

_____ 4. In HIV disease, the virus has an affinity for attaching to <u>plasma</u> cells.

_____ 5. <u>CD4+ T cell counts</u> are reported as copies per milliliter.

_____ 6. The presence of the virus in the bloodstream is detected by a <u>Western blot</u> test.

_____ 7. After a patient has a positive ELISA test, a <u>viral load</u> is completed.

_____ 8. The most potent class of antiretroviral drugs are the <u>nonnucleoside reverse transcriptase inhibitors.</u>

_____ 9. Current protocols for the management of HIV and AIDS are called <u>viral loads.</u>

_____ 10. Two classes of drugs that affect the same enzyme in two different ways are the <u>nucleoside reverse transcriptase inhibitors</u> and the <u>nonnucleoside reverse transcriptase inhibitors.</u>

DECISIONS, DECISIONS

Essay

1. What are the potential benefits of early antiretroviral therapy?

2. What are the potential risks of early antiretroviral therapy?

3. Why is monotherapy contraindicated for the treatment of HIV disease and AIDS?

CORE DRUG KNOWLEDGE: JUST THE FACTS

Multiple choice

Circle the option that best answers the question or completes the statement.

1. What is the difference in the mechanism of action between nucleoside reverse transcriptase inhibitors (NRTI) and nonnucleoside reverse transcriptase inhibitors (NNRTI)?

   a. The mechanism of action occurs in a different site within the virus.

   b. NRTI drugs inhibit replication by binding to reverse transcriptase, and NNRTI drugs cause chain termination by incorporation into the viral DNA.

   c. NRTI drugs cause chain termination by incorporation into the viral DNA, and NNRTI drugs inhibit the end production of the virus before being expelled from the CD4+ T cell.

   d. NRTI drugs cause chain termination by incorporation into the viral DNA, and NNRTI drugs inhibit replication by binding to reverse transcriptase.

2. To decrease the potential for maternal transmission of HIV to the fetus, which of the following drugs should be administered to mom during pregnancy?

   a. zidovudine (Retrovir)

   b. stavudine (Zerit)

   c. delavirdine (Rescriptor)

   d. ritonavir (Norvir)

3. Zidovudine (Retrovir) therapy has many adverse reactions. In which of the following body systems do the most serious effects occur?

   a. CNS

   b. respiratory

   c. endocrine

   d. hematologic

4. Zidovudine (Retrovir) should be taken

   a. with a low-fat meal.

   b. with a high-fat meal.

   c. 1 hour before meals.

   d. at bedtime only.

5. Which of the following adverse effects are associated most frequently with didanosine (Videx) and zalcitabine (Hivid) therapy?

   a. nausea and vomiting

   b. peripheral neuropathy and pancreatitis

   c. myalgias and thrombocytopenia

   d. seizures and vomiting

6. Stavudine (Zerit) and lamivudine (Epivir) are usually administered

   a. BID.

   b. TID.

   c. QD.

   d. QID.

7. To increase the bioavailability of protease inhibitors such as saquinavir (Invirase, Fortovase), the medication should be administered

   a. 1 hour before meals.

   b. 2 hours after meals.

   c. with a high-fat meal.

   d. with a low-fat meal.

8. Which of the following statements concerning drug–drug interactions with saquinavir (Invirase, Fortovase) is correct?

   a. There are multiple interactions, and many may produce subtherapeutic levels of saquinavir.

   b. There are multiple interactions, but they are insignificant.

   c. There are very few interactions, and some are very significant.

   d. There are very few interactions, and they are all insignificant.

9. Nevirapine (Viramune) should be taken

   a. with meals.

   b. on an empty stomach.

   c. It does not matter.

10. A very serious adverse effect that may occur with nevirapine therapy is

   a. cardiac arrhythmias.

   b. pulmonary edema.

   c. pulmonary emboli.

   d. Stevens-Johnson syndrome.

11. Patients receiving antiretroviral therapy should have serial laboratory tests done. These include

   a. CBC.

   b. renal and hepatic function.

   c. T cell count and viral load.

   d. all of the above.

12. The drug of choice for prophylaxis of *Pneumocystis carinii* pneumonia is

   a. atovaquone (Mepron).

   b. sulfamethoxazole-trimethoprim (Bactrim, Septra).

   c. pentamidine (NebuPent).

   d. pyrimethamine (Daraprim).

13. Adefovir (Preveon) may induce toxicity to which of the following body systems?

   a. cardiovascular

   b. respiratory

   c. urinary

   d. CNS

14. The drugs of choice for *Mycobacterium avium* complex (MAC) prophylaxis include

   a. dapsone (Avlosulfon).

   b. azithromycin or clarithromycin (Biaxin).

   c. pyrimethamine (Daraprim).

   d. sulfamethoxazole-trimethoprim (Bactrim, Septra).

CORE PATIENT VARIABLES: PATIENTS, PLEASE

Multiple choice

Circle the option that best answers the question or completes the statement.

1. Clark Williams has AIDS. He is currently taking zidovudine (Retrovir), nevirapine (Viramune) and saquinavir (Invirase, Fortovase). Clark has been diagnosed with CMV retinitis and prescribed ganciclovir (Cytovene). Due to this combination of drugs, which of the following lab tests should be closely monitored?

   a. intraocular pressure

   b. CBC

   c. hepatic enzymes

   d. renal enzymes

2. Michael is taking zidovudine (Retrovir). What diet education should be done with Michael?

   a. high carbohydrate, moderate protein, low fat

   b. low carbohydrate, high protein, low fat

   c. moderate carbohydrate, moderate protein, high fat

   d. low carbohydrate, low protein, high fat

3. Angela Lewis, age 12, has HIV disease. Which of the following drugs is not approved for use in children?

   a. zidovudine (Retrovir)

   b. saquinavir (Invirase, Fortovase)

   c. lamivudine (Epivir)

   d. didanosine (Videx)

4. Jeffrey Davis is taking saquinavir for HIV disease. Jeffrey has been diagnosed with tuberculosis. Which of the following drugs would be contraindicated for use with Jeffrey?

   a. isoniazid (INH)

   b. ethambutol (Myambutol)

   c. spectinomycin

   d. rifampin (Rifadin)

5. Davis Thompson, age 30, is taking ritonavir (Norvir) for HIV disease. It is important to include which of the following statements in patient teaching for Mr. Thompson?

   a. Shield the medication from light.

   b. Refrigerate the medication.

   c. Keep the medication in a warm cabinet.

   d. Keep the medication in a damp place, such as the bathroom.

6. Leslie Thompson, age 26, is also taking ritonavir (Norvir). Because of her age and gender, what additional instructions should be given to Mrs. Thompson?

   a. Use a method other than birth control pills for contraception.

   b. This medication may induce amenorrhea.

   c. This medication may induce menorrhagia.

   d. This medication may increase breast tenderness.

7. Mr. and Mrs. Thompson should be advised to take the ritonavir (Norvir)

   a. with a high-fat diet.

   b. twice a day with meals.

   c. every 8 hours on an empty stomach.

   d. once a day at bedtime.

8. Richard Wright is taking triple antiretroviral therapy for HIV disease. Richard comes to the clinic for a routine checkup. His labs include a CD4+ T cell count of 455 and an undetectable viral load. Richard states, "Shouldn't I be taking more medications to keep me from getting other diseases?" Which of the following would be the best response?

   a. "You probably should, but this is an HMO."

   b. "Yes, but then you run the risk of inducing more adverse effects."

   c. "You might develop drug resistance if we add any more drugs."

   d. "At this point, your immune system is capable of providing that protection."

NURSING MANAGEMENT: EVERY GOOD NURSE SHOULD . . .

Multiple choice

Circle the option that best answers the question or completes the statement.

1. To maximize the effectiveness of zidovudine, the nurse should

   a. administer with meals.

   b. administer one time a day.

   c. instruct the patient to avoid fatty foods.

   d. do all of the above.

   e. do none of the above.

2. To maximize the therapeutic effects of saquinavir, the nurse should

   a. administer 30 minutes after meals.

   b. skip a dose if the patient complains of mild nausea.

   c. instruct the patient to avoid fatty foods.

   d. do all of the above.

   e. do none of the above.

3. To minimize the risk of rash developing from the use of nevirapine, the nurse should

   a. administer with food.

   b. administer with milk.

   c. administer drug in one daily dose.

   d. administer therapeutic dose gradually by dose escalation.

4. Anthony Pascale has HIV infection. He recently was diagnosed and treated for an oral yeast infection (candidiasis). The nurse would expect to administer which of the following to Anthony?

   a. isoniazid

   b. rifampin

   c. amphotericin B

   d. sulfamethoxazole-trimethoprim

5. Tamara Sheperd is receiving zidovudine and saquinavir to treat her HIV infection. Patient education for Tamara regarding these drug therapies should include

   a. these drugs should not be taken at the exact same time.

   b. GI upset may occur; the effects may resolve after being on therapy for 3 to 4 weeks.

   c. drug resistance can develop if doses are skipped or drugs are taken intermittently.

   d. all of the above

   e. none of the above

CASE STUDY

Lisa Brown is 21 years old. She has a history of IV drug abuse and alcohol abuse. She states she hasn't used drugs or alcohol in 6 months since she was diagnosed with HIV. She is being treated with saquinavir and zidovudine. She was admitted to the hospital this time with *Pneumocystis carinii* pneumonia and was treated with sulfamethoxazole-trimethoprim (SMZ-TMP) IV successfully. She will be going home on oral SMZ-TMP. In report, you learn that she frequently refuses her medications, and the nurses need to go in three or four times to get her to take everything. The nurse giving report says, "I don't know why we bother. When she leaves the hospital, she'll be noncompliant and then will be right back in here. What else can you expect?"

Consider the core drug knowledge and Lisa's core patient variables. What teaching do you think Lisa might need?

CRITICAL THINKING CHALLENGE

1. What additional questions do you think you should ask Lisa to more fully assess her?

2. How might this knowledge alter your teaching plan or teaching strategies?

CHAPTER 55

Drugs for Treating Parasites

TOP TEN THINGS TO KNOW ABOUT DRUGS FOR TREATING PARASITES

1. Parasites include protozoa, helminths, and arthropods. Pharmacologic intervention for parasites must be specific not only to the type of parasite, but also to the stage of its life cycle.

2. Chloroquine is used to treat malaria. It is also used in rheumatoid arthritis and discoid lupus. It is taken up inside the infected erythrocyte and interrupts the synthesis of RNA and DNA. In treating rheumatoid arthritis, it antagonizes histamine and serotonin, inhibiting prostaglandin synthesis; this creates an anti-inflammatory effect.

3. Common adverse effects of chloroquine are hypotension, ECG changes, nausea, vomiting, diarrhea, and abdominal pain. Give drug at same day of week if given on weekly basis. Have patient take with food to minimize gastrointestinal (GI) problems. Encourage patients to change positions slowly to minimize symptoms of hypotension.

4. Metronidazole, a synthetic antibacterial and antiprotozoal drug, is used to treat various organisms causing infection. It works by entering anaerobic bacteria and inhibiting DNA synthesis, causing bacterial cell death. Avoid use in pregnancy (at least through first trimester) and in alcoholics (disulfiramlike reaction can occur). Common adverse effects are GI and central nervous system (CNS).

5. Give PO metronidazole with food to minimize GI effects; give intravenous (IV) metronidazole slowly over 1 hour. Monitor for thrombophlebitis and secondary infections. Educate patients that sex partners need to be treated simultaneously for trichomonal infections.

6. Pentamidine is used to prevent or treat *Pneumocystis carinii* pneumonia (PCP). Its action is unclear, but it appears to interfere with nucleotide, phospholipid, and protein synthesis of the parasite. Pentamidine is given through aerosolization for prophylaxis and IV for treatment of PCP.

7. Sudden, severe effects may develop after a single dose of pentamidine. Cough and bronchospasm, and sudden severe hypotension are the most frequent adverse effects. Other adverse effects are thrombocytopenia, leukopenia, anemia, arrhythmias, tachycardia, acute hypoglycemia (especially in diabetics), pancreatitis, and elevated liver enzymes (especially in patients with preexisting hepatic disease).

8. Keep patient in bed while administering pentamidine, monitor blood pressure carefully throughout therapy, give a bronchodilator before inhaled pentamidine, protect IV solution from light, and use respiratory precautions.

9. Mebendazole is an oral, broad-spectrum, synthetic antihelminthic that treats a variety of worms, especially nematodes. It acts by damaging the cells of the helminth but not the host. Common adverse effects are transient GI, CNS, and fever during expulsion of worms. Potential serious adverse effects are blood abnormalities and hepatotoxicity. Avoid use in pregnancy (teratogenic and embryo toxic). Monitor blood counts and liver function test if long-term therapy. Instruct patient to chew the drug or crush and mix with food.

10. Lindane, an antiectoparasitic drug, is used to treat scabies and pediculosis. It is applied topically where it is absorbed through the exoskeleton of parasites. CNS overstimulation occurs, followed by death. Avoid use in abraded skin to prevent systemic absorption into the patient. Teach patient how to apply and how to prevent reinfection.

KEY TERMS

Crossword puzzle

Use the definitions in the list provided below to complete the crossword puzzle.

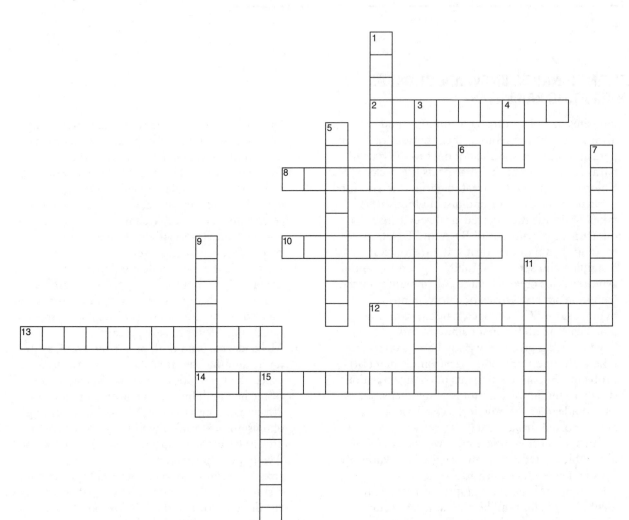

Across

2. Vectors of disease such as mites
8. Flukes
10. Infection with a protozoan parasite that causes diarrhea, dyspepsia, and occasionally malabsorption
12. Sexually active organism that produces active amebiasis
13. Disease caused by infection with a species of protozoa of the genus *Trichomonas* or related genera
15. Type of parasite that infects external body surfaces

Down

1. Disease spread by the bite of an infected mosquito
3. Disease caused by the protozoan parasite
4. Abbreviation for type of pneumonia that affects many people with AIDS
5. Disease caused by the microorganism *Entamoeba histolytica*
6. Worms
7. Roundworm
9. Organism that lives on or in another and draws its nourishment therefrom
11. Unicellular organism
15. Tapeworm

CORE DRUG KNOWLEDGE: JUST THE FACTS

Multiple choice

Circle the option that best answers the question or completes the statement.

1. In addition to the treatment of malaria, which of the following is a pharmacotherapy of chloroquine (Aralen)?
   a. scabies
   b. lice
   c. rheumatoid arthritis
   d. *Pneumocystis carinii* pneumonia

2. Which of the following body systems can be affected by chloroquine therapy?
   a. genitourinary
   b. endocrine
   c. hematologic
   d. sensory

3. Which of the following procedures should be done before initiating chloroquine therapy?
   a. pulmonary function test
   b. coronary stress test
   c. breast examination
   d. ophthalmologic examination

4. Which of the following drugs would be INAPPROPRIATE for the treatment of malaria?
   a. hydroxychloroquine (Plaquenil)
   b. pyrimethamine (Daraprim)
   c. metronidazole (Flagyl)
   d. mefloquine (Lariam)

5. What is the drug of choice for the radical cure of *Plasmodium vivax* and *Plasmodium ovale* malaria?
   a. primaquine
   b. mefloquine (Lariam)
   c. quinine
   d. hydroxychloroquine (Plaquenil)

6. Which of the following is NOT a disorder treatable with metronidazole (Flagyl)?
   a. Crohn's disease
   b. trichomonas
   c. amebiasis
   d. *Pneumocystis carinii* pneumonia

7. Metronidazole (Flagyl) is contraindicated for which of the following patients?
   a. Nancy, with alcoholism
   b. Beth, with anemia
   c. Tom, with prostatic hypertrophy
   d. Nelson, with bipolar disease

8. Hiliary Jones, age 21, has been diagnosed with vaginal trichomonas and is prescribed metronidazole (Flagyl) 2 g to be taken one time. Before administration of metronidazole, which of the following laboratory tests should be completed?
   a. complete blood count
   b. pregnancy test
   c. liver function tests
   d. kidney function tests

9. For patients with an allergy to sulfa drugs, the drug of choice for *Pneumocystis carinii* pneumonia (PCP) prophylaxis is
   a. co-trimoxazole (Bactrim, Septra).
   b. pentamidine (NebuPent).
   c. atovaquone (Mepron).
   d. any of the above.

10. Which of the following is an approved route of administration for pentamidine?
    a. inhalation
    b. enteral
    c. intravenous
    d. a and c
    e. a and b

11. Which of the following interventions for the administration of pentamidine is INCORRECT?
    a. shield IV pentamidine from light
    b. administer pentamidine within 24 hours of preparation
    c. administer bronchodilator before pentamidine by inhalation
    d. dilute IV pentamidine with normal saline

12. Atovaquone (Mepron) should be administered
    a. with a fatty meal.
    b. 1 hour before meals.
    c. 2 hours after meals.
    d. at bedtime.

13. Mebendazole (Vermox) is administered by which of the following routes?

    a. subcutaneous

    b. intravenous

    c. enteral

    d. all of the above

14. In which of the following patients would mebendazole (Vermox) be administered with caution?

    a. Cathy, with peptic ulcers

    b. Theresa, with asthma

    c. Allison, with cardiac arrhythmias

    d. James, with ulcerative colitis

15. Which of the following drugs would be used in the treatment of flukes and tapeworms?

    a. mebendazole (Vermox)

    b. praziquantel (Biltricide)

    c. thiabendazole (Mintezol)

    d. niclosamide (Niclocide)

16. Vicky Fountain is breast-feeding her 2-month-old daughter. How long should Vicky refrain from breast-feeding when she uses lindane (Kwell) to resolve scabies?

    a. She does not need to stop breast-feeding.

    b. 1 week

    c. 24 hours

    d. 48 hours

17. Lindane (Kwell) shampoo should be applied to

    a. clean, dry hair.

    b. oily, dry hair.

    c. clean, wet hair.

    d. oily, wet hair.

18. Which of the following statements is correct concerning crotamiton (Eurax) use?

    a. A second application should be done in 1 week.

    b. Only one application is necessary.

    c. A second application is needed in 24 hours.

    d. If symptoms remain, a second application can be done in 3 days.

CORE PATIENT VARIABLES: PATIENTS, PLEASE

Multiple choice

Circle the option that best answers the question or completes the statement.

1. Andrew Newmeyer, age 66, has recently returned from a trip and is diagnosed with malaria. Which of the following disorders would contraindicate the use of chloroquine (Aralen)?

    a. hypertension

    b. retinopathy

    c. peptic ulcer disease

    d. Crohn's disease

2. Aracelli Thomas has just returned from a vacation in a malaria-endemic country. Ms. Thomas took chloroquine (Aralen) 2 weeks before leaving and once a week during her vacation. She is symptom-free and asks if she can stop the medication. Which of the following is the best response?

    a. "You can stop the medication because you have no symptoms."

    b. "Take the medication one more week, then you can stop."

    c. "Take the remainder of the medication at bedtime tonight."

    d. "No, you need to continue the medication for an additional 4 weeks."

3. Penny Williams is taking chloroquine (Aralen) for malaria. Which of the following instructions should be given to Mrs. Williams?

    a. "Be sure to keep this medication out of the reach of your children."

    b. "Take the medication on the same day each week."

    c. "The medication can make you dizzy; be sure to change positions slowly."

    d. all of the above

4. Henry Davis is taking metronidazole (Flagyl) for trichomoniasis. Mr. Davis asks you what type of adverse effects may occur. Which of the following groups of symptoms is correct?

    a. xerostomia, dysgeusia, nausea, and vomiting

    b. chest pain, nausea, and vomiting

    c. constipation, dysgeusia, and vomiting

    d. urinary frequency, xerostomia, and vomiting

5. Jack Palmer, age 52, has multiple medical problems. Mr. Palmer has a history of congestive heart failure (CHF) and takes digoxin (Lanoxin) and furosemide (Lasix). He also has a history of deep vein thrombosis and takes warfarin (Coumadin). Mr. Palmer has been diagnosed with *Helicobacter pylori* and is prescribed metronidazole (Flagyl) for 3 weeks. In light of Mr. Palmer's history, what interventions should be done while taking metronidazole?

a. monitor for disulfiram reaction

b. perform an exercise stress test before initiation of therapy

c. monitor for signs of bleeding

d. monitor for pancreatitis

6. Leslie Victor calls the clinic concerned that her urine has discolored. She states she is being treated for trichomoniasis and is taking metronidazole (Flagyl). Which of the following statements is most appropriate?

a. "Trichomoniasis is a sexually transmitted disease, maybe you have another type as well."

b. "Perhaps you have a urinary tract infection."

c. "I would stop the medication immediately and come to the clinic."

d. "This is an common occurrence with this medication, but it is harmless."

7. Petra Olson has just been diagnosed with PCP. Ms. Olson is to receive pentamidine (NebuPent) IV. Which of the following precautions should be taken with Ms. Olson immediately after the infusion? Monitor for

a. hypotension

b. anemia

c. headache

d. GI distress

8. Lee Channing has HIV disease and seizures. Lee is prescribed carbamazepine (Tegretol) for seizures and receives pentamidine (NebuPent) by inhalation every month. Lee should be advised to call the health care provider if which of the following symptoms occur?

a. increased urine output

b. spontaneously resolved abdominal pain

c. anemia

d. cough

9. Melanie Cross has brought Chase, age 4, to the clinic because of rectal itching. Chase is diagnosed with pinworms. Which of the following instructions should be given to Mrs. Cross?

a. "Keep Chase away from the other children in the family until he is no longer contagious."

b. "It's best to treat all members of the family at the same time because pinworms are so contagious."

c. "This is not an easy disease to acquire, so you do not have to worry about it."

d. "Give this medication to Chase on an empty stomach."

10. Marla Wyman has brought her children, ages 1½, 10, and 12, to the clinic. They are diagnosed with scabies and prescribed lindane (Kwell), with the exception of the youngest. Mrs. Wyman asks why the baby cannot use the same medication as the other children. Which of the following responses is correct?

a. "Children under the age of 2 absorb more of the drug because of their skin and run the risk of toxicity."

b. "The medication does not work for them because their liver is not mature."

c. "You are right, you can use the medication for all of the children."

d. "The scabies die without treatment because the skin of babies does not have enough nutrients to keep them alive."

NURSING MANAGEMENT: EVERY GOOD NURSE SHOULD . . .

Multiple choice

Circle the option that best answers the question or completes the statement.

1. Janet Goodway, 19 years old, will be traveling out of the country with her church group to a region known to have malaria. She is given a prescription for chloroquine. Teaching regarding chloroquine therapy should include instructions to

a. begin drug therapy 2 weeks before the planned travel schedule.

b. discontinue drug therapy when leaving the malarial area.

c. take the drug every day at the same time.

d. take the drug on an empty stomach.

2. Patients taking metronidazole for a giardiasis infection should be taught to avoid which of the following?

    a. milk

    b. over-the-counter (OTC) liquid cold medicines

    c. OTC antipyretics

    d. rice

3. Brenda Wisner, 22 years old, is being treated for a *Trichomonas* infection with metronidazole. The nurse should ask Brenda

    a. whether she has a current sexual partner.

    b. whether she could be pregnant.

    c. whether she is taking anticoagulants.

    d. all of the above.

    e. none of the above.

4. Damon Wilson is to receive IV pentamidine to treat a current PCP infection. To minimize adverse effects from the drug, the nurse should

    a. mix the drug in a saline solution.

    b. monitor temperature every hour during infusion.

    c. administer IM morphine before infusion.

    d. do all of the above.

    e. do none of the above.

5. Patient teaching regarding the use of mebendazole to treat a pinworm infection should include which of the following?

    a. Chew the tablets.

    b. Take with milk.

    c. All family members should be treated.

    d. all of the above

    e. none of the above

CASE STUDY

Aaron Silber, 33 years old, is a diabetic and has AIDS. He is admitted from the emergency room to the floor with a diagnosis of PCP. His vital signs are 101.5–92–32. 138/80. He has a nonproductive cough and is short of breath. He is ordered to receive pentamidine 250 mg IV per day for 14 days. By the time Aaron's pentamidine arrives from the pharmacy, it is 10:30 at night. The nurse hangs the drug.

1. What parameters should the nurse monitor while administering the pentamidine?

2. What other actions should the nurse perform to minimize adverse effects?

CRITICAL THINKING CHALLENGE

Aaron's infusion of pentamidine goes well, and the evening nurse reports off duty to the night nurse at 11:30 PM. When the night nurse gets in to Aaron's room on her rounds at 12:30 AM, she finds him ashen, diaphoretic, and hard to arouse.

Consider the core drug knowledge and the core patient variables. What assessment might you make of Aaron's current status?

Answer Key

Chapter 1

KEY TERMS

Essay

1. desired effect of the drug
2. changes that occur to the drug when it is inside the body
3. effects of the drug on the body
4. when the drug should not be used, or when it should be used with caution
5. effects that are not intended, or may be undesirable
6. effects that occur when a drug is given along with another drug, food, or substance
7. grouping of pharmacologic facts: pharmacotherapeutics, pharmacokinetics, pharmacodynamics, contraindications and precautions, adverse effects, and drug interactions
8. assessment of patient-centered variables
9. chronic conditions causing system or organ dysfunction
10. age, physiologic development, reproductive state, ability to read and write, and gender
11. amount of activity and exercise; sleep–wake patterns; occupation; use or abuse of such substances as nicotine, alcohol, and illegal drugs; use of nonprescribed or over-the-counter (OTC) drugs; use of alternative health practices; and eating preferences and patterns
12. location where drug therapy will be administered; physical environment that may influence aspects of drug therapy, exposure to potentially harmful substances, lighting that may affect the drug or the person receiving the drug, cost of the drug
13. religious and ethnic backgrounds that may alter the effect of the drug or reduce the person's receptiveness to drug therapy
14. anticipated therapeutic and adverse effects of a drug
15. application of knowledge in the administration of drug therapy
16. drug that is representative of a drug class
17. method of learning and remembering a vast amount of information concerning drugs

CORE DRUG KNOWLEDGE: JUST THE FACTS

Multiple choice

1. c   2. a   3. b   4. a

CORE PATIENT VARIABLES: PATIENTS, PLEASE

Multiple choice

1. a   2. d   3. d   4. a

CASE STUDY

1. Health status: Are you allergic to any medication? Do you take any other medications routinely? Do you take any OTC drugs? Do you have any history of kidney or liver disease? Do you have any other chronic illnesses? What difficulties are you having with urination?
   Life span and gender: Are you postmenopausal? Do you take hormone replacement therapy?
   Lifestyle, diet, and habits: Do you smoke cigarettes, use alcohol, or use recreational drugs? Do you drink caffeinated beverages? If yes to above, how much? What is your usual diet? How many meals do you usually eat? Do you use herbs, vitamins, or other alternative therapies? Do you have health insurance? Does it include prescription drugs? Environment: Do you live alone? Do you have stairs in your home?
   Culture: What is your religion?
2. How often do you garden? At what time of the day are you in the sun? How long do you remain in the sun? What type of protective clothing do you wear? Do you wear sunscreen when you garden?

CRITICAL THINKING CHALLENGE

Essay

Because this drug can induce photosensitivity, the patient is at risk for sunburn. The nurse should teach the patient about the potential for photosensitivity, as well as the need to limit her sun exposure and to wear sunscreen when sun exposure is unavoidable.

Chapter 2

KEY TERMS

Matching

1. h	2. l	3. a	4. k	5. b
6. c	7. j	8. d	9. e	10. i
11. g	12. f	13. m		

1. l	2. j	3. e	4. c	5. k
6. d	7. m	8. a	9. g	10. i
11. h	12. f	13. b		

Chapter 3

KEY TERMS

1. enteral
2. intradermal
3. parenteral
4. topical
5. local effect
6. systemic
7. emulsion
8. enteric coating
9. suspension
10. intrathecal
11. sublingual
12. buccal
13. troche
14. tablet
15. intravenous
16. sustained-release
17. capsule
18. syrup
19. intramuscular
20. elixir
21. intravenous push; intravenous piggyback
22. subcutaneous
23. intra-articular
24. intra-arterial

CORE DRUG KNOWLEDGE: JUST THE FACTS

Multiple choice

1. d   2. b   3. c   4. c   5. a

Essay

1. **Pros:** has immediate effect; allows administration of a large volume of drug; avoid tissue irritation or injury; acceptable when no other route is possible; circumvents impaired circulation; potential for prolonged, continuous administration of solution
   Cons: unable to retrieve once given; distribution cannot be slowed or stopped
2. Intradermal
   Intra-articular
   Intra-arterial
   Intrathecal
3. An enteric-coated tablet resists the acid environment of the stomach to protect acid-labile drugs, to provide a sustained-release dose, or to guard against local adverse effects from a drug.
4. The layers of enteric coating dissolve in response to changes in the pH of fluids. The drug is released in a steady, controlled manner from a matrix of drug encased in a slowly dissolving substance such as wax. The drug may be bound to ion-exchange resins or to chemical compounds that form insoluble complexes within the capsule.
5. Transdermal patches, ointments, creams, drops, suppositories, foams, liquid vaginal tablets, sprays, inhalers

CORE PATIENT VARIABLES: PATIENTS, PLEASE

Essay

1. Vastus lateralis
2. Patient is vomiting, uncooperative, or unconscious; NPO status; patient unable to swallow or has difficulty swallowing
3. Crush the pill and mix with few milliliters of water; mix in a tablespoon of jelly, applesauce, or pudding; contact the health care provider to substitute a liquid formulation
4. Verify placement of the tube; for an NG tube, elevate the head of the bed, unless contraindicated; assess if the drug can be administered in the presence of food (tube feeding); flush the tube with normal saline; administer the medication; flush the tube again with normal saline
5. Skin is abraded or denuded; drug is added to a specific solvent; skin is covered by an occlusive dressing after the drug is applied
6. Wear gloves when applying topical drugs; use an applicator to administer; use sterile technique when the skin is broken or denuded; remove the patch immediately if adverse reactions occur
7. Right patient, right drug, right dose, right time, right route, right documentation
8. Is Mrs. Jones a diabetic? If so, monitor glucose levels.
   Assess for gingivitis.
   Assess for dental caries.
9. Lying on left side
10. Central access device

NURSING MANAGEMENT: EVERY GOOD NURSE SHOULD . . .

Labeling

a. Vastus lateralis, dorsal gluteal, or ventrogluteal
b. Deltoid, vastus lateralis, rectus femoris, dorsal gluteal, ventrogluteal (with deltoid preferred site)
c. All sites but deltoid
d. Vastus lateralis and rectus femoris
e. Back of arms, abdomen, anterior, medial midthigh

CASE STUDY

1. Does he have difficulty swallowing his medicines? Does he have more difficulty with some of his drug therapies than others (eg, he might have great difficulty with the dry tablets, only some difficulty with the enteric tablet and the capsules, and no difficulty with the suspension)? If he has difficulty swallowing his drug therapies, does this mean that he doesn't take all of his prescribed therapies? What methods assist him to swallow?

2. Do any of the drugs come in liquid forms? (This is especially important for the enteric-coated tablet because it cannot be crushed or broken to promote ease of swallowing.) If not, can another drug or another brand of this same drug be substituted for the drug therapy?

3. How to crush tablets and mix with a small amount of fluid or soft food, such as applesauce or jelly. Not to crush enteric-coated tablets and rationale for this. How to open capsules and mix with fluid or soft food to swallow. Why to mix in only a small volume of fluid or food. Necessity for shaking suspension well before measuring. The importance of using a medication cup or dosage spoon or cup rather than household teaspoon or tablespoon to measure correct dose of the suspension. If he is able to swallow some or all of his drug therapies but has some difficulty (complains that they stick in his throat, for example), instructing him to take a sip of water before placing the tablets or capsules in his mouth can assist in swallowing. Also, he may be more successful swallowing one item at a time rather than attempting to swallow two or more items at one time.

CRITICAL THINKING CHALLENGE

a. Does Mr. Johnson have the ability (cognitive ability, physical dexterity, sight) to self-administer his drugs through the gastroscopy tube? Will a family member or other caregiver be involved in administering the drug therapies to Mr. Johnson some or all of the time? If yes, they need to be involved in teaching also.

b. How to crush tablets finely into powder that can be mixed with water to administer. Enteric tablets cannot be crushed; an alternative form of the drug must be used. Capsules may be opened and mixed with water to administer through the tube. How to check that the tube is properly placed before administering drugs through the tube. How to flush the tube before and after drug administration to prevent obstruction of the tube. Whether tube feedings will interfere with drug administration or absorption. If yes, how long before or after an intermittent tube feeding should the drugs be administered. If a continuous tube feeding is used, how long should the feeding be shut off before and after drug administration.

Chapter 4

KEY TERMS

Matching

1. d	2. j	3. f	4. k	5. b
6. i	7. l	8. g	9. a	10. c
11. h	12. e	13. m		

1. c	2. e	3. b	4. j	5. m
6. k	7. i	8. l	9. d	10. f
11. a	12. g	13. h		

CORE DRUG KNOWLEDGE: JUST THE FACTS

Multiple choice

1. c	2. a	3. b	4. b	5. c
6. b	7. a	8. d	9. c	

ESSAY

1. sweat and salivary glands
   GI tract
   liver
   lungs
   skin

2. In active reabsorption, a carrier mechanism is involved, energy is consumed, and the drug or metabolite may be moved from a high concentration in the filtrate to a low concentration in the efferent arteriolar blood. In passive reabsorption, lipid-soluble drugs and some water-soluble drugs diffuse down a concentration gradient back into the blood.

CORE PATIENT VARIABLES: PATIENTS, PLEASE

Multiple choice

1. b	2. a	3. a	4. b	5. c

NURSING MANAGEMENT: EVERY GOOD NURSE SHOULD . . .

Multiple choice

1. a. Patients who have difficulty swallowing may not be able to swallow oral medication, depending on the drug form. Circulatory impairment will not affect a patient who has difficulty swallowing, although it will decrease the distribution of the drug. Skin integrity is not relevant for orally administered drugs, only those administered topically. Visual acuity might be important to assess if the drug caused an adverse effect of visual impairment, but this is not relevant here.

2. b. A smaller dose than normal to achieve the desired effect would be expected. A patient with renal disease will have kidneys that don't work as well as someone without renal disease. If the kidneys don't work optimally, then the drug will be excreted at a slower rate. This will increase the circulating level of the drug and place the patient at increased risk of developing adverse effects from the drug, if the dose is not decreased. A larger dose than normal would be the opposite of what you would expect because it would further increase the risk of adverse effects and toxicity. Giving the drug more frequently does not alter half-life of the drug, which is related to the time required for half of the drug to be eliminated.

3. b. Risk for injury related to potentially high drug serum levels would be an appropriate nursing diagnosis and relates most directly to drug therapy.

4. b. Drug toxicity. Because her albumin (protein) levels are below normal, more drug will be free and active than would usually be expected from this dose. Therefore, she will be more likely to have adverse effects, in addition to having increased therapeutic effects from the drug. Low albumin levels are hypoalbuminemia, not hyperalbuminemia. Low potassium levels (hypokalemia) are not related to protein levels. CNS depression would only be a concern if the drug could produce CNS depression as an adverse effect.

5. c. Drug B induces the isoenzyme P-450; this will increase the metabolism of Drug A. As the drug is more rapidly metabolized, blood levels of Drug A will fall and this may produce a decreased therapeutic effect from Drug A. The effects (both therapeutic and adverse) of Drug B are not altered by this interaction.

CASE STUDY

1. Absorption may be decreased due to removal of part of the stomach and small intestine. Distribution may be diminished due to her peripheral vascular disease.
2. She may need an increased dose, because not as much drug is available.
3. Does she show improvement in her peripheral vascular disease? Is the color better? Is there more warmth? Is there an improved pulse?

CRITICAL THINKING CHALLENGE

Steady state should have been achieved in five half-lives or 7.5 hours. An assessment of effectiveness was made before the drug was at steady state. Therefore, the drug was increased too early, causing an excessive increase in coagulation time in 8 hours.

Chapter 5

KEY TERMS

True/false

1.	True	
2.	False	Receptor
3.	False	Agonists
4.	False	Antagonists
5.	False	Competitive agonists
6.	True	
7.	False	Mixed agonists
8.	False	Affinity
9.	False	Potency
10.	False	Efficacy
11.	False	Loading dose
12.	False	Maintenance dose
13.	True	

CORE DRUG KNOWLEDGE: JUST THE FACTS

Multiple choice

1. c   2. d   3. b

Essay

Two factors predict the quantitative aspect of a drug's margin of relative safety. These factors are known as the effective dose 50% (ED_{50}) and lethal dose 50% (LD_{50}). The ratio of effective dose to lethal dose is called the therapeutic index (TI).

CORE PATIENT VARIABLES: PATIENTS, PLEASE

Multiple choice

1. b   2. a

NURSING MANAGEMENT: EVERY GOOD NURSE SHOULD . . .

Multiple choice

1. d.   Potency refers to how much of a drug is needed to produce an effect. Unless the increased dose increases the size of the pill or tablet to a size that is difficult or impossible to swallow, potency is not the most important consideration when comparing different drugs designed to treat the same condition. How well the drug works, or its efficacy, is the most important consideration.

2. b.   Liver disease will decrease the rate of drug metabolism. This will cause an increase in the circulating drug. Unless the dose is decreased some, the patient is likely to have adverse effects from the drug therapy. A smaller than usual dose given to a patient with liver disease will produce the same response as the standard dose in a patient with normal liver function.

3. a.   Tolerance develops when a drug is used for an extended period. Less effect comes from the same dose of the drug. Neither potency, receptor agonists, nor efficacy is being demonstrated here, and information about them is not pertinent in this situaton.

4. a.   When a patient has developed tolerance to a drug, a larger dose will be needed to achieve the same desired effect. A smaller dose would be even less effective. Giving the same dose more frequently will increase the dose received in 24 hours and may be helpful. However, this is not an independent nursing decision. Giving less drug in 24 hours will be even less effective.

CASE STUDY

1. The IV route will achieve a faster onset of action than the oral route. The faster route was chosen today to quickly bring down the heart rate. The oral route can be used tomorrow once the heart rate has decelerated some.

2. The large dose today is a loading dose. It is designed to quickly bring the drug into therapeutic level without waiting for steady state to occur. The smaller dose beginning tomorrow is the maintenance dose; it will keep the drug at a therapeutic level.

CRITICAL THINKING CHALLENGE

Ann Faraday is at risk of toxicity and adverse effects from the digoxin during digitalization with the loading dose. The nurse should monitor closely for signs of adverse effects during this time period.

Chapter 6

KEY TERMS

Anagrams

1. interaction		2. adverse
3. side		4. toxicity
5. anaphylaxis		6. idiosyncratic
7. chelation		8. additive
9. synergistic		10. antagonistic
11. potentiation		12. radiopharmaceutical
13. neurotoxicity		14. immunotoxicity
15. hepatoxicity		16. neurotoxicity
17. ototoxicity		18. cardiotoxicity

CORE DRUG KNOWLEDGE: JUST THE FACTS

1. Drug interaction
2. Rash, hives, redness, swelling, and itching
3. Antibiotics, diagnostic agents, biologicals, aspirin, gold salts, iron dextra, phenothiazines, topical anesthetics, and tranquilizers
4. Dyspnea, bronchospasm, laryngeal edema, cardiac dysrhythmias, hypotension, and acute cardiovascular collapse
5. Drowsiness, auditory or visual disturbances, restlessness, nystagmus, and tonic-clonic seizures
6. Hepatitis, jaundice, elevated liver enzyme levels, fatty infiltration of the liver
7. Tinnitus, sensorineural hearing loss, light-headedness, vertigo, nausea and vomiting
8. Drug binding, alteration in GI motility, alteration in gastric pH, alteration in intestinal flora, and an alteration within the walls of the intestine
9. Non-narcotic analgesic with a narcotic analgesic Diuretic with a beta blocker to combat hypertension Anticholinergic with dopaminergic to treat Parkinson's disease
10. Synergism is an interaction in which the effects of both of the interacting drugs is enhanced, whereas in potentiation only one of the two interacting drugs has an increased effect.
11. Physical incompatibility of the two drugs

CORE PATIENT VARIABLES: PATIENTS, PLEASE

Multiple choice

1. d   2. c   3. a   4. b   5. b
6. b   7. c   8. c

NURSING MANAGEMENT: EVERY GOOD NURSE SHOULD...

Multiple choice

1. b.   Intake and output levels indicate one parameter of renal function. Renal function is impaired by a nephrotoxic drug. ALT and AST levels measure hepatic function. Balance is altered when ototoxicity occurs. Cognitive function is altered in neurotoxicity.

2. c.   Liver disease will decrease the metabolism of the drug, and this will increase the circulating blood levels of the drug. More circulating drug means that the patient is at higher risk of developing adverse effects. Although more therapeutic effect may also be evident, this is not generally a problem. When excessive therapeutic effects occur, they are usually considered an adverse effect (e.g., drugs to treat hypertension are supposed to lower the blood pressure; excessive lowering of the blood pressure produces hypotension, which is an adverse effect of the drug therapy). Allergic effects and idiosyncratic effects are both related to patient-specific conditions and not elevated drug levels. These effects occur with normal dosing.

3. c.   Drug therapy is often prescribed using more than one type of drug class to treat one disease or pathology. The drugs will work in different ways to bring about an additive response to therapy. Almost all drugs used this way can be administered at the same time because the goal is for them to achieve their effect together.

4 d.   Patients and their families need to have a thorough understanding of the risks involved in drug therapy and what they need to do to decrease these risks. They also need to understand possible drug interactions that may decrease the effectiveness of the drug therapy or produce adverse effects.

5. a.   Older adults have physiologic changes in their body systems that decrease the effectiveness of organs (e.g., decreased renal and hepatic function). These changes place the older adult at increased risk of adverse effects. Decreased therapeutic effects and pharmacodynamic effects, while possible, are generally not a major concern for older adults receiving drug therapy (see Life Span: Older Adults, Chapter 9). Allergic responses are not accentuated by age.

CASE STUDY

Both of these drug therapies may cause ototoxicity. Teach Amy that tinnitus and hearing loss are signs of ototoxicity. Other signs are light-headedness, vertigo, and nausea and vomiting. If these signs occur, she should contact her health care provider. She should take the drugs as prescribed and not take extra doses on her own, unless directed to do so by the health care provider. Dosages should be taken at prescribed intervals. If a dose is missed, she should not double the dose. Regularly scheduled hearing tests may need to be part of health maintenance if drug therapy is prolonged, dosage is high, or if the patient is unable to detect auditory changes easily.

CRITICAL THINKING CHALLENGE

HEALTH STATUS

Does she exhibit any other symptoms of gastric ulcer or gastric reflux?
Is she taking any over-the-counter drugs to treat the acidity?
Is she taking regular aspirin or enteric-coated aspirin?
Is she taking the prescribed dose of aspirin?

LIFESTYLE, DIET, AND HABITS

Is she taking the aspirin with an acidic beverage, such as orange juice, that may be contributing to excess stomach acidity?
Is she taking the aspirin on an empty stomach?

MINIMIZING ADVERSE EFFECTS

Suggest taking the aspirin on a full stomach or with food.
Enteric forms of aspirin may help decrease gastric distress.
Avoid drinking large amounts of acidic beverages, especially when taking drug doses.
Avoid self-medicating with large doses of antacids, especially sodium bicarbonate because acid rebound may occur.
If these suggestions do not eliminate the problem, she should see her physician or nurse practitioner because she may be developing a gastric ulcer from the aspirin.

Chapter 7

KEY TERMS

Matching

1. b   2. c   3. d   4. a   5. e

CORE DRUG KNOWLEDGE: JUST THE FACTS

1. Immature body systems, greater fluid composition, smaller size
2. Appropriate drug dosages
3. $\text{BSA} = \dfrac{\text{weight in kg} \times \text{height in cm}}{3{,}600}$
4. 1 year old
5. Water content, fat content, immature liver function, immature blood–brain barrier
6. Generic and trade names of drugs
Rationale for therapy
Anticipated therapeutic effects
Route
Frequency and duration of therapy
Potential adverse effects
Precautions or restrictions

Matching

1. b   2. c   3. d   4. a   5. e

CORE PATIENT VARIABLES: PATIENTS, PLEASE

Multiple choice

1. b   2. c   3. c   4. a   5. d

NURSING MANAGEMENT: EVERY GOOD NURSE SHOULD . . .

Multiple choice

1. c.   In this case, a 25-gauge needle would be appropriate. The correct site is the vastus lateralis because it is the most developed at birth. The ventrogluteal site is difficult to find on an infant. The needle length should be 5/8 inch or shorter. Aspiration should always occur before administering an IM injection to prevent accidental administration into the vein.

2. d.   Use the measuring dropper, found with the medicine, to measure an accurate dosage of this drug. Avoid mixing the drug into an infant's formula to prevent rejection of future feedings due to memory of bad taste. Infants are not cognitively developed to be able to understand explanations and willingly comply with drug administration. Infants, however, will respond to a soothing voice and calm attitude.

3. b.   This will prevent Brenda from playing with the pump settings and accidentally increasing the dose received. A pump should always be used to regulate IV infusions; they should not run by gravity. Enough volume should be placed in the microdrip calibrated chamber (e.g., metriset, buretrol, or volutrole) to last for 1 hour only to prevent overdosage if the pump malfunctions. IV insertion sites should be checked every hour in pediatric patients for patency.

4. a.   This offers preschoolers a true choice and allows them to have some control. They are, therefore, likely to be cooperative. Asking preschoolers if they want to take the medicine at all is not an appropriate choice because the child might say no. You would then have to coax or force the child to take the prescribed drug therapy. Children should never be threatened regarding taking their drug therapy. Preschoolers fear punishment and bodily harm. Threatening them will make then fearful and uncooperative. Children should not be called "bad" if they are hesitant to take the drug therapy. This creates more unpleasant feelings and anxiety and will reduce cooperation.

5. c.   The adolescent needs to be involved in the therapy and have an accurate understanding of it. Understanding will promote cooperation. Although the parents need to be involved, the adolescent needs to have an active role in the therapy, unlike with younger children for whom the parent is the primary person responsible for answering questions and voicing concerns. Adolescents need support but should not be treated like younger children. The nurse needs to relinquish some control to the adolescent, as appropriate. The sense of control and ability to make choices will promote cooperation in the adolescent.

CASE STUDY

1. To maximize therapeutic effect, assess Jordan's lifestyle, diet, and habits. It is important to determine if he smokes either cigarettes or marijuana. If he uses these substances after discharge, he will likely have a drop in theophylline levels and, therefore, will not achieve therapeutic effects from the theophylline drug therapy.

2. To minimize adverse effects, assess another aspect of Jordan's lifestyle, diet, and habits: his use of caffeine. How many caffeinated sodas does he drink in a day? Does he drink coffee or tea? Does he drink hot chocolate regularly? How much chocolate candy does he eat? Because theophylline is similar to caffeine, it produces similar CNS stimulant effects. High intake of caffeinated products will increase the risk of tachycardia, palpitations, insomnia, and other CNS effects in Jordan.

CRITICAL THINKING CHALLENGE

Marshall is at risk of CNS depression and toxicity from the morphine his mother receives. This is because the blood–brain barrier is not fully developed in the newborn. Additionally, the liver and kidneys do not function optimally yet. Drugs are not metabolized or excreted as fast as they would be in an older child, so more drug is available to cause adverse effects.

Chapter 8

KEY TERMS

1. preeclampsia
2. organogenesis
3. hyperemesis gravidarum
4. fetal alcohol syndrome
5. lactation
6. eclampsia
7. gestational diabetes
8. teratogenic
9. fetal hydantoin syndrome

CORE DRUG KNOWLEDGE: JUST THE FACTS

Multiple choice

1. c   2. b   3. a   4. c   5. c

Matching

1. c   2. e   3. b   4. a   5. d

CORE PATIENT VARIABLES: PATIENTS, PLEASE

Multiple choice

1. a   2. d   3. d   4. a

NURSING MANAGEMENT: EVERY GOOD NURSE SHOULD . . .

Multiple choice

1. d.   Metabolic needs will vary during the course of the pregnancy, and, therefore, insulin requirements will also vary. Oral hypoglycemics are contraindicated in pregnancy because they cross the placenta. Insulin is used to keep the blood glucose levels in a normal range because elevated glucose levels may cause fetal deformities. Patients who develop gestational diabetes may return to normal glucose levels after delivery, so insulin may only be needed during the pregnancy.

2. b. Piperazines have not been found to be teratogenic. The patient has concerns that injury may occur to her baby while she is taking a drug, and the correct information needs to be provided to reduce anxiety. Greatest risk for fetal injury from drug therapy is in the first trimester, not second. Because this drug has not been found to be teratogenic, an effective dose should be taken. Hyperemesis gravidarum has deleterious effects on the mother and fetus due to risk for dehydration, and fluid and electrolyte imbalance.

3. d. All of the above are necessary before giving the first dose.

4. d. Instruct the patient to rest with her feet elevated several times a day. This is a nonpharmacologic intervention for swelling, a common occurrence in pregnancy. Drug therapy should be avoided if possible to reduce risk of adverse effects to mother and fetus. Extra sodium in the diet will cause the patient to retain more fluid, so this is not an appropriate response. Although caffeine produces a mild diuresis, large doses of caffeine are not recommended in pregnancy, and this would not be an appropriate suggestion.

5. b. Patient education should include that heroin and cocaine are contraindicated in breast-feeding because they will be transferred in the breast milk to the infant. Because the patient abuses both of these drugs, this is critical information to share with the patient. Breast milk has significant advantages over commercial formula (not the other way around), among them the fact that antibodies are passed to the child from the mother and the ease of digestion of the breast milk. However, due to the possibility that the mother may continue to abuse drugs, encouraging the use of commercial formula may be more prudent in this situation. Because breast-feeding is not the best choice for this patient, teaching positions for breast-feeding is not appropriate. Although postpartum rest is important, it is not the priority in this situation.

CASE STUDY

Anita needs to have blood levels of aminophylline drawn at regular intervals while on drug infusion and after dose increases. This is because aminophylline can reach toxic levels, causing adverse effects in both the mother and the fetus. Breath sounds and vital signs should be assessed at regular intervals to determine effectiveness of the drug. Also, Anita should be assessed for signs of adverse effects (tachycardia, insomnia, GI distress). The aminophylline should be discontinued as soon as possible to help minimize risk to the fetus. Therapeutic effect for Anita should be attained, however.

CRITICAL THINKING CHALLENGE

Although it is unknown whether ipratropium is excreted in breast milk, it is unlikely to be of concern. Little of the drug is absorbed systemically when it is administered through an inhaler. Assess Anita's lifestyle to determine if she smokes because this may be contributing to her bronchitis. Smoking cigarettes would also counteract the effect of the inhaler. Assess her home environment. Does another person who smokes live with her? Second-hand smoke is also irritating and can cause respiratory problems for Anita and her baby. Also, consider whether environmental pollutants may be contributing to her bronchitis.

Chapter 9

KEY TERMS

True/false

1.	False	risk–benefit ratio
2.	True	
3.	False	paradoxical
4.	True	
5.	False	polypharmacy
6.	False	frail elderly

PHYSIOLOGY AND PATHOPHYSIOLOGY: THE BODY HUMAN

Essay

1. Increased gastric pH levels; slowed blood flow; decreased GI motility; reduced surface area of the GI tract

2. Decreased body mass; reduced levels of plasma albumin; less effective blood–brain barrier; declining cardiac output; extreme changes in body weight; poor nutrition or dehydration; inactivity or extended bed rest

3. decreased size of the liver; decreased number of metabolically active hepatocytes; decreased blood flow to the liver; decreased ability to remove many byproducts; overall efficiency of the liver is reduced

4. decreased glomerular filtration rate; decreased renal tubular secretion; decreased renal blood flow

CORE DRUG KNOWLEDGE: JUST THE FACTS

Multiple choice

1. a   2. b   3. a   4. c   5. a

CORE PATIENT VARIABLES: PATIENTS, PLEASE

Multiple choice

1. c   2. c   3. a   4. d

Essay

- Identify the *etiology* of the nonadherence first
- Advocate with the provider to keep the medication regimen as simple as possible
- Coordinate the orders of all providers to minimize the number of drugs needed
- Create memory aids
- Facilitate the ability to open medications
- Write all instructions in simple terms
- Print in large letters as needed

NURSING MANAGEMENT: EVERY GOOD NURSE SHOULD . . .

Multiple choice

1. d. Oral drugs may need to be crushed or in liquid form. Mr. Goodwin can swallow, but large pieces of food pose difficulty for him. Therefore, it may be assumed that he may have trouble with large pills, tablets, or capsules. Crushing the medication or providing it in a liquid oral form will make the medications easier to swallow. It is not necessary to avoid the oral route as long as he can swal-

low without choking. Drug absorption and elimination are not affected by his difficulty swallowing.

2. b.   How does Mrs. Thomas usually obtain prescriptions and refills? Is there a regular plan in place, such as a relative, neighbor, or friend who takes her to the store, or does she drive herself? Does she walk to a neighborhood store? Buy her prescriptions by mail? If Mrs. Thomas is unsure how she will obtain the prescription, she may have trouble obtaining it and being adherent with the drug regimen. Although knowledge about her ability to get out of the house and her fluid intake may provide more data about her, neither directly relates to potential adherence problems. Renal and hepatic disease may alter pharmacokinetics, but they don't have an effect on her adherence with drug therapy.

3. b.   Ms. Humphreys is an older adult, and her renal function is most likely not as good as in younger adults. She is receiving a drug that may cause further renal damage. A smaller dose would be expected, and possibly also given at less frequent intervals, to decrease the risk of renal damage from the gentamicin.

4. d.   These are signs of adverse effects from the drug therapy. Older adults are more sensitive to the CNS effects of drugs that depress the CNS, such as phenytoin. Excessive sleepiness and difficulty concentrating are signs of CNS depression. Although normal aging may include some of these symptoms, the new onset of the symptoms tends to dispute that they are age-related changes.

5. a.   4 mg. Begin drug dosage with the minimal effective dose and titrate upward with older adults. This is especially important with drugs that depress the CNS. Additionally, she has received anesthesia, also a CNS depressant, and may still be having some CNS effects from that.

CASE STUDY

1. All of the drugs should have their first dose of the morning given early in the day, such as 8 AM, because a dose would not have been taken since the previous evening. Instruct Mr. Vibaldi to take the first dose "with breakfast" to be a memory aid. The captopril, being dosed three times a day, will need a second dose late afternoon to distribute the day's dosing. A recommended time would be 4 PM. Ideally, the second dose of furosemide, nicardipine, and potassium would be early evening, such as 6 PM with dinner. Administration of furosemide, a diuretic, should be avoided in the late evening because it will create nocturia in Mr. Vibaldi. If a drug at 4 PM and others at 6 PM prove to be too difficult to remember, the furosemide, captopril, nicardipine, and potassium could all be given together at 4 PM. The theophylline is due at 8 PM. To limit the dosage times, consult with the prescriber to confirm that the second dose may be given at a different time. Pharmacokinetics of the theophylline, a sustained-release drug, indicate that a 2-hour swing either way most likely should not cause significant problems with therapeutic blood levels. Therefore, ask the provider if the theophylline may be taken at 6 PM with the second dose of furosemide, nicardipine, and potassium. Or, if those drugs were given at 4 PM, consider giving the theophylline at 10 PM with the last dose of the captopril.

2. Written instructions should be given to Mr. Vibaldi regarding the dosing of each medicine. (He was missing one dose of nicardipine every day.) Having dosages given around mealtime and bedtime will be memory prompts to take the drugs as prescribed. Also, a daily pill organizer, in which all the doses for the day are placed would be helpful. An egg crate could also be used. If he has a watch with an alarm setting, he could set the alarm to go off when his doses are due. The 4 PM dose especially is likely to be forgotten because it is not taken at a time when an activity (eating, going to bed) will help jog his memory. Other aids, such as pictures that show a clock, the time of the dose, and the correct drug, could also be used.

CRITICAL THINKING CHALLENGE

HEALTH STATUS

Does he have a clear understanding of why he takes these drugs for his health problems?

Does he understand why they need to be taken regularly?

Does he have adequate short- and long-term memory to take the different drugs at the correct times and remember taking them?

Does he have arthritis or any trouble with the fine hand movement needed to open the bottle caps?

If yes, are his drugs being dispensed in a child-resistant package?

LIFESTYLE, DIET, AND HABITS

Is he having adverse effects from one or more of the drugs he takes?

ENVIRONMENT

Does he have the income or health insurance to afford the drug therapies?

Does he have physical difficulty getting to the drugstore?

CULTURE

Are there any cultural issues that may be causing him to be hesitant or resistant to taking the prescribed drug therapies?

If yes to any of the above, he may not be taking the drug therapies as prescribed.

Chapter 10

KEY TERMS

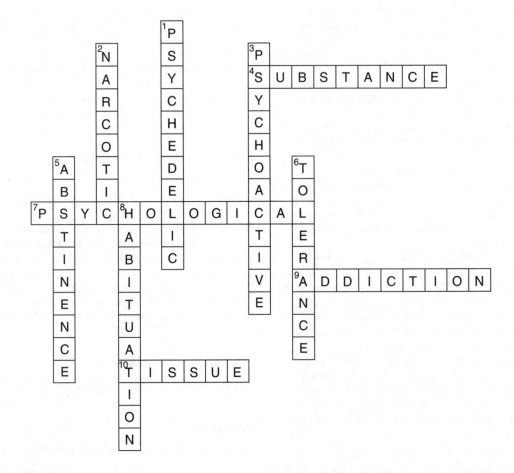

PHYSIOLOGY AND PATHOPHYSIOLOGY: THE BODY HUMAN

Matching

1. d   2. b   3. c   4. a

Matching

1. c   2. b   3. a   4. d

CORE DRUG KNOWLEDGE: JUST THE FACTS

True/false

1. False
2. True
3. False
4. False
5. True
6. True
7. False
8. True
9. True
10. False

CORE PATIENT VARIABLES: PATIENTS, PLEASE

Multiple choice

1. a   2. b   3. c   4. b   5. d
6. c   7. a   8. c

NURSING MANAGEMENT: EVERY GOOD NURSE SHOULD . . .

Multiple choice

1. d. Nicotine (in cigarettes), alcohol, and street drugs are all substances that may be abused and may interact with prescribed drug therapy.
2. c. Disulfiram interacts with alcohol, producing feelings of acute illness and unpleasant sensations. Any alcohol intake will produce this response. The drug needs to be taken regularly. It does not decrease craving.
3. c. Staying with the patient and speaking in a calm and soothing manner will help alleviate fear and anxiety from the "bad trip." Patients should be placed in a quiet room to decrease sensory stimulation, not the middle of a busy emergency room. Phenothiazines should not be administered because they cause hypotension, confusion, or increased panic reactions. Contact the physician for orders for tranquilizers, barbiturates, or benzodiazepines.

4. b. Patients who have intoxication from inhalants may experience hypoxia from CNS depression; therefore, oxygen may be required. Maintenance of respiratory function is a priority. Lee is already short of breath. Epinephrine is contraindicated; this is not an allergic reaction and the cardiac stimulation from the epinephrine (a vasopressor) may interact with the inhalant causing cardiac arrhythmias. A defibrillator should not be needed as long as vasopressors have not been administered, although significant overdosage may produce cardiac arrest secondary to CNS depression. An emesis basin is not a priority item in this situation.

CASE STUDY

This patient abuses alcohol. It is likely that there was still alcohol in his system when he underwent surgery. This may have created an additive CNS effect with the anesthesia and narcotics he received. He may have also required a larger dose of anesthesia and analgesia due to a cross tolerance to the CNS depressant effects of these drugs from his alcohol abuse.

CRITICAL THINKING CHALLENGE

1. He may be demonstrating signs of alcohol withdrawal. He needs to be monitored carefully for further changes. The physician should be notified regarding these findings. Consult with the physician regarding drug orders to prevent complications of withdrawal.
2. He is well educated and a professional. He does not meet the image of an alcoholic being a "skid row bum." The documentation that he "drinks socially on weekends" is vague and can be interpreted in different ways. Alcohol use is an accepted practice in the United States. The difficulty to arouse him after surgery may have been attributed to individual variation from anesthesia and analgesia if additional questions had not been asked regarding his drinking.

Chapter 11

KEY TERMS

Essay

1. Alternative therapies and complementary therapies include supplements of basic food elements, vitamins, and minerals, as well as the use of herbs and botanicals. Initially, they were called alternative therapies because they were viewed as "non-Western." Today, they are viewed as augmentations or supplements to Western health care, thus the term "complementary."
2. Herbal and botanical preparations are those substances derived from a plant source used either as a dietary supplement or as a medication.
3. The major mineral cations include calcium, magnesium, potassium, and sodium.
4. Phytomedicines are therapeutic agents derived from plants or a preparation derived from a plant.
5. The most important trace elements include chromium, copper, iron, selenium, and zinc.

6. A vitamin is an organic compound needed by the body to maintain health, regulate metabolism, assist in the biochemistry of food digestion, and act as cofactors for enzymes.

CORE DRUG KNOWLEDGE: JUST THE FACTS

Multiple choice

1. c   2. c   3. a   4. c

CORE PATIENT VARIABLES: PATIENTS, PLEASE

Multiple choice

1. b   2. d   3. c

NURSING MANAGEMENT: EVERY GOOD NURSE SHOULD . . .

Multiple choice

1. e. All of the above should be assessed. It is important to consider all nutritional supplements that the patient is taking because these may interact with current drug therapy or therapy that will be prescribed. It is also important to ask if the patient is taking the supplement on their own or on a prescriber's recommendation as patients may self-medicate without knowing of potential drug interactions.
2. d. Older adults with chronic health problems and who take multiple medications are more at risk of having drug-induced nutritional deficiencies. Asking what is the patient's typical daily diet provides some information as to whether any foods or beverages taken may interact with drug therapy. Knowing when the patient normally takes medications may indicate if drug absorption might be impaired from taking a drug with food when it should be taken on an empty stomach, or vice versa.
3. c. Echinacea is an immune stimulant. Taking it with drug therapy designed to suppress the immune system will counteract the purpose of the drug therapy. Because the intended effect is not achieved from the drug, the patient may have disease-related complications. Although vitamin C may be helpful to prevent infections, it should not be taken with Echinacea. The nurse should encourage patients to buy herbs from a reputable source because purity and strength can vary; however, this patient should not be encouraged to buy Echinacea.

CASE STUDY

Because the patient is malnourished, it is likely that he has low serum albumin (protein) levels. As heparin is highly protein bound, the low protein levels cause him to have higher than expected blood levels of heparin. This would cause the additional anticoagulant effect from the heparin. A blood test measuring his protein levels would confirm this.

CRITICAL THINKING CHALLENGE

The chamomile and the garlic may both potentiate the action of anticoagulants, like warfarin. Taken together, they have significantly increased the coagulation time.

Chapter 12

KEY TERMS

Matching

1. c   2. a   3. e   4. b   5. d

CORE DRUG KNOWLEDGE: JUST THE FACTS

1. Acute care hospitals, acute rehabilitative units, transitional care units, outpatient units, long-term care facilities, and the home or community environment.
2. In addition to the setting, other major considerations include trained personnel and the ability to safely monitor the patient.
3. Heat, light, moisture, and sudden temperature changes
4. Industrial solvents, polycyclic aromatic hydrocarbons, pesticides, and ethanol
5. Smoking and diet

CORE PATIENT VARIABLES: PATIENTS, PLEASE

Multiple choice

1. a   2. c   3. b   4. c

NURSING MANAGEMENT: EVERY GOOD NURSE SHOULD...

Multiple choice

1. d.   How long the patient is outdoors and in the sunlight will determine how much risk the patient has to develop a photosensitivity reaction. Assessing if there is refrigeration, where medications are usually stored, and other people in the house to assist the patient can be important questions to ask concerning other drug therapies interacting with the environment, but they are not especially relevant here.
2. b.   Heat from hot water in a hot tub will cause vasodilation. Because the patient is prescribed a vasodilator, hypotension may occur from excessive vasodilation. You would not recommend that a hot tub be used every day, and patients need to be aware of this interaction with the environment.
3. a.   Exposure to polychlorinated biphenyls, among other environmental pollutants and chemicals, is known to alter drug metabolism occurring in the liver. If the drug is not metabolized as well, more drug may be circulating than would normally be expected, placing the patient at increased risk of adverse effects from drug therapy. The patient should be well aware of the potential adverse effects and notify the physician if they occur. Telling a patient he cannot work due to a potential drug environment interaction would not be appropriate.

CASE STUDY

No, the obstetrician would not start oxytocin to induce labor in her office suite, even if she has a nurse to be with Janice. Oxytocin needs to be administered in an environment where the patient and baby can be continuously monitored, specifically a labor and delivery unit of a hospital.

CRITICAL THINKING CHALLENGE

You need to refuse to accept this patient for admission to your floor. A general medical surgical unit is not equipped to adequately monitor a woman and baby during induction of labor. Contact the nurse manager, nursing supervisor, and the attending obstetrician for assistance if necessary. The induction may have to be postponed for a short time until the labor and delivery suite can attend to Janice.

Chapter 13

KEY TERMS

Anagrams

1. Biocultural ecology
2. Stereotyping
3. Culture
4. Ethnocentrism
5. Ethnicity
6. Cultural competence
7. Cultural blindness

CORE DRUG KNOWLEDGE: JUST THE FACTS

Multiple choice

1. a   2. c   3. b   4. d   5. a
6. c

Essay

Overview: heritage and residence
Communication
Family roles and organization
Workforce issues
Biocultural ecology
High-risk health behaviors
Nutrition
Pregnancy and childbearing practices
Death rituals
Spirituality
Health care practices
Health care practitioners

CORE PATIENT VARIABLES: PATIENTS, PLEASE

Multiple choice

1. c   2. c   3. b   4. b   5. a
6. c

NURSING MANAGEMENT: EVERY GOOD NURSE SHOULD...

Multiple choice

1. d.   All of the above are important reasons to consider a patient's culture.
2. b.   Evenly spaced daily doses will help to maintain an effective blood level. Teaching with present-oriented people should emphasize current or present situations as opposed to possible complications that may occur in the future.

3. d.   Ask Mr. Lee about other herbs he uses regularly. These may have an interaction with prescribed drug therapy. Teasing, verbal "put downs," and insistence that Western medicine is the only correct approach are examples of ethnocentrism.
4. a.   Albert Clark, the white American, is more likely to be a slow metabolizer of isoniazid than the men of the other cultural backgrounds. Thus, he is more at risk for adverse effects from the drug. To prevent this, the doses are likely to be spaced further apart, providing less milligrams of drug in a 24-hour period.

CASE STUDY

Chinese Americans tend to have thalassemia, an inherited disorder of hemoglobin metabolism, more often than other cultures. This makes Susan more at risk for developing anemia. Sulfonamides have the possible adverse effect of anemia. The risk of developing anemia from sulfonamide use is increased in Chinese Americans with thalassemia. Additionally, Chinese Americans may have G_6PD deficiency, which results in anemia; again, the risk of developing anemia is increased if taking sulfonamides.

CRITICAL THINKING CHALLENGE

Health status: Low or low-normal hemoglobin before the start of the drug
Life span and gender: Her hemoglobin may be normally low due to loss of blood from menstruation.
Lifestyle, diet, and habits: Diet may be poor in iron-rich foods

Chapter 14

KEY TERMS

Fill in the blanks

1. central nervous system
2. peripheral nervous system
3. autonomic nervous system
4. agonists
5. antagonists
6. neurotransmitters
7. synaptic transmission
8. nonselective-acting drugs
9. selective-acting drug
10. sympathetic nervous system; parasympathetic nervous system
11. adrenergic nervous system

PHYSIOLOGY AND PATHOPHYSIOLOGY: THE BODY HUMAN

Matching

1. c	2. a	3. d	4. a	5. b
6. c	7. a	8. a	9. d	10. d

CORE DRUG KNOWLEDGE: JUST THE FACTS

Multiple choice

1. a	2. c	3. e	4. b	5. d
6. b	7. b	8. a	9. c	10. d

CORE PATIENT VARIABLES: PATIENTS, PLEASE

Multiple choice

1. d	2. c	3. d	4. a	5. b
6. d	7. b	8. a	9. d	10. c

NURSING MANAGEMENT: EVERY GOOD NURSE SHOULD . . .

Multiple choice

1. b.   The first priority is to limit the vasoconstrictive damage done by the drug by limiting the drug that gets into the tissues. To limit the blood flow to the area, the arm should be elevated, not lowered. A tourniquet placed below the area of extravasation will cause further venous constriction to the arm and hand. Blood pressure should be assessed, because the drug was being given to treat hypotension, but this is not the priority.
2. c.   Phentolamine is an alpha blocker and is the antidote for overdosage or extravasation of phenylephrine. It should be injected subcutaneously into the affected tissue. Epinephrine is not appropriate because it also causes vasoconstriction.
3. b.   Changes in rhythm may occur from epinephrine use. Hypertension is possible after epinephrine administration, not hypotension. Decreased urinary output and fever are not related to epinephrine use.
4. d.   Beta agonists will increase the heart rate. If the patient is already tachycardic, this may cause serious arrhythmias.
5. c.   Avoid driving for 4 hours after the first dose. First dose of prazosin may cause sedation or syncope. To avoid dizziness and weakness related to orthostatic hypotension, the patient should avoid quick position changes, drinking alcohol, and activities that cause more vasodilation, such as hot showers. Taking the drug at night, at least the first dose, will minimize the recognition of the adverse effects of sedation and syncope.
6. b.   Abrupt stopping of propranolol, and other beta blockers, will cause a reflex tachycardia, resulting in angina, and possibly even myocardial infarction. Depression can be a significant adverse effect from propranolol and other beta blockers. The depression will go away when the drug is stopped. An increased dose should not be given because this may worsen depression and/or cause other adverse effects.

CASE STUDY

LIFESTYLE, DIET, AND HABITS

Does she shake the canister thoroughly before administration? If not, active drug may not be dispersed into the aerosol spray.

Does she place her mouth properly on the mouthpiece? Can she perform the proper respiratory sequence when administering the drug? (Exhale slowly, trigger inhaler while slowly inhaling, holding the breath, and then exhaling.) If not, she may not be inhaling the drug. Accurate assessment of these issues may require Judy to demonstrate her technique to you; she may not realize she is making errors.

How long does she use the drug before obtaining a refill? Does she keep track of how many doses are used in the inhaler? If not, she may be using an empty canister sometimes.

Are there financial problems for her family in obtaining the prescription refills? If yes, she may be trying to stretch the dosages out of the inhaler and sometimes may be using an empty or near empty inhaler; this would cause the drug to appear less effective.

CRITICAL THINKING CHALLENGE

1. Although abrupt cessation of beta blockers can cause tachycardia and angina, skipping or delaying one dose is not the same as abrupt cessation. Although drug levels will fall, possibly to subtherapeutic levels, some of the drug will remain in circulation. Because it is expected that the patient will be able to take oral fluids after surgery, he could receive the next dose at that time. Mark the chart to make sure that the anesthesiologist is aware of the hypertension, the use of propranolol, and the dose that was withheld this morning in case the patient experiences hypertension during surgery.

2. Yes. Plan on giving the propranolol when the patient is fully recovered from surgery and allowed oral intake.

Chapter 15

KEY TERMS

Matching

1. h   2. f   3. c   4. e   5. i
6. a   7. g   8. b   9. d

PHYSIOLOGY AND PATHOPHYSIOLOGY: THE BODY HUMAN

True/false

1.	False	constriction
2.	False	decreases
3.	True	
4.	False	hypotension
5.	False	increase
6.	False	retention
7.	True	
8.	False	antagonize
9.	False	high
10.	True	

CORE DRUG KNOWLEDGE: JUST THE FACTS

Multiple choice

1. a   2. d   3. b   4. d   5. a
6. b   7. b   8. c   9. a   10. b

Essay

1. The major actions of atropine include a reduction in salivary, bronchial, and sweat gland secretions; mydriasis; cycloplegia; changes in heart rate; contraction of the bladder detrusor muscle and of the GI smooth muscle; decreased gastric secretion; and decreased GI motility.

2. Symptoms of a cholinergic crisis include nausea and vomiting, diarrhea, increased salivation, sweating, peripheral vasodilation, bronchial constriction, and respiratory arrest.

CORE PATIENT VARIABLES: PATIENTS, PLEASE

Multiple choice

1. c   2. b   3. b   4. a   5. d
6. c   7. b   8. a

Essay

Respiratory status
Presence of ptosis
Diplopia
Ability to chew and swallow
Strength of hand grip bilaterally
Gait

NURSING MANAGEMENT: EVERY GOOD NURSE SHOULD . . .

Multiple choice

1. a. Pilocarpine will cause pupil constriction, which makes it difficult to see in the dark. Eyedrops should be administered into the conjunctival sac rather than directly over the eyeball. Pilocarpine will increase saliva; actions to relieve dry mouth are not indicated.

2. b. Starting at the higher dose will prevent abrupt withdrawal and minimize craving. The patches should be used in the sequence recommended by the manufacturer. Because the drug is slowly absorbed through the skin, the patch is worn continuously to achieve a steady state and therapeutic level of the drug. Patients should not smoke while wearing a nicotine patch because this may cause them to overdose on nicotine.

3. c. Onset of action is within 75 minutes, so 1.5 hours after administration the drug will be working. Duration is up to 4 hours after onset. After this period, the drug's effectiveness is diminished, so tiring activities should be avoided. Earlier than this period and the drug will not have taken effect, so again, tiring activities should be avoided.

4. b. Pilocarpine is a cholinergic agonist. Excessive cholinergic stimulation will increase salivation (thus the drooling) and will cause abdominal cramps, nausea, vomiting (from increased GI tone), flushing (vasodilation), and sweating.

5. b. Atropine, an anticholinergic, is the direct antidote to cholinergic overdose.

CASE STUDY

HEALTH STATUS

Does Mr. Fitzsimmons have glaucoma?
Does he have a history of urinary retention or difficulty voiding?
Does he have constipation or signs of intestinal obstruction?
Any cardiac history?
All of these would be aggravated by the use of anticholinergics.

LIFE SPAN AND GENDER

How old is Mr. Fitzsimmons? Older adults are more likely to be sensitive to the adverse effects of anticholinergics. Older males are more likely to have some urinary retention from an enlarged prostate.

CRITICAL THINKING CHALLENGE

Mr. Fitzsimmons appears to be demonstrating excessive anticholinergic effects. Verify that he only used one patch per day because using more could lead to overdosage. Question whether he washed his hands after removing the patch. There is still drug left in the patch after it has been worn. It is likely that he removed the patch, got some scopolamine on his fingers, and then rubbed his eyes. This would have gotten scopolamine into his eyes, causing adverse effects such as blurred vision.

Chapter 16

KEY TERMS

True/false

1. False narcoanalysis
2. False nondepolarizing
3. False local
4. False paralysis
5. True
6. False anesthesia
7. False neuroleptanesthesia
8. False depolarizing
9. False balanced
10. True
11. False general

PHYSIOLOGY AND PATHOPHYSIOLOGY: THE BODY HUMAN

Matching

1. d   2. a   3. c   4. b

CORE DRUG KNOWLEDGE: JUST THE FACTS

Multiple choice

1. c   2. d   3. b   4. c   5. c
6. b   7. d   8. d   9. c   10. a
11. d   12. b   13. a   14. b

Essay

Esters are relatively unstable in solution and are rapidly hydrolyzed in the body by plasma cholinesterase and other esterases. One of the main breakdown products is para-amino benzoate (PABA), which is associated with allergic phenomena and hypersensitivity reactions. In contrast, amides are relatively stable in solution and are slowly metabolized by hepatic amidases, and hypersensitivity reactions to amide local anesthetics are rare. In current clinical practice, esters have largely been superseded by the amides.

CORE PATIENT VARIABLES: PATIENTS, PLEASE

Multiple choice

1. a   2. b   3. d   4. a   5. c
6. c   7. a   8. b   9. c   10. b
11. b   12. c   13. b

NURSING MANAGEMENT: EVERY GOOD NURSE SHOULD . . .

1. d. A relaxed patient will have an easier and smoother induction into anesthesia. Active conversations will stimulate the patient, possibly causing stress, and will not promote relaxation. The environment should be quiet, not a busy hallway where noise and activity occur. Thorough preoperative teaching, including what to expect during induction of anesthesia, will decrease anxiety because the patient does not have to contend with "fear of the unknown."

2. d. Because isoflurane may cause hypotension and cardiovascular depression, vital signs need to be carefully assessed to be stable and to have returned to the patient's baseline. The patient should void before leaving the recovery room to demonstrate return of urinary function. As isoflurane is a general, inhaled anesthetic, residual drowsiness may occur after initial recovery. For safety, the patient should not be driving or engaging in activities requiring full alertness and concentration.

3. d. While on tubocurarine, Mr. Brooks will not be able to speak, move, or breathe for himself. Turning and repositioning him will help prevent venous pooling and ulcer formation. Keeping the skin clean and dry will also prevent skin breakdown. Although he cannot talk, he can hear and think. It is important for the nurse to speak to Mr. Brooks while providing care and offer explanations of what is being done to reduce fear and anxiety that may accompany being paralyzed from tubocurarine.

4. c. Succinylcholine causes intense muscle fasciculations before muscle paralysis. This may produce severely sore muscles. The presence of sore muscles is not a dangerous finding, or a sign that the patient was injured through negligence or drug error. Contacting the anesthesiologist is not necessary, and an incident sheet is inappropriate. Another dose of succinylcholine is inappropriate as it is used for rapid endotracheal intubation and short procedures such as endoscopy and ECT.

CASE STUDY

1. The lidocaine would be administered subcutaneously to provide local anesthesia around the tissues where the chest tube is to be inserted.
2. Lidocaine comes in several concentrations. Consult with the physician as to the strength of lidocaine desired, if it is not in the orders.

CRITICAL THINKING CHALLENGE

Mr. Kornevitz is showing signs of lidocaine toxicity. This may have been from a large dose, and/or the physician may have inadvertently administered it into a vessel.

Chapter 17

KEY TERMS

Definitions

1. *Anxiety* is an uncomfortable feeling that may be a response to a normal stressor or may be pathologic.
2. *Neurotransmitters* are chemicals that facilitate electrical impulse transmission from neuron to neuron.
3. A *synapse* is the space between two neurons.

ESSAY

Generalized anxiety disorder (GAD), obsessive-compulsive disorder (OCD), panic disorder, phobias (including agoraphobia and social phobia), posttraumatic stress disorder (PTSD), and eating disorders are the most common types of pathologic anxiety.

PHYSIOLOGY AND PATHOPHYSIOLOGY: THE BODY HUMAN

Essay

1. The thalamus functions as a central relay station for ascending sensory impulses from other parts of the CNS to the cerebral cortex; all sensory pathways, except the olfactory, are connected to thalamic nuclei.
2. The limbic system works with the cerebral cortex, brain stem, and hypothalamus to normalize the expression of emotions, such as anxiety, anger, fear, pleasure, sorrow, and sexual feelings.
3. The RAS motor function receives input from higher brain regions that control skeletal muscles. The RAS sensory function alerts the cortex to incoming sensory signals. It also is responsible for maintaining consciousness and for awakening the person from sleep.
4. Dopamine (DA), serotonin (5-HT), histamine, norepinephrine (NE), noradrenaline, acetylcholine, GABA, glutamate, and neuropeptides.
5. Sleep stages 3 and 4 are also known as delta or slow wave sleep. These stages allow deep restorative sleep, during which time immune function is fortified and growth hormone is secreted.

CORE DRUG KNOWLEDGE: JUST THE FACTS

Multiple choice

1. d   2. a   3. c   4. c   5. b
6. a   7. c   8. d

CORE PATIENT VARIABLES: PATIENTS, PLEASE

Multiple choice

1. a   2. b   3. a   4. d   5. d
6. b   7. c   8. b

NURSING MANAGEMENT: EVERY GOOD NURSE SHOULD . . .

Multiple choice

1. d.   Phenobarbital decreases the effectiveness of oral contraceptives, therefore the patient is at risk for pregnancy. A common adverse effect of phenobarbital is sedation, especially when the drug is first used. Drinking alcohol while taking phenobarbital may cause additive CNS depression.
2. b.   These muscles are large muscles and can best accommodate IM phenobarbital. A 5/8-inch, 25-gauge needle is appropriate for subcutaneous injections, not for intramuscular injections. A 90-degree angle is needed to give an injection intramuscularly.
3. d.   Initial use of lorazepam may cause drowsiness, so driving should be avoided until the effects of the drug on the individual patient are known. Alcohol and other CNS depressants will cause additive CNS depressant effects. Lorazepam is a pregnancy class D drug and may cause birth defects.
4. c.   Older adults usually have age-related deterioration of the liver, which can slow metabolism of lorazepam. They tend to be more sensitive to the CNS depressant effects so dosage should be started with a low dose and titrated upward if needed.
5. d.   Because sedation and ataxia are common adverse effects, Mrs. Farrow is at risk for falling when going down the stairs of her house, so she should be instructed to hold the hand railing. Taking the evening dose at bedtime will allow the sedation that occurs from the drug to be beneficial and promote sleep. If she is having significant daytime sedation from the drug, the 24-hour dose should be divided into unequal halves (if possible), and the larger half taken at night so the sedation is helpful, rather than an adverse effect.

CASE STUDY

Tell Mr. Williamson not to be concerned. The IV lorazepam often causes amnesia of events that occurred after receiving the drug. This is a temporary effect and will not alter his permanent memory.

CRITICAL THINKING CHALLENGE

Mr. Williamson may be experiencing digoxin toxicity due to a drug interaction with lorazepam. Check his blood level of digoxin to determine if it is elevated. See Chapter 27 for more information on digoxin.

Chapter 18

KEY TERMS

Anagrams

1. antidepressants
2. depression
3. mood stabilizers
4. mood
5. bipolar disorder
6. neurotransmitters

PHYSIOLOGY AND PATHOPHYSIOLOGY: THE BODY HUMAN

Essay

1. norepinephrine (NE), dopamine (DA), and serotonin (5-HT). acetylcholine (ACh), gamma-aminobutyric acid (GABA), norepinephrine (NE), dopamine (DA), and serotonin (5-HT)
3. Flulike symptoms (eg, fatigue, myalgia, loose stools, nausea), light-headedness/dizziness, uneasiness/restlessness, sleep and sensory disturbances, headache

CORE DRUG KNOWLEDGE: JUST THE FACTS

Multiple choice

1. d   2. b   3. a   4. d   5. b
6. c   7. c   8. d   9. b   10. a
11. b   12. c

CORE PATIENT VARIABLES: PATIENTS, PLEASE

Multiple choice

1. a   2. c   3. b   4. a   5. d
6. b   7. b   8. b   9. a   10. c

NURSING MANAGEMENT: EVERY GOOD NURSE SHOULD . . .

Multiple choice

1. a.   Cured meats and aged cheeses are high sources of tyramine, which can precipitate hypertensive crisis when taking MAOI like phenelzine; they should be avoided. Semolina pasta, apples, and orange juice are not foods with high tyramine levels and do not cause an adverse effect when taken with phenelzine.
2. b.   A dry mouth is one anticholinergic effect that is common with tricyclic antidepressants. Most patients will develop a tolerance to this adverse effect over time and it will be less bothersome. Tricyclic antidepressants require several weeks to months to be fully effective. She needs to tolerate the adverse effects for awhile, until the therapeutic effects are known. Coping strategies might be suggested such as sucking on hard candy. Dry mouth is not a sign of an allergic response, and the drug therapy should not be stopped.
3. a.   SSRIs, like fluoxetine, can stimulate the CNS. Drinking coffee and other caffeinated beverages, with fluoxetine can create enough CNS stimulation to cause insomnia. Carbohydrates do not increase the antidepressant effect from fluoxetine. Although a very slight risk of weight gain or weight loss is possible with fluoxetine, no emphasis on calorie restriction is normally required.
4. b.   Susan is presenting with depression and suicidal tendencies. Desipramine and other tricyclics are potentially life threatening, especially in overdose. The prescription should provide a limited amount of drug to minimize risk of fatal overdose. She should not be told to expect a relief of depression within 1 week; several weeks are needed to see the full therapeutic effect. Psychotherapy or counseling is an important aspect of managing and treating depression, and it should be continued during drug therapy. This is especially important as she may be suicidal and is given drug therapy that will not be effective for several weeks.
5. a.   Lithium levels should be monitored because the drug has a narrow therapeutic index, and toxicity is likely. Also monitor sodium levels. Potassium levels are not relevant to adverse effects from lithium. Foods with tyramine, including dairy products, interact with MAOI, not lithium.

CASE STUDY

Health status

Is he taking an anxiolytic or antipsychotic with the lithium? These are needed to control some of the symptoms until the lithium achieves its desired effects.

Lifestyle, diet, and habits

Does he take a caffeinated beverage (coffee, tea, hot chocolate, cola) in the morning? The caffeine may be decreasing the effectiveness of the lithium and aggravating mania. Is he abusing drugs or alcohol? These may also reduce the effectiveness of lithium. Does he eat breakfast? Does he take his lithium on an empty stomach? If yes, have him take it with food to minimize GI upset.

CRITICAL THINKING CHALLENGE

Larry is showing signs of lithium toxicity, based on symptoms and elevated blood levels. His significant decrease in salt (sodium) content has contributed to the toxicity. Because the body interprets a lithium ion to be similar to a sodium ion, it treats them the same way. When his sodium level declined from its usual state, the body tried to conserve sodium. Unfortunately, it mistakenly conserved lithium, leading to increased drug levels in the blood.

Chapter 19

KEY TERMS

Fill in the blanks

1. antipsychotic agents
2. neuroleptics
3. typical antipsychotics
4. extrapyramidal side effects
5. tardive dyskinesia
6. neuroleptic malignant syndrome
7. atypical antipsychotics
8. dementia
9. Alzheimer's disease
10. schizophrenia
11. D2
12. psychosis

PHYSIOLOGY AND PATHOPHYSIOLOGY: THE BODY HUMAN

Essay

1. The left hemisphere appears to be dominant controlling comprehension, logic, rational thinking, and speech. The right hemisphere, often referred to as the "creative" brain, is associated with affect, behavior, and spatial-perceptual functions.

2. The frontal lobes control voluntary body movement, expression of feelings, perceptual interpretation of information, and thinking.

3. The extrapyramidal system is responsible for muscle coordination; the limbic system is responsible for the emotions of anger, anxiety, fear, pleasure, sorrow, and learning and memory; and the reticular activating system is responsible for consciousness, and filtering and alerting to stimuli.

4. ACh, DA, NE, and 5-HT increase and decrease the rate of neuron stimulation, thus regulating changes in thought processes, mood states, and psychomotor responses.

CORE DRUG KNOWLEDGE: JUST THE FACTS

Multiple choice

1. a 2. c 3. c 4. d 5. b
6. a 7. b 8. d 9. b 10. a
11. c 12. a 13. b 14. b 15. a
16. c

CORE PATIENT VARIABLES: PATIENTS, PLEASE

Multiple choice

1. a 2. d 3. b 4. c 5. c
6. d 7. c 8. b 9. a 10. d
11. b 12. c 13. a 14. d 15. b
16. d

NURSING MANAGEMENT: EVERY GOOD NURSE SHOULD . . .

Multiple choice

1. b. Hard candies or gum will help promote formation of saliva to reduce dry mouth. Drinking extra water is also helpful. Hydrogen peroxide rinses will not decrease dryness of the mouth, neither will increased sodium intake.

2. a. Chlorpromazine causes photosensitivity and protective measures need to be used to prevent severe sunburn. The goal of antipsychotic drug therapy is to have the patient's affective behavior stabilized so that he can interact appropriately in society. If he is well enough, he should work. Urine may turn pink or reddish brown while on chlorpromazine, not blue.

3. d. Taking the drug at bedtime will help eliminate daytime sedation. The patient should stand up more slowly and gradually to prevent orthostatic hypotension, not stand up quickly. Increased appetite and weight gains are common adverse effects from chlorpromazine. Eating 6 large meals a day will make this problem worse and not correct daytime sedation. Increasing the dose of chlorpromazine is not an appropriate response of the nurse as it is not an independent action of the nurse and it will most likely make adverse effects worse.

4. b. More fluid intake will help keep stool soft and alleviate constipation. Exercise should be encouraged, not limited, to promote peristalsis and regular bowel movements. More fiber and roughage are needed in the diet to promote regular bowel movements, bland, soft foods, may contribute to constipation.

5. a. Uncorrected hearing problems or vision problems may exacerbate the confusion the patient is exhibiting. These factors should be corrected first so that the full effect of rivastigmine can be determined. Eyeglasses should not be taken from the patient, as this will contribute to confusion if the patient doesn't see well. Patient's with Alzheimer Disease have memory loss and are not reliable to be in charge of their own medication schedule. The memory loss is the reason drug therapy is prescribed.

CASE STUDY

Chlorpromazine increases appetite and this is an adverse effect of chlorpromazine. Teach Marty that his increase in appetite is drug related and that he may need to control his eating. Assess his normal, daily dietary intake for adequate calories for his age and size. If necessary, contact the halfway house and see if any additional calories can be given to Marty. If this is not possible, a referral to a food bank or a soup kitchen may be indicated to help provide needed calories during the day.

CRITICAL THINKING CHALLENGE

Chlorpromazine causes thermoregulation problems where the patient is more sensitive to the temperature in the environment and less able to self regulate their internal temperature. This is especially true for older adults like Marty. Marty is outside all day in the summmer sun. The combination of unusual daytime temperatures, his being outside all day and his use of chlorpromazine have contributed to his developing heat stroke.

Chapter 20

KEY TERMS

1. International Classification of Epileptic Seizures
2. ictal
3. generalized seizure
4. postictal
5. absence
6. seizure
7. partial seizure
8. tonic-clonic seizure
9. epilepsy
10. GABA
11. epileptogenesis
12. status epilepticus
13. glutamate

PHYSIOLOGY AND PATHOPHYSIOLOGY: THE BODY HUMAN

1. pH, levels of oxygen, glucose, amino acids, calcium, sodium, and potassium
2. GABA
3. hyperexcitability due to increased release of neurotransmitters at the excitatory synapses

CORE DRUG KNOWLEDGE: JUST THE FACTS

Multiple choice

1. b   2. a   3. d   4. d   5. c
6. b   7. c   8. b   9. b   10. a
11. a   12. d   13. c   14. a   15. c
16. a

CORE PATIENT VARIABLES: PATIENTS, PLEASE

Multiple choice

1. c   2. b   3. c   4. a   5. d
6. c   7. c   8. d   9. b   10. c
11. a   12. c   13. b

NURSING MANAGEMENT: EVERY GOOD NURSE SHOULD . . .

Multiple choice

1. c.   Verify if drug interactions exist between the drugs. Phenytoin interacts with a long list of drugs. Before starting any new drug therapy, the nurse should assess if there is a potential drug interaction. Administering the drugs on opposite days is not an acceptable practice; it will decrease the effectiveness of both therapies considerably and may precipitate seizures. Antacids, although they may be helpful adjuncts to cimetidine therapy, should not be administered with phenytoin due to interference with absorption. There is no need for seeking this order.

2. a.   Monitor blood phenytoin levels for a drop compared to before theophylline therapy. As metabolism of phenytoin is increased due to the introduction of theophylline, there is less active phenytoin available for the patient. If blood levels fall below therapeutic range or patient shows increased seizure activity, contact the prescriber.

3. c.   Before Alma attempts to become pregnant, she should consult with her provider about the possibility of being weaned off the drug as she has been seizure free for 5 years. Phenytoin is a pregnancy Category D drug and causes teratogenic effects in the fetus. Fetal phenytoin syndrome is not related to dose toxicity and may occur with normal therapeutic drug levels, although the majority of women receiving this drug deliver normal babies. She should not abruptly stop taking her phenytoin, because this may bring about recurring seizures or status epilepticus. Additionally, fetal injury may occur if she stops and thus induces seizures.

4. c.   Turn the tube feeding off for 1 hour before and 1 hour after administering phenytoin. Tube feedings interfere with the absorption of phenytoin. Phenytoin should not be mixed with tube feedings. Daily doses of phenytoin cannot be combined; overdosage may result.

5. b.   Administer the drug slowly. Too rapid administration of IV phenytoin may produce cardiovascular collapse, hypotension, and life-threatening arrhythmias. Have resuscitation equipment nearby when administering phenytoin IV. Status epilepticus is an emergency situation, and drug therapy needs to be instituted immediately. Blood levels would be expected to be below therapeutic if the patient is currently experiencing status epilepticus. Gingival hyperplasia is a long-term adverse effect of phenytoin. Oral hygiene is important with chronic use. Warning the patient that he may be drowsy from therapy is inappropriate during emergency use of the drug while the patient continues to have seizures.

6. a.   Initially, he may have drowsiness, but this should go away after he has been on the drug awhile. CNS depressant effects are common adverse effects from ethosuximide and other AEDs. Fever and other signs of infection, however, may indicate that a blood dyscrasia is occurring. Fatal blood dyscrasia, although not common, has occurred. Doses should never be doubled due to the likelihood of inducing overdosage. There are no known drug–food interactions with ethosuximide; fried foods do not need to be avoided.

7. a.   As carbamazepine can cause fatal blood dyscrasias (aplastic anemia and agranulocytosis) it is very important that a complete blood count be measured regularly. Carbamazepine does not alter urinary elimination, requiring additional fluid intake. Like all AEDs, carbamazepine may cause CNS depression, including drowsiness when it is first started. She should avoid driving, and other potentially dangerous activities where alertness is needed, until she knows how the carbamazepine will affect her.

CASE STUDY

1. Elizabeth is toxic from the phenytoin.
2. Question the mother closely about dosing. Was the drug given exactly as prescribed? Were there any double doses? What type of spoon is used to measure the dose? (A household "teaspoon" may be larger than 5 cc.) Was there a change in the measuring spoon? Is there any chance that Elizabeth took doses on her own? Did anyone else beside the mother give doses? Overdosage may have occurred from these methods. Was the suspension shaken well before each dose? If not, the early doses may have had little or no active drug in them, thus the low blood levels; and the last doses were pure drug, leading to overdosage.

CRITICAL THINKING CHALLENGE

1. Ted appears to be having adverse effects and is possibly showing signs of early toxicity to the phenytoin.
2. Although most people need a drug level between 10 and 20 μg/mL to be in the therapeutic range, Ted apparently was therapeutic when his blood levels were at 8. Increasing the dose to put him in the "normal" range made him toxic. Drug blood levels are only one parameter of therapeutic effect from drug therapy. In this case, they were misleading. The dose should have been maintained at the original level because it was controlling seizures effectively.

Chapter 21

KEY TERMS

Matching

1. g   2. c   3. f   4. e   5. d

6. b   7. a

PHYSIOLOGY AND PATHOPHYSIOLOGY: THE BODY HUMAN

Essay

1. Actin and myosin
2. When muscle contracts, the sarcomere shortens and the Z lines move closer together. The filaments slide together because myosin attaches to actin and pulls on it. The myosin head attaches to actin filament, forming a crossbridge. After the crossbridge is formed, the myosin head bends, pulling on the actin filaments and causing them to slide. The end result is the Z lines move closer together, the I band becomes shorter, and the A band stays the same.
3. Localized skeletal muscle injury from acute trauma, hypocalcemia, hypo- or hyperkalemia, chronic pain syndromes, or epilepsy
4. Spasticity is usually caused by damage to the portion of the brain or spinal cord that controls voluntary movement. It may occur in association with spinal cord injury, multiple sclerosis, cerebral palsy, anoxic brain damage, brain trauma, severe head injury, some metabolic diseases such as adrenoleukodystrophy, and phenylketonuria.
5. Symptoms may include hypertonicity (increased muscle tone), clonus (a series of rapid muscle contractions), exaggerated deep tendon reflexes, muscle spasms, scissoring (involuntary crossing of the legs), and fixed joints.

CORE DRUG KNOWLEDGE: JUST THE FACTS

Multiple choice

1. c   2. d   3. a   4. b   5. d

6. b   7. b   8. b   9. b   10. d

CORE PATIENT VARIABLES: PATIENTS, PLEASE

Multiple choice

1. c   2. b   3. a   4. a   5. c

6. d   7. c   8. d

NURSING MANAGEMENT: EVERY GOOD NURSE SHOULD...

Multiple choice

1. b.   Dry mouth is a common adverse effect of cyclobenzaprine due to the anticholinergic properties of the drug. Although this adverse effect is not dangerous to the patient, it is uncomfortable and the nurse should recommend some general strategies for dealing with a dry mouth. A dry mouth is not a sign of a drug interaction, an allergy, or a normal therapeutic response to cyclobenzaprine therapy.
2. d.   To prevent withdrawal symptoms, Mr. Andrews should be slowly tapered off of the drug over 2 weeks.

Giving two pills a day initially cuts the dose by one third. Reducing the dose to one pill next cuts the dose in half again. Because this tablet is not scored, the dose cannot be decreased to less than one pill or less than 10 mg. This drug should not be discontinued abruptly, but it does not need to be tapered over 2 months.

3. a.   Baclofen causes sedation, dizziness, weakness, lightheadedness, lethargy, and fatigue, among other CNS effects, as adverse effects. Until the effects on Mr. Ford are known, he should be assisted in ambulation so he does not fall. Doing toe touches may increase feelings of dizziness or light-headedness and should be avoided. Alcohol may potentiate the CNS effects of baclofen and should be avoided, especially in the early period of drug therapy. GI distress often occurs with baclofen; smaller, frequent meals may be indicated.
4. b.   This will promote ease of swallowing. The dantrolene helps to control the muscle spasms with multiple sclerosis and should be continued if possible. However, because Barbara is having some choking episodes, she should not be forced to try to swallow the capsule because she may choke on it. Cutting the capsule in half changes the prescribed dose and may not eliminate difficulty in swallowing; it is not an appropriate nursing intervention.

CASE STUDY

1. When did the fatigue and weakness begin in relation to starting drug therapy? Was it a rapid change or a progressive deterioration? Are the fatigue and weakness getting worse or have they improved at all? These questions will help to sort out whether the fatigue and weakness are adverse effects of baclofen or signs of disease progression of the ALS. Sudden onset after the start of baclofen and gradual improvement indicates drug-related effects.

    Are you taking the Miglitol as prescribed? Are you following the prescribed diabetic diet?

    Elevated blood glucose levels may be responsible for the urinary frequency.
2. Assess the blood glucose levels, preferably fasting. Baclofen may increase blood glucose levels in diabetics. If the levels are normal and the patient reports using drug and diet therapy as prescribed to control his diabetes, the increased urinary frequency may be an adverse effect of the baclofen.

CRITICAL THINKING CHALLENGE

1. Additive CNS depression has occurred from the combination of the antidepressant, amitriptyline, and the baclofen. He may accommodate to these effects if he stays on both drugs.
2. Teach the wife to assist Mr. Carlisle with ambulation and to correct environmental factors that might promote falls, such as removing scatter rugs and arranging furniture so items are not in the traffic pathway. Suggest that he take the amitriptyline at night instead of in the morning to help minimize daytime sedation. If this is not effective in the next few days, the nurse should contact the physician regarding decreasing the dose of the amitriptyline. Also contact the physician regarding whether the depression could be related to the baclofen and perhaps this dose should be decreased.

Chapter 22

KEY TERMS

Anagrams

1. paralysis agitans
2. bruxism
3. bradykinetic episodes
4. basal ganglia
5. akinesia
6. ballismus
7. substantia nigra
8. dopaminergic
9. neuroleptic malignant syndrome
10. corpus striatum
11. bradykinesia
12. parkinsonism

PHYSIOLOGY AND PATHOPHYSIOLOGY: THE BODY HUMAN

Essay

1. Basal ganglia; cortical areas of the brain projecting to the basal ganglia; cerebellar areas of the brain projecting to the basal ganglia; parts of the reticular formation; thalamic nuclei connecting to the basal ganglia
2. Dopamine is an inhibitory neurotransmitter, whereas acetylcholine is an excitatory neurotransmitter. These two neurotransmitters work in balanced antagonism allowing for the initiation, modulation, and completion of smooth, coordinated movement.
3. Trauma, bacteria, viruses, and environmental factors can induce diseases. In this disease, the loss of dopamine occurs with the natural aging process and is not induced by other factors. This means all of the elderly are at risk for this disease.
4. Muscle rigidity, tremor at rest, akinesia, bradykinesia
5. Parkinsonism is a syndrome of similar characteristics of Parkinson's disease. Parkinsonism, however, is not naturally occurring. It is secondary to other conditions that have structurally damaged the dopaminergic pathway or interfere with the action of dopamine within the basal ganglia.
6. ALS begins in the distal neurons and progresses in a centripetal but asymmetric direction. Ultimate neuronal cell death results in muscular weakness, muscle atrophy and fasciculations, spasticity, dysarthria, dysphagia, and respiratory compromise.

CORE DRUG KNOWLEDGE: JUST THE FACTS

Mulitple choice

1. c
2. c
3. a
4. c
5. c
6. a
7. b
8. c
9. a
10. a

CORE PATIENT VARIABLES: PATIENTS, PLEASE

Multiple choice

1. a
2. a
3. c
4. b
5. a
6. c
7. c
8. b

NURSING MANAGEMENT: EVERY GOOD NURSE SHOULD

The patient receiving both benztropine and carbidopa-levodopa needs to receive care to maximize the therapeutic effects and to minimize the adverse effects from both of these drugs. Maximize therapeutic effects of benztropine by administering it regularly as ordered. To maximize the therapeutic effect of carbidopa-levodopa, administer it on an empty stomach (to promote absorption), limit intake of dietary protein (high protein slows or prevents absorption), and limit intake of foods high in pyridoxine (e.g., avocados, bacon, beans, beef liver, dry skim milk, oatmeal, peas, pork, sweet potatoes, tuna), because pyridoxine increases the breakdown of levodopa in the peripheries (i.e., there is less available to cross the blood–brain barrier). Constipation may occur from both benztropine (as an anticholinergic) and carbidopa-levodopa, thus actions to prevent constipation are essential to minimize the adverse effects of these drugs. Provide a diet high in dietary fiber with at least 2000 cc of fluid intake per day, and encourage moderate daily exercise to minimize constipation.

Benztropine, like other anticholinergics, will also cause dry mouth, so frequent mouth care is important. Offer the patient hard candy to suck on; chewing gum may also relieve a dry mouth, if this is appropriate for the patient. To minimize the other anticholinergic adverse effects, caution patients against driving, especially at night, because they may have blurred vision or enlarged pupils. If their eyes are sensitive to the light, they should be instructed to wear sunglasses. If their eyes are dry, administer artificial tears. Urinary retention from benztropine can be minimized by having male patients stand to void, and having female patients sit upright on a bedpan or commode seat. Monitor patients' output and for any signs of retention

Carbidopa-levodopa may cause nausea or vomiting, so the dose should be titrated upwards slowly. This action will also minimize the adverse effect of orthostatic hypotension from carbidopa-levodopa.

CASE STUDY

1a. The nurse should do a complete physical exam to establish a baseline to monitor the progression of the disease. It is especially important to assess Mrs. Wade's ability to perform activities of daily living.
1b. Drug therapy for Parkinson disease loses effectiveness over time. It is not started until the symptoms become distressing for the patient and interfere with normal activities.
2. Assess for blurred vision, dry mouth, constipation, and urinary retention. Assess for a decrease in tremors. Assess for any other signs of progression of Parkinson disease.
3. The nurse should advise Mrs. Wade that carbidopa-levodopa will not cure Parkinson's disease but will help control symptoms. She should be cautioned that the onset of action is slow and she will not see immediate results. She should be instructed to take the medication exactly as prescribed and to never abruptly stop the medication. Mrs. Wade should be given dietary instructions to limit or avoid excessive vitamin B_6 and ingestion of alcohol. She should also be cautioned to take the medication with a low-protein meal. Additionally, she should be advised to contact the

clinic immediately if she experiences uncontrolled movements of her face, eyelids, mouth, tongue, neck, arms, hands, or legs. She should also contact the clinic if she experiences any mood or mental changes, irregular heart beat or palpitations, difficulty urinating, severe or persistent nausea or vomiting, appetite loss, difficulty swallowing, or taste distortion. Mrs. Wade should be given information about the "on-off effect" which may occur. She should be taught not to perform any activities that require mental alertness until she sees how the medication affects her. The nurse should demonstrate to Mrs. Wade how to change positions slowly to avoid falling from dizziness or fainting.

4. Mrs. Wade should be told about the potential for bradykinetic episodes and the slow decline in efficacy of anti-Parkinson drugs with long-term use. Caution Mrs. Wade to sit down immediately if she experiences a feeling of weakness to avoid injury from falls.

CRITICAL THINKING CHALLENGE

Riluzole can elevate liver enzymes. This may be a transient effect while the body accommodates to the drug therapy. Repeated blood work will determine if accommodation has occurred (and enzymes are returned to normal or near normal levels) or if liver damage is occurring and the therapy cannot be continued in this patient.

Chapter 23

KEY TERMS

Fill in the blanks

1. attention deficit-hyperactivity disorder
2. cataplexy
3. narcolepsy
4. sleep paralysis
5. obesity
6. hypercapnia
7. analeptic
8. anorectic
9. hypnogogic hallucinations

PHYSIOLOGY AND PATHOPHYSIOLOGY: THE BODY HUMAN

Multiple choice

1. c   2. b   3. d   4. b

CORE DRUG KNOWLEDGE: JUST THE FACTS

Essay

1. advanced arteriosclerosis, symptomatic cardiovascular disease, moderate to severe hypertension, hyperthyroidism, previous idiosyncratic reactions to sympathomimetic drugs glaucoma, history of drug abuse, concurrent use of MAOI drugs pregnancy
2. restlessness, dizziness, insomnia, agitation
3. palpitations, tachycardia, increased BP
4. Cachexia and hypoproteinemia may alter the pharmacokinetics of other drugs, thus increasing the risk for adverse reactions, subtherapeutic levels, or toxicity.

5. Acidic juices and fruits must be limited. Foods containing caffeine, such as cola, tea, coffee, chocolate, must be limited.
6. Sibutramine inhibits the central reuptake of dopamine, norepinephrine, and serotonin. It is thought that the serotonin mechanism enhances satiety, whereas the norepinephrine mechanism raises the metabolic rate.
7. The most common adverse reactions are anorexia, constipation, insomnia, headache, and xerostomia.
8. This combination may result in "serotonin syndrome" characterized by CNS irritability, motor weakness, shivering, myoclonus, and altered consciousness.

CORE PATIENT VARIABLES: PATIENTS, PLEASE

Multiple choice

1. d   2. b   3. a   4. d   5. b
6. a   7. c   8. d

NURSING MANAGEMENT: EVERY GOOD NURSE SHOULD . . .

Multiple choice

1. d.   Symptomatic cardiovascular disease will be aggravated by the use of CNS stimulants such as dextroamphetamine. In hyperthyroidism, the CNS is already stimulated; adding a CNS stimulant may cause significant adverse effects. A patient with a history of drug abuse is more at risk of abusing dextroamphetamine.
2. b.   Caffeine is also a CNS stimulant and may produce signs of CNS overstimulation when taken with dextroamphetamine. To minimize insomnia from dextroamphetamine, take in the morning and/or at least 6 hours before bedtime. Sustained-release capsules should never be chewed or crushed. Never take double doses, because signs of CNS overstimulation may develop.
3. d.   Dottie appears to be having adverse effects from the dextroamphetamine, so you will contact the prescriber. Insomnia and restlessness are signs of CNS overstimulation. Sleeping aids will treat her symptoms but not address the real issue of overstimulation. Contact the health care provider concerning decreasing the dosage to avoid adverse effects.
4. c.   An increase in activity levels or exercise will assist in raising metabolism and promoting the weight loss effects from silbutramine. Additionally, diet changes that incorporate a low-calorie and low-fat approach will increase the effectiveness of silbutramine. This may not be what the patient is currently following. Further assessment is needed here. Peak levels of the drug are achieved when the drug is taken on an empty stomach, not a full stomach. Because the drug may cause insomnia, it should not be taken at bedtime.
5. d.   Signs of intolerance or overdose from caffeine in newborns include tachypnea (rapid breathing), fever, and hyperglycemia.

CASE STUDY

Prescription anorexics are indicated when the patient is clinically obese and other methods have been unsuccessful. Mrs. Clemson does not meet these requirements. Over-the-counter anorexiants do help to suppress the appetite by stimulating the satiety center in the brain. However, these agents are not recommended during breast-feeding because they will enter breast milk and thus the infant. Safety has not been established in children.

CRITICAL THINKING CHALLENGE

Mrs. Clemson would be best advised to use nonpharmacologic methods to lose weight. She should drink plenty of fluids to promote breast milk production. Drinking water will also help promote feelings of satiety and help with weight loss. She should also be advised to cut down on calories while maintaining balanced nutrient intake, and to increase her exercise to lose weight.

CORE DRUG KNOWLEDGE: JUST THE FACTS

Multiple choice

1. d   2. c   3. d   4. c   5. c
6. d   7. b   8. c   9. a   10. c

CORE PATIENT VARIABLES: PATIENTS, PLEASE

Multiple choice

1. a   2. c   3. b   4. a   5. c
6. a   7. c   8. b

Chapter 24

KEY TERMS

Matching

1. f   2. e   3. j   4. a   5. i
6. h   7. c   8. d   9. b   10. g
11. l   12. m   13. q   14. p   15. k
16. r   17. s   18. n   19. o

PHYSIOLOGY AND PATHOPHYSIOLOGY: THE BODY HUMAN

Essay

1. CNS depressants may provoke a decreased release of neurotransmitters or an increased reuptake and inhibition of the postsynaptic enzymes.
2. A-delta fibers are fast-traveling, myelinated, and responsive to mechanical stimuli. They sense sharp, stinging, cutting, or pinching pain. C fibers are slow-traveling, unmyelinated, and responsive to mechanical, chemical, hormonal, or thermal stimuli. They sense dull, burning, or aching pain.
3. Anxiety, fear, apprehension, attention, motivation, and cognitive processes
4. Pain threshold appears related to stimulation of the anterior cingulate cortex, frontal inferior cortex, and thalamus. Pain intensity is related to stimulation of the periventricular gray and posterior cingulate cortex. The feelings of unpleasantness or suffering associated with pain are from the posterior sector of the anterior cingulate cortex
5. Delay healing and rehabilitation, prolong other symptoms, induce dysfunctional behavior such as drug abuse, result in immunocompromise, cause other comorbid states

NURSING MANAGEMENT: EVERY GOOD NURSE SHOULD . . .

Decision tree

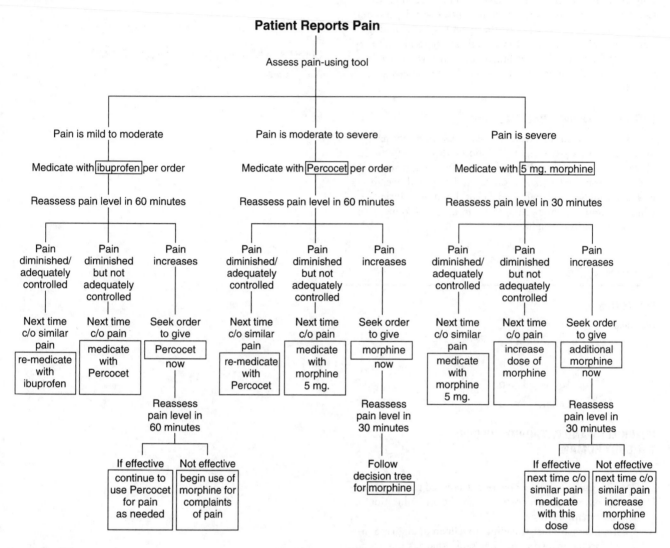

Patient Reports Pain

CASE STUDY

1. Yes. Pain is subjective, and the patient reports he has severe pain. It is not unexpected that he has pain because he is postoperative.
2. Does he obtain any relief from the one Percocet? How long does the relief last? What does the pain level become when the drug is working? What nonpharmacologic methods are effective for Gordon in dealing with pain and reducing sensation of pain?
3. Medicate him with two Percocet now, repeat the dose in 4 hours, not 6 hours. (One tablet was not effective; do not repeat an ineffective dose.) If two are not effective, begin use of morphine 8 mg IM every 3 hours.

CRITICAL THINKING CHALLENGE

Gordon has a history of opioid and alcohol abuse, which may have created a cross tolerance to the opioid analgesics, requiring him to have a higher dose for pain relief. His tolerance for substances that depress the CNS will minimize the sedation, an adverse effect, of morphine. Tyler does not have a history of substance abuse and, therefore, may be more sensitive to the CNS depressant effects of the morphine. Additionally, because he is only 2 hours postsurgery, the anesthetics, also CNS depressants, may have created an additive effect with the morphine.

Chapter 25

KEY TERMS

Matching

1. g   2. c   3. h   4. e   5. f

6. i   7. b   8. a   9. d

PHYSIOLOGY AND PATHOPHYSIOLOGY: THE BODY HUMAN

Essay

1. Swelling, heat, redness, pain, and loss of function

2. Initial vasoconstriction of the surrounding vessels then vasodilation to allow increased blood flow to the area; increased capillary permeability and release of chemical mediators

3. Margination, emigration, chemotaxis, phagocytosis

4. PSIs work by the inhibition of prostaglandins. There are many different types of prostaglandins, many of which have opposing function. When PSIs inhibit prostaglandins, they not only inhibit the cells that cause inflammation, but also inhibit the cells that provide the body's protective mechanisms.

CORE DRUG KNOWLEDGE: JUST THE FACTS

Multiple choice

1. d   2. c   3. b   4. b   5. a

6. c   7. a   8. b   9. d   10. c

11. a   12. d   13. c   14. d

CORE PATIENT VARIABLES: PATIENTS, PLEASE

Multiple choice

1. c   2. a   3. a   4. d   5. c

6. b   7. a   8. b   9. d   10. d

NURSING MANAGEMENT: EVERY GOOD NURSE SHOULD . . .

Multiple choice

1. c.   Return for laboratory tests every 6 months. Aspirin may cause bleeding disorders due to the inhibition of platelet aggregation. Agranulocytosis and aplastic anemia are also possible. Additionally, aspirin may cause hepatic or renal toxicity. Laboratory blood work on a regular basis will help to detect early signs of these problems. Due to its gastric-irritating effects, aspirin should not be taken on an empty stomach. Moisture causes aspirin to lose its effectiveness. Because there is frequently a good bit of steam in bathrooms, the bathroom medicine cabinet is not usually the best choice as a storage location for aspirin. Crushing coated tablets intended for extended release will cause the aspirin to be released more rapidly into the bloodstream, possibly causing excessively high levels, and adverse effects. Additionally, the action will only be for a short duration if the tablets are crushed.

2. a.   Unusual bruising. This is a sign of excessive interference with platelet aggregation. Tachycardia is a sign of serious adverse effects, as it relates to internal bleeding. Upset stomach and slight dizziness are common adverse effects and are not significant problems that need to be reported immediately.

3. b.   Administer acetylcysteine. This is the only antidote for acetaminophen and should be administered as soon as possible. Acetylsalicylic acid is aspirin and would not be given. Acetaminophen does not have an effect on platelet aggregation. CT scan of the abdomen would not be relevant.

4. b.   Ashley is demonstrating flulike symptoms and should not be treated with aspirin due to the possibility of developing Reye's syndrome. Dosage of acetaminophen for children is based on height and weight. The most appropriate dose can be calibrated with a children's formula.

5. c.   Because of Ms. Scarpio's history of GI ulceration, she is at risk for developing GI complications from either aspirin or ibuprofen. Neither of these should be substituted for the celecoxib, although they are effective in treating arthritis pain. Celecoxib works in a different way than aspirin and ibuprofen. It is not the same as aspirin or a prescription-strength aspirin.

CASE STUDY

1. Ibuprofen was ordered for its analgesic and anti-inflammatory effects.

2. Yes, it is safe for Mr. Brooks to receive both ibuprofen and oxycodone. The ibuprofen acts on the peripheral nervous system, and the oxycodone acts on the central nervous system. Combined use of an opioid and NSAID is recommended by the U.S. Department of Health and Human Service's Clinical Practice Guidelines. This combination provides more pain relief, while minimizing the dose of the opioid and, therefore, the adverse effects from the opioid.

3. Round-the-clock dosing maintains a therapeutic blood level and prevents pain from escalating. Round-the-clock dosing should be used during periods when acute pain can be anticipated, such as immediately after surgery.

CRITICAL THINKING CHALLENGE

1. Mr. Brooks may be having water retention and acute renal failure related to his use of ibuprofen.

2. Mr. Brooks' age puts him at higher risk for adverse effects from the ibuprofen. He may also have had some renal insufficiency or diminished renal blood flow, possibly also related to his age.

3. Hold the next dose of ibuprofen and contact the physician. Monitor intake and output and blood pressure closely. Assess for signs of fluid overload.

Chapter 26

KEY TERMS

Matching

1. f   2. d   3. g   4. a   5. e
6. i   7. c   8. h   9. b

PHYSIOLOGY AND PATHOPHYSIOLOGY: THE BODY HUMAN

Essay

1. Rheumatoid factor (RF) interacts with IgG or other antibodies to form immune complexes that activate the complement system, resulting in an inflammatory response. Leukocytes, monocytes, and lymphocytes are attracted to the area and phagocytize the immune complexes. When the immune complexes are destroyed, lysosomal enzymes are released. These enzymes are capable of destroying joint cartilage, resulting in an inflammatory process that starts the cycle again.
2. Symptoms include morning stiffness that lasts more than 1 hour, symmetric involvement of joints, and rheumatoid nodules over bony prominences or extensor surfaces.
3. Gout occurs when the hyperuricemia forms monosodium urate crystals, which precipitate into the synovial fluid and initiate an inflammatory response.

CORE DRUG KNOWLEDGE: JUST THE FACTS

Multiple choice

1. c   2. b   3. a   4. d   5. d
6. c   7. a   8. b   9. c   10. c
11. b   12. c

CORE PATIENT VARIABLES: PATIENTS, PLEASE

Multiple choice

1. b   2. a   3. b   4. d   5. c
6. a   7. b   8. a   9. d   10. a
11. b   12. d

NURSING MANAGEMENT: EVERY GOOD NURSE SHOULD . . .

Multiple choice

1. d.   All of the above. GI effects are common and can be minimized with food or milk intake. Diarrhea frequently occurs but should not last more than 3 days. Steady state is not reached for 8 to 12 weeks, when full therapeutic effect will be realized.
2. b.   Take this drug at the first sign of a gout attack. This will most minimize the pain from the gout attack. Taking colchicine when the pain is most severe will not control as much pain. Taking colchicine near the end of the gout attack will offer minimal decrease of pain. Colchicine is taken on an as-needed basis; it does not prevent gout attacks.
3. b.   Take the probenecid with milk. Probenecid may cause gastric upset, and this will minimize it. Cranberry juice should be avoided because it acidifies the urine, and probenecid is excreted more easily in alkaline urine. Water intake should be encouraged, at least 10 glasses a day, to help reduce the risk of kidney stones forming while the patient is on probenecid. Alcoholic beverages should be avoided because they can cause stomach problems and increase uric acid in the blood, predisposing the person to a gout attack.
4. a.   Foods such as organ meats, oily fish, seafood, beans, peas, oatmeal, spinach, asparagus, cauliflower, and mushrooms should be avoided because these foods are high in purines. Uric acid levels are a product of purine metabolism. None of the other foods are high in purines and do not need to be avoided.

Chapter 27

KEY TERMS

Word find exercise

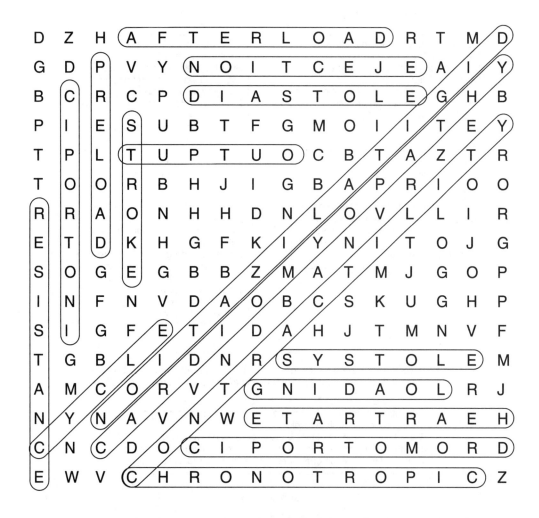

PHYSIOLOGY AND PATHOPHYSIOLOGY: THE BODY HUMAN

Essay

1. Blood flows from the vena cava to the right atrium, through the tricuspid valve to the right ventricle through the pulmonary valve to the pulmonary artery to the lungs to the pulmonary vein to the left atrium, through the mitral valve to the left ventricle and through the aortic valve to the aorta.
2. Preload, contractility, and afterload
3. Right-sided failure induces systemic symptoms such as edema, jugular vein distention, and a third heart sound. Left-sided failure induces pulmonary symptoms such as rales, rhonchi, and shortness of breath.

CORE DRUG KNOWLEDGE: JUST THE FACTS

Multiple choice

1. d   2. c   3. b   4. a   5. c
6. a   7. b

CORE PATIENT VARIABLES: PATIENTS, PLEASE

Multiple choice

1. c   2. c   3. a   4. d   5. c
6. c

NURSING MANAGEMENT: EVERY GOOD NURSE SHOULD . . .

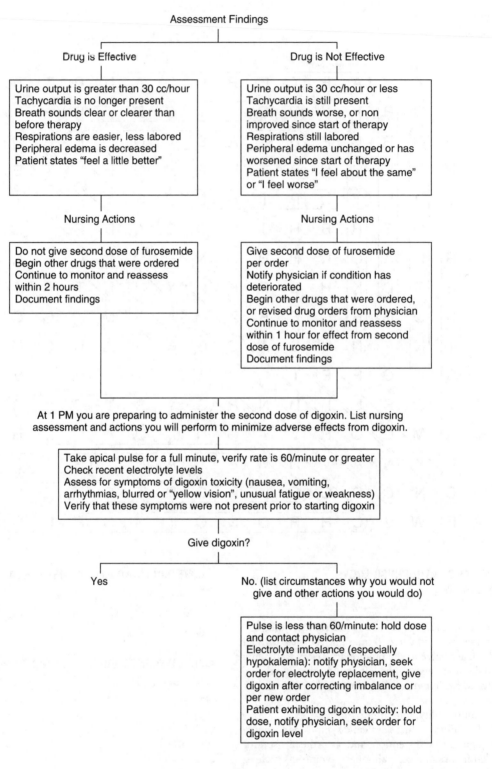

Assessment Findings

Drug is Effective

Urine output is greater than 30 cc/hour
Tachycardia is no longer present
Breath sounds clear or clearer than before therapy
Respirations are easier, less labored
Peripheral edema is decreased
Patient states "feel a little better"

Drug is Not Effective

Urine output is 30 cc/hour or less
Tachycardia is still present
Breath sounds worse, or non improved since start of therapy
Respirations still labored
Peripheral edema unchanged or has worsened since start of therapy
Patient states "I feel about the same" or "I feel worse"

Nursing Actions

Do not give second dose of furosemide
Begin other drugs that were ordered
Continue to monitor and reassess within 2 hours
Document findings

Nursing Actions

Give second dose of furosemide per order
Notify physician if condition has deteriorated
Begin other drugs that were ordered, or revised drug orders from physician
Continue to monitor and reassess within 1 hour for effect from second dose of furosemide
Document findings

At 1 PM you are preparing to administer the second dose of digoxin. List nursing assessment and actions you will perform to minimize adverse effects from digoxin.

Take apical pulse for a full minute, verify rate is 60/minute or greater
Check recent electrolyte levels
Assess for symptoms of digoxin toxicity (nausea, vomiting, arrhythmias, blurred or "yellow vision", unusual fatigue or weakness)
Verify that these symptoms were not present prior to starting digoxin

Give digoxin?

Yes

No. (list circumstances why you would not give and other actions you would do)

Pulse is less than 60/minute: hold dose and contact physician
Electrolyte imbalance (especially hypokalemia): notify physician, seek order for electrolyte replacement, give digoxin after correcting imbalance or per new order
Patient exhibiting digoxin toxicity: hold dose, notify physician, seek order for digoxin level

CASE STUDY

The furosemide is a diuretic to pull excess fluid out of the lungs and the periphery. This will help her to breathe easier and keep her heart from working so hard. It is a powerful diuretic and works quickly, especially when given by IV push. The ACE inhibitor (captopril) blocks the creation of a sub-stance that constricts the blood vessels. Constricted blood vessels mean the heart works harder to pump the blood. The ACE inhibitor, therefore, allows the blood vessels to become relaxed and allows the blood to leave the heart more easily. The diuretic that is a pill (hydrochlorothiazide) is not as strong and does not work as fast as the furosemide. Once the excess fluid has been quickly eliminated, this will keep the circulating volume low to make an easier workload for the heart. The digoxin slows the rate the heart beats, but makes each contraction stronger, so more blood is pushed out with each beat. Because it takes a while for the full effect of the digoxin to occur, a loading dose is given. This is a larger-than-normal dose, given in three increments. This helps the drug to reach a therapeutic level faster. A smaller, maintenance dose is then given daily.

CRITICAL THINKING CHALLENGE

Another dose of furosemide IV may be ordered. For the persistent dyspnea, hydralazine (a vasodilator) and/or nitrates may be added. For the persistent hypertension, a direct vasodilator or an alpha blocker may be added. Because she is no longer tachycardic, the digoxin dose is apparently effective. You would not expect to see this changed. The dose of the ACE inhbitor and the thiazide diuretic might also be increased.

Chapter 28

KEY TERMS
Matching

1. c   2. g   3. f   4. a   5. b
6. d   7. e

PHYSIOLOGY AND PATHOPHYSIOLOGY: THE BODY HUMAN

Essay

1. Angina occurs when the oxygen demands of the heart exceed the oxygen supply available to the heart. This can be due to blockage, increased workload of the heart, or vasospasms.
2. Cardiac troponin T and cardiac troponin I.
3. Three main drug groups are used to treat angina—beta blockers, calcium channel blockers, and nitrates.
4. Antianginal drugs work by slowing the heart rate, depressing AV conduction, decreasing cardiac output, or reducing systolic and diastolic blood pressure at rest and during exercise.

CORE DRUG KNOWLEDGE: JUST THE FACTS

Multiple choice

1. b   2. d   3. d   4. b   5. a
6. c

CORE PATIENT VARIABLES: PATIENTS, PLEASE

Multiple choice

1. b   2. c   3. a   4. b   5. d
6. a

NURSING MANAGEMENT: EVERY GOOD NURSE SHOULD . . .

Multiple choice

1. c.   Nitroglycerin given SL (sublingually) is administered under the tongue so it is absorbed by the vascular system there. For chest pain, administer up to three doses, each 5 minutes apart, if the previous dose is not effective. Administering the tablet into the patient's mouth does not allow for rapid absorption of the drug, because it will be dissolved and some of it swallowed, losing effectiveness. Although three doses may be administered, they are not administered all at one time. There is no need to contact the physician immediately. The patient was admitted with chest pain and has orders to treat chest pain. Notify the physician if three tablets do not relieve chest pain.

2. c.   Pulse and blood pressure indicate how the heart is functioning during the chest pain, and will also show effect from the nitroglycerin. They should be measured before and during therapy. Additionally, hypotension and tachycardia are possible from nitroglycerin, and you should assess for these adverse effects. Lung sounds are not a priority assessment during an episode of acute chest pain. Although urinary output gives some information about cardiac output, this is also not the priority at this time.

3. d.   A patient with a history of stable chronic angina who develops acute chest pain should be treated with the quick-acting sublingual form of nitroglycerin. Nitrol ointment is not used in acute situations. Furthermore, you would not want to administer a standing dose, which was to be given every 6 hours, 4 hours early. Excessive vasodilation may occur from this short interval of dosing. Also this would mean that 10 hours would elapse until the next dose, and the patient may develop chest pain from altered scheduling. Nitrol ointment is not applied to the foot, because this is the most distal point from the heart. The chest wall or upper arm is normally used. The patient who has developed acute chest pain should not be left untreated for 4 hours because this may be an MI and not angina.

4. d.   Active ingredient remains in the used patches, which can be very harmful to small children or to pets. It is important to safely dispose of patches to prevent accidental poisoning. Patches should be folded with the medicated side inward and flushed down the toilet. Transdermal patches of nitroglycerin are impregnated with active drug; the patient does not need to measure the dose. To minimize the risk of nitrate tolerance, the patient should not wear the patch 24 hours a day but should remove it for 10 to 12 hours a day. Transdermal patches of nitroglycerin are used routinely to manage chronic angina, not for acute episodes of angina.

5. a.   Nitroglycerin tablets lose their potency when exposed to light. Keeping them in the original brown bottle minimizes light exposure. The bottles should not be left with the cap off because this exposes the tablets to moisture and light, which decrease the effectiveness of the nitroglycerin. Activity should not be encouraged during an episode of chest pain; rather, the person should sit or lie down to decrease the oxygen demands on the heart. Because she has a diagnosed history of angina and is prescribed nitro-

glycerin for it, she should take her tablets immediately. If three pills in 15 minutes offer no relief of chest pain, she would then call 911 because she might be having a MI.

6. d. All of the above are necessary. The patient needs to have blood pressure and pulse continuously monitored during IV infusion of nitroglycerin. The use of IV glass bottles and non-PVC tubing, supplied by the manufacturer, prevents the loss of active drug during infusion.

CASE STUDY

A family history of coronary artery disease and diabetes are significant risk factors for Mr. Thomlinson's cardiovascular disease progressing and causing a second MI. It is important to treat him aggressively with multiple drug therapies at this time.

The transdermal nitroglycerin will provide vasodilation and decrease peripheral resistance and blood pressure, decreasing the workload on the heart. The propranolol will slow the heart rate, depress AV conduction, decrease cardiac output, and reduce blood pressure These effects decrease the oxygen demands of the heart and thereby decrease angina. The antianginal effects will be compounded because the different drugs work in different ways. Aspirin is used for its anticoagulant effects. This prevents thrombus formation and the occurrence of another MI. The sublingual nitroglycerin is to treat any acute episodes of chest pain that may develop.

CRITICAL THINKING CHALLENGE

If Mr. Thomlinson had asthma, beta blockers would not be used because they constrict the bronchioles, worsening asthma. Instead, a calcium channel blocker, such as verapamil, would be used.

Chapter 29

KEY TERMS

True/false

1.	F	dysrhythmia
2.	F	arrhythmia
3.	F	diastole
4.	F	systole
5.	T	
6.	F	transmembrane potential
7.	F	depolarization
8.	T	
9.	F	automaticity
10.	F	repolarization
11.	F	reentry phenomena
12.	F	atrial fibrillation
13.	F	proarrhythmia
14.	F	ectopic foci
15.	F	action potential
16.	F	ventricular fibrillation
17.	T	

PHYSIOLOGY AND PATHOPHYSIOLOGY: THE BODY HUMAN

Essay

1. The progression of the electrical impulse that produces the heartbeat starts in the SA node. The action potential leaves the SA node traveling through the atria, causing them to contract. The impulse is slowed at the AV node so that the atria and the ventricles do not contract simultaneously. The impulse then travels through the bundle of His to the bundle branches and then through the Purkinje fibers.

2. **Phase 0:**
Depolarization occurs rapidly and "fast sodium channels" open and sodium rushes into the cell, changing the inside of the cell, to a positive charge.
Phase 1:
Immediately after the interior positive charge is achieved, the movement toward repolarization begins. The initial downward movement toward zero is phase 1 of the action potential.
Phase 2:
In this plateau phase, the calcium channels open slowly. These "slow channels" allow calcium ions to enter the cell. The positively charged calcium channels close, potassium channels open, and potassium again moves into the cell.
Phase 3:
When potassium moves into the cell, a rapid acceleration of repolarization begins.
Phase 4:
Full polarization is achieved, and the cell is capable of depolarization again.

3. The plateau phase allows for a slower repolarization of cardiac muscle and, thus, is a protective mechanism of the heart. Repolarization of skeletal muscle occurs rapidly after depolarization, allowing the muscle to be stimulated to contract again almost immediately. Tetany, or constant contractions, may occur in skeletal muscles. This process would be life threatening if it occurred in the heart because no effective contractions would be present.

4. Initially after depolarization, the cell is in the absolute refractory period and cannot be stimulated to fire, no matter how great the stimulus. As repolarization continues, the cell enters the relative refractory period and is able to respond to a stimulus, although the intensity of the stimulus needs to be much greater than when the cell is in the resting state.

5. The electrolytes may induce arrhythmias in one of three ways: through a disorder with impulse formation (the automaticity of the heart), through a disorder of the impulse conduction system, or through a combination of both.

CORE DRUG KNOWLEDGE: JUST THE FACTS

Multiple choice

1. c   2. a   3. b   4. c   5. b

6. d   7. a   8. c   9. d   10. b

11. d   12. a

CORE PATIENT VARIABLES: PATIENTS, PLEASE

Multiple choice

1. c   2. d   3. a   4. c   5. b
6. d   7. a   8. b   9. c   10. b

NURSING MANAGEMENT: EVERY GOOD NURSE SHOULD . . .

Multiple choice

1. c.   Serum levels of quinidine will be needed to determine that a therapeutic and nontoxic drug level has been reached and maintained. Blood tests for potassium levels, liver enzymes, renal function, and complete blood counts will be needed to monitor for adverse effects. Potassium levels need to be in normal range to prevent decreased effectiveness and increased adverse effects of quinidine; thus, dietary intake should not be limited. Oral quinidine should be taken with food to minimize GI upset. Sustained-release tablets should never be chewed because this alters the absorption time, allowing more drug to be active at a time, which may cause adverse effects and overdosage.

2. b.   Hypotension is a common adverse effect when giving amiodarone IV. It is a sign that the infusion is too fast and needs to be slowed. Patients with life-threatening arrhythmias, such as ventricular fibrillation, are not ambulated but maintained on bed rest. Amiodarone is not given by the IM route. Constipation is not an adverse effect of amiodarone.

3. b.   Beta blockers and verapamil both suppress contractility and AV conduction of the heart and, thus, should not be given together, because significant decreases in cardiac output may then occur. Digoxin is used with verapamil in atrial flutter to prevent the ventricles from developing tachycardia. Potassium and diuretics have no known interaction with verapamil.

4. a.   This will clear the tract of stool so that when the drug is administered into the rectum the exchange of sodium for potassium ions will be facilitated. The suspension is administered by gravity. Pulse and ECG should be monitored for adverse effects of hyperkalemia. Liver enzymes are not affected by the drug therapy or hyperkalemia.

5. c.   Beta blockers will constrict the bronchioles making it even more difficult for the patient to breathe. Beta blockers are used to treat hypertension and angina, as well as arrhythmias.

CASE STUDY

1. Assess his pulse and blood pressure. Verapamil will also reduce blood pressure and, thus, should be monitored as well as pulse for rhythm.
2. Renal disease will mean that he will excrete the drug more slowly. Blood levels may build up, creating an increased risk of adverse effects.

CRITICAL THINKING CHALLENGE

Any drug used to treat an arrhythmia may also induce an arrhythmia. Because Mr. Thomas has renal disease and doesn't eliminate verapamil as rapidly as other people, this may have contributed to his development of a secondary arrhythmia, although arrhythmias may occur with normal doses and blood levels of antiarrhythmics.

Chapter 30

KEY TERMS

Fill in the blanks and word find exercise

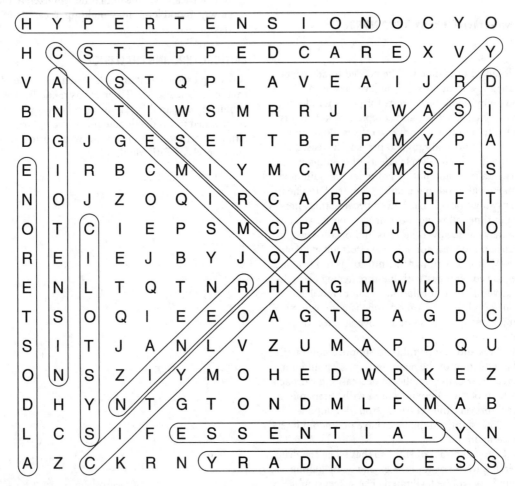

PHYSIOLOGY AND PATHOPHYSIOLOGY: THE BODY HUMAN

Essay

1. Systolic
2. Generally speaking, decreased cardiac output would result in a decreased blood pressure, however, other factors such as peripheral resistance, stimulation of the adrenergic system, or stimulation of the renin-angiotensin-aldosterone system could mediate that response.
3. Alpha-1 and beta-1 generate a sympathomimetic response, whereas alpha-2 and beta-2 generate a sympatholytic response.
4. Alpha-1 in the vasculature, alpha-2 in the brain, beta-1 in the heart, and beta-2 in the bronchial and vascular musculature.
5. This system vasoconstricts as well as increases circulating volume by retention of sodium and water. These actions result in an elevation of blood pressure.

CORE DRUG KNOWLEDGE: JUST THE FACTS

Multiple choice

1. d	2. a	3. c	4. b	5. a
6. c	7. b	8. c	9. d	10. a
11. a	12. c	13. c	14. b	15. a
16. d	17. b	18. b	19. a	20. b
21. d	22. c	23. c	24. d	

CORE PATIENT VARIABLES: PATIENTS, PLEASE

Multiple choice

1. c	2. b	3. d	4. a	5. c
6. a	7. c	8. b	9. c	10. c
11. a	12. a	13. d		

NURSING MANAGEMENT: EVERY GOOD NURSE SHOULD...

Multiple choice

1. b. Hypotension can occur during the 2 hours after the first dose of Captopril. Taking the drug at bedtime will minimize

the effects of the hypotension because the patient will be lying down during this time. Captopril should be taken on an empty stomach to promote absorption. Position changes should be gradual to minimize any orthostatic hypotension or dizziness felt from the drug therapy. Sodium intake should be kept the same or limited. Increased sodium intake would be counterproductive to the drug action.

2. c. Monitor blood glucose levels more closely. Tachycardia (a sign of hypoglycemia) is not experienced due to the beta-blocking actions of labetalol; therefore, patients need to rely not on how they feel but on their blood glucose levels to determine if they are experiencing hypoglycemia. Hyperglycemia is also possible. Beta blockage reduces insulin release in response to elevated blood glucose. Increasing dietary sugar is not appropriate in diabetic patients. Hot baths or showers will increase peripheral vasodilation and promote orthostatic hypotension. These should be avoided while on labetalol. Rapid discontinuation of the drug may cause angina, myocardial infarction, or ventricular arrhythmias in patients with cardiovascular disease. The drug should be slowly stopped instead.

3. a. This promotes a constant therapeutic level of clonidine. The patch should be applied to a new site each time, and to a site that has minimal hair. If the patch becomes loose during the 7 days, extra adhesive overlays may be used to maintain a seal.

4. d. Hydralazine causes reflex tachycardia from the vasodilation; beta blockers, like atenolol, counteract this. Hydralazine also causes an increase in angiotensin II, which promotes the retention of sodium and water; diuretics, like hydrochlorothiazide, promote excretion of excess sodium and water. Both beta blockers and diuretics may be used alone to treat hypertension. The combination therapy is indicated to prevent possible complications from the use of hydralazine alone and to make the hydralazine therapy more effective rather than due to the severity of the patient's hypertension.

5. d. Nitroprusside can be inactivated by reactions with trace contaminants that will cause the nitroprusside to appear blue, green, or red or brighter than its normal faint brown appearance. It should not be used if this discoloration is seen. Nitroprusside is never given directly by IV push; it must be further diluted and administered by IV infusion. Nitroprusside should be protected from light after dilution.

6. a. Patients of child-bearing age should be cautioned about becoming pregnant. Losartan is associated with fetal and neonatal deaths and morbidity. Dietary sodium should not be increased with hypertension because this can cause retention of fluid and increase peripheral resistance. Fluid loss is not a problem with losartan, although fluid retention may occur. Losartan is used to treat hypertension, it does not cause hypertension.

CASE STUDY

1. The nurse should slow the infusion rate. If symptoms do not disappear, the infusion may need to be stopped for a while.
2. Abdominal pain and nausea are two signs that the blood pressure has been reduced too quickly. These symptoms will disappear if the infusion is slowed or stopped.

CRITICAL THINKING CHALLENGE

1. It appears that Mr. Mohammed is experiencing cyanide poisoning.
2. The infusion should be stopped, and the doctor should be notified immediately. The nurse should consult with the physician regarding new orders to counteract the cyanide poisoning, usually sodium nitrate followed by sodium thiosulfate. Additional blood work, such as blood gases to assess whether acidosis has occurred, and cyanide level assay, may also be ordered.

Chapter 31

KEY TERMS

Anagrams

1. glomerular filtration
2. tubular secretion
3. oliguria
4. edema
5. diuresis
6. hypervolemia
7. tubular reabsorption
8. hypertension
9. hypokalemia
10. osmolality
11. diuretic
12. hyperkalemia

PHYSIOLOGY AND PATHOPHYSIOLOGY: THE BODY HUMAN

Essay

1. The kidneys are responsible for filtering and purifying the body; ridding the body of impurities and waste by producing urine and excreting water, electrolytes, and other substances; regulating the body's acid–base balance; maintaining blood pressure; influencing circulating fluid volume; assisting in the production of red blood cells; and contributing to calcium metabolism.
2. Kidneys, ureters, and bladder
3. Glomerular filtration, renal tubular reabsorption, and renal tubular secretion
4. Less than 2 L in 24 hours
5. Excretion of hydrogen ions or reabsorbing bicarbonate
6. Synthesis, storage, and release of renin
7. Secretes erythropoietin, which stimulates bone marrow to produce red blood cells
8. Chemically transforms precursors of vitamin D to an active form

CORE DRUG KNOWLEDGE: JUST THE FACTS

Multiple choice

1. b   2. c   3. c   4. a   5. c
6. c   7. a   8. a   9. c   10. b
11. a   12. d   13. c   14. c

CORE PATIENT VARIABLES: PATIENTS, PLEASE

Multiple choice

1. c   2. a   3. d   4. b   5. b
6. a   7. d   8. c   9. b   10. a
11. b   12. d

NURSING MANAGEMENT: EVERY GOOD NURSE SHOULD...

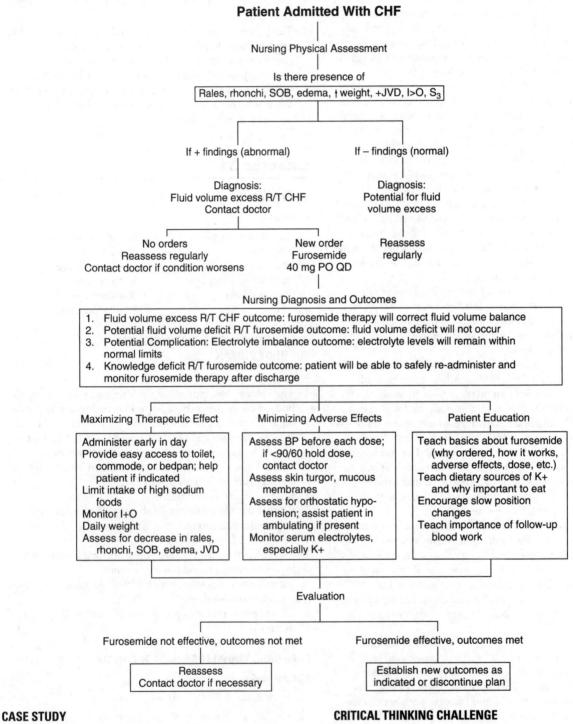

Patient Admitted With CHF

Nursing Physical Assessment

Is there presence of

Rales, rhonchi, SOB, edema, ↑ weight, +JVD, I>O, S_3

If + findings (abnormal)

If − findings (normal)

Diagnosis:
Fluid volume excess R/T CHF
Contact doctor

Diagnosis:
Potential for fluid
volume excess

No orders
Reassess regularly
Contact doctor if condition worsens

New order
Furosemide
40 mg PO QD

Reassess
regularly

Nursing Diagnosis and Outcomes

1. Fluid volume excess R/T CHF outcome: furosemide therapy will correct fluid volume balance
2. Potential fluid volume deficit R/T furosemide outcome: fluid volume deficit will not occur
3. Potential Complication: Electrolyte imbalance outcome: electrolyte levels will remain within normal limits
4. Knowledge deficit R/T furosemide outcome: patient will be able to safely re-administer and monitor furosemide therapy after discharge

Maximizing Therapeutic Effect

Administer early in day
Provide easy access to toilet, commode, or bedpan; help patient if indicated
Limit intake of high sodium foods
Monitor I+O
Daily weight
Assess for decrease in rales, rhonchi, SOB, edema, JVD

Minimizing Adverse Effects

Assess BP before each dose; if <90/60 hold dose, contact doctor
Assess skin turgor, mucous membranes
Assess for orthostatic hypotension; assist patient in ambulating if present
Monitor serum electrolytes, especially K+

Patient Education

Teach basics about furosemide (why ordered, how it works, adverse effects, dose, etc.)
Teach dietary sources of K+ and why important to eat
Encourage slow position changes
Teach importance of follow-up blood work

Evaluation

Furosemide not effective, outcomes not met

Furosemide effective, outcomes met

Reassess
Contact doctor if necessary

Establish new outcomes as
indicated or discontinue plan

CASE STUDY

1. The vial of mannitol should be warmed in a warm water bath to dissolve the crystals. The drug should be no warmer than body temperature. An IV administration set with a filter should be used.
2. Mannitol is not absorbed via the GI route so it must be given IV.
3. Hourly urinary output should be measured to see if the mannitol is effective. Output should increase and be at least 30 cc per hour. An indwelling urinary catheter is needed to accurately determine hourly output.

CRITICAL THINKING CHALLENGE

1. The nurse should administer a test dose of 0.2 g/kg in 3 to 5 minutes before beginning the main infusion. If urine output remains less than 30 cc/hour after the test dose, the infusion should be held and the doctor contacted. A second test dose may be ordered.
2. Mr. Button's age was a risk factor for him having decreased renal function.

Chapter 32

KEY TERMS

Crossword puzzle

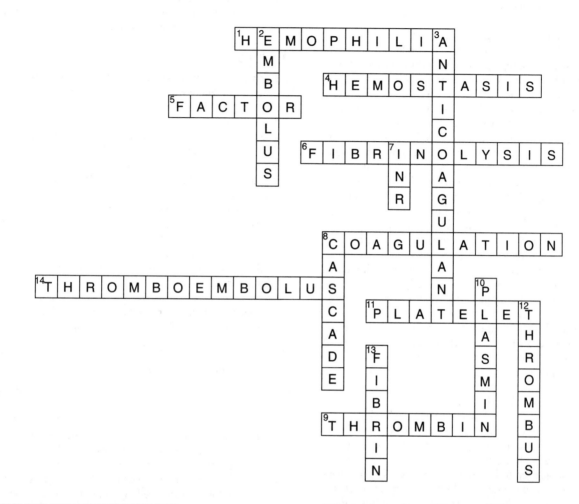

PHYSIOLOGY AND PATHOPHYSIOLOGY: THE BODY HUMAN

Essay

1. Anticoagulant drugs "thin" the blood by interrupting the clotting cascade. Antiplatelet drugs decrease the ability of the blood to clot by interfering with platelet membrane function and platelet aggregation. Hemorrheologics reduce blood viscosity, increase the flexibility of the RBC, and decrease platelet aggregation. Thrombolytics have the ability to dissolve existing clots.
2. The clotting cascade is initiated by the tissue damage and platelet activation, which mobilize the clotting factors circulating in the blood. Once active, these clotting factors work with calcium to form fibrin. At this point, blood coagulation is completed and blood loss stops.
3. Factors are plasma components that are an integral part of the clotting cascade.
4. Plasmin is the substance that lyses a blood clot.

CORE DRUG KNOWLEDGE: JUST THE FACTS

Multiple choice

1. d	2. a	3. a	4. b	5. c
6. a	7. c	8. d	9. a	10. b
11. a	12. d	13. d	14. c	15. a
16. c	17. b	18. a	19. c	20. d
21. c	22. a			

CORE PATIENT VARIABLES: PATIENTS, PLEASE

Multiple choice

1. b	2. c	3. d	4. c	5. c
6. d	7. b	8. a	9. a	10. a
11. d	12. c	13. d	14. b	15. b
16. d	17. d			

NURSING MANAGEMENT: EVERY GOOD NURSE SHOULD . . .

Multiple choice

1. d.   Intravenous heparin infusions should not be stopped to run other drugs through the IV site because this lowers the blood level of heparin and will alter the therapeutic response. Many other drugs are incompatible with heparin, and they should not be piggybacked or added to heparin infusions. Use of a separate IV site for the antibiotics will allow continuous infusion of heparin and appropriate dosing of the antibiotics.

2. b.   Research has shown that a 3-cc syringe produces less hematoma formation than a 1-cc syringe. To further prevent hematomas, do not aspirate before injection and do not massage the insertion site after injection. The scapula is not a recommended site for heparin administration.

3. c.   Warfarin causes a known pattern of fetal changes, known as fetal warfarin syndrome. Precautions should be taken to prevent pregnancy while on warfarin. Vitamin K is the antidote to warfarin, and increases in dietary sources, such as green leafy vegetables, should be avoided. Potassium does not have an effect on warfarin. The symbol for potassium is "K," but it is not the same thing as vitamin K. Doses should be taken regularly; however, a double dose should not be taken because it may produce bleeding.

4. a.   Food helps to increase the absorption of ticlopidine and also decreases the GI problems that may occur with drug therapy. Blood work will be needed every other week, starting in the second week of therapy, until the end of the third month to check the CBC to detect neutropenia. This drug will lengthen the bleeding time experienced by patients, and they and their families need to know to put pressure on wounds until bleeding stops.

5. c.   Although onset of therapeutic effect begins in 2 to 4 weeks, full effect is delayed. Patients need to realize this and be encouraged to be patient to see results. Drug therapy needs to be continued until full therapeutic effect is achieved. There is always individual variation in response to drug therapy; however, the patient needs to hear reinforcement regarding the delayed onset of action to prevent discouragement and stopping the drug prematurely.

6. a.   For the next 8 hours, assess vital signs every 15 to 30 minutes depending on patient's condition. Streptokinase is always administered with an infusion pump, never by gravity flow, to prevent overdosage. Avoid IM injections because this may cause internal bleeding. Coffee ground emesis is a sign of internal bleeding and the infusion should be stopped.

7. d.   Diluted drug is rotated, not shaken, to prevent gel formation in the antihemophilic factor. The drug is administered by the IV route to deliver it directly into the bloodstream where it can act. IM routes are avoided to prevent bleeding into the muscle. Coagulation studies are monitored during therapy to assess for therapeutic effect of the drug. Additional antihemophilic factor may be needed if bleeding is not controlled or coagulation studies show subtherapeutic levels of the factor.

8. b.   This is to determine that an appropriate amount of aminocaproic acid has been administered to control bleeding. The fresh incision is a likely source for bleeding. Aminocaproic acid is administered by the IV route. It should not be mixed with other drugs. The patient should be connected to a cardiac monitor throughout therapy to detect any cardiac arrhythmias that may occur.

CASE STUDY

1. Heparin is an anticoagulant used to treat DVT. It is safe to use in pregnancy because it does not cross the placenta.
2. Some heparin is ordered to be given by IV push as a bolus of the drug. This brings about a quick rise in blood levels and helps to achieve a therapeutic level more quickly.
3. The aPTT done before the heparin is started is the baseline measurement. Repeated measurements will determine if the drug has reached therapeutic levels. If the blood level is not in therapeutic range, the nurse needs to seek an order to increase the heparin dosage. If the blood level is above therapeutic range, the nurse needs to seek an order to decrease the heparin dosage.
4. Heparin does not break down the formed clot. It prevents further clots from forming while the body naturally walls off the clot and allows it to be broken down. Heparin also prevents the extension of the clot. Ambulating before the clot has lysed makes it more likely that the clot will break off from the vein wall and travel, lodging perhaps in the heart, lungs, or brain.

CRITICAL THINKING CHALLENGE

The nurse should immediately turn off the infusion and disconnect the pump from the infusion tubing. The nurse should then contact the physician and seek orders for STAT aPTT levels. Because Ms. Lopez is stable and is not showing any evidence of bleeding, protamine sulfate is not indicated immediately, although the nurse may obtain an order for the drug at this time to be given later if needed. Ms. Lopez must be monitored closely for signs of bleeding. In another 6 to 8 hours, the aPTT should be reassessed to determine if she has recovered from the overdosage. The heparin infusion may be restarted after it is determined that blood levels have returned to a preoverdose level. A different IV pump should be used, and the defective pump should be returned for servicing. The nurse should write an incident sheet detailing the pump's malfunction and the effect on the patient. Additional protocols may need to be followed depending on the institution's policies for equipment malfunctions, and the nurse should check her hospital's policies.

Chapter 33

KEY TERMS

Matching

1. j   2. f   3. g   4. i   5. b
6. d   7. a   8. c   9. k   10. e
11. h

1. f   2. e   3. i   4. g   5. b
6. j   7. c   8. k   9. d   10. h
11. a

1. j   2. h   3. f   4. k   5. b
6. i   7. c   8. a   9. d   10. e
11. g

PHYSIOLOGY AND PATHOPHYSIOLOGY: THE BODY HUMAN

Essay

1. The essential components of the immune system are hematopoietic cells, barrier defenses, the nonspecific immune response, the specific immune response, and immunity.
2. Skin, mucus, and the GI tract
3. Granulocytes, monocytes, and lymphocytes
4. T cells and B cells
5. Effector or cytotoxic, T helper cells, T suppressor cells
6. Thymosin

CORE DRUG KNOWLEDGE: JUST THE FACTS

Multiple choice

1. b   2. d   3. a   4. c   5. c
6. a   7. d   8. d   9. b   10. a
11. c   12. d

CORE PATIENT VARIABLES: PATIENTS, PLEASE

Multiple choice

1. b   2. c   3. d   4. a   5. b
6. c   7. d   8. c   9. a   10. b

NURSING MANAGEMENT: EVERY GOOD NURSE SHOULD ...

Multiple choice

1. d. All of the above. Interferon alfa-2a is only administered by injection. The patient is at risk for infections due to possible bone marrow suppression. Bone marrow depression and elevated liver enzymes can occur as adverse effects, and blood work should be monitored carefully to prevent serious problems.
2. c. Epoetin alfa is administered subcutaneously. It can also be administered IV. Shaking will denature the protein in epoetin alfa and make the drug less effective, so should be avoided. The single-dose, 1-mL vials have no preservative in them and should be discarded after being opened

and medication should be withdrawn to prevent contamination and infection.

3. a. Although at 10 days there should be an increase in the reticulocyte count (immature red blood cell count), it takes 2 to 6 weeks for the hematocrit, hemoglobin, and red cell count to rise. It is appropriate to continue with the same dose because it is too soon to determine that she needs a larger dose. A smaller dose would be inappropriate at this time. Because it is an expected finding for the hematocrit to be unchanged at this time, the physician does not need to be notified immediately, although the physician should be made aware of the lab results at some point in time.

4. d. Patients with decreased white blood cell counts are at increased risk of contracting an infection. Frequent hand washing by the patient and family members is an important method of preventing infection. The patient needs to avoid crowds and people with illnesses to minimize the risk of incurring an infection. Filgrastim will make the neutrophil count rise 1 to 2 days after starting therapy, but this is a transient increase. Filgrastim must be continued until the full nadir (lowest point) of marrow-suppressing activity from the antineoplastic has occurred. This varies by the antineoplastic used. Medullary bone pain occurs in about one fourth of the patients on filgrastim.

5. b. Rituximab is administered by slow IV infusion. Using an IV pump will regulate the infusion rate and keep it at the prescribed rate. Antipyretics, such as acetaminophen, should be administered before the first dose. Because infusion reactions appear to be dose related, the infusion should be started with a fairly small dose and then titrated upward.

6. d. Turn off the infusion because she is experiencing an infusion reaction. Keep the infusion off until the symptoms resolve, and then resume the infusion at half the rate that produced the reaction. Turning down the infusion might be helpful, but it is not the best choice. Blankets and ice chips are not the priority initial action. The patient should have been premedicated with acetaminophen; another dose would not be the priority now.

7. c. Elevated BUN levels indicate that kidney function is impaired. This is a concern because cyclosporine has a significant risk of causing nephrotoxicity. The damage to the kidney may persist even if the cyclosporine is discontinued. Hyperkalemia may occur from cyclosporine, but a small elevation is not a sign of significant problem. A slightly lower white cell (neutrophil) count would be expected; only significant neutropenia would be a concern.

CASE STUDY

1. Lydia needs to know how to reconstitute the interferon alfa-2a, draw up the proper dose in the syringe, locate injection sites, administer by correct technique, rotate sites of injection, and store the reconstituted drug.
2. Concerns would be related to Lydia's eyesight. Can she see well enough to read the labels? Read the syringes? Locate an appropriate injection site? Is she capable of performing the injection herself? If not, does her husband's arthritis preclude him from being able to help her? Would the daughter be available to help with the administration of the drug if necessary?

CRITICAL THINKING CHALLENGE

Is there a refrigerator to store the reconstituted drug?
Is there a place to safely store the needles and syringes? How about used syringes?
Are there environmental risks for falls in the home? (Are there stairs? Is a handrail present on the stairs? Are there scatter rugs? Is there adequate lighting in hallways and stairwells?)

Chapter 34

KEY TERMS

Essay

1. Atherosclerosis is a narrowing of the arterial interior due to buildup of hard, thick deposits, and a loss of elasticity of the arterial wall
2. This is another name for atherosclerosis.
3. Hyperlipidemia is an elevation of blood lipid levels.
4. Serum lipids are the fats found in the bloodstream. These lipids include cholesterol, cholesterol esters (compounds), phospholipids, and triglycerides.

PHYSIOLOGY AND PATHOPHYSIOLOGY: THE BODY HUMAN

Essay

1. Chylomicrons; very low-density lipoproteins (VLDL); intermediate-density lipoproteins (IDL); low-density lipoproteins (LDL); and high-density lipoproteins (HDL)
2. Low-density lipoprotein (LDL) is the major cholesterol carrier in the blood. LDL has a structure that can vary, based on its size and density. LDL includes VLDL and IDL. (The intermediate-density lipoprotein [IDL] is considered an abnormal lipoprotein.) Lp(a) is a type of LDL and is considered a genetic variation. About one third to one fourth of blood cholesterol is carried by high-density lipoprotein (HDL). Chylomicrons are the largest and least dense of the lipoproteins. Triglycerides are transported primarily by the chylomicrons and the very low-density lipoproteins (VLDL), a subgroup of LDL.
3. It has been hypothesized that triglyceride-rich lipoproteins move into macrophages in the bloodstream, then interact with small, dense LDL and HDL particles to form arterial thromboses.
4. Lowering serum lipid levels decreases the risk for atherosclerosis, hypertension, and coronary heart disease. Lowering cholesterol levels can stop or reverse atherosclerosis in all vascular beds.
5. The antihyperlipidemics are composed of the HMG Co A reductase inhibitors, the fibric acid derivatives, nicotinic acid, the bile acid sequestrants, and miscellaneous agents.

CORE DRUG KNOWLEDGE: JUST THE FACTS

Multiple choice

1. d   2. b   3. d   4. a   5. b
6. c   7. b

CORE PATIENT VARIABLES: PATIENTS, PLEASE

Multiple choice

1. a   2. a   3. c   4. b   5. d
6. b   7. c

NURSING MANAGEMENT: EVERY GOOD NURSE SHOULD . . .

Multiple choice

1. c. Lovastatin should not replace a low-fat diet, but supplement it to achieve the greatest effect in lowering cholesterol levels. Dosages of lovastatin should not be randomly increased by the patient because adverse effects may occur. The goal is to lower dietary fat intake, not to raise it. Raising fat intake will not prevent adverse effects from lovastatin but will counteract some of its therapeutic effect.

2. b. Lovastatin is metabolized by the hepatic enzyme CYP3A4. Many drugs interact with this pathway. Because Mr Hudson receives multiple drug therapies, it is likely that one or more of the drugs may interact with lovastatin and inhibit this hepatic enzyme pathway. This will slow down metabolism of lovastatin, increasing circulating blood levels, and increasing the risk for adverse effects. An increase in therapeutic response is also possible, not a decrease. Anaphylactic reactions and electrolyte imbalances are not adverse effects from lovastatin.

3. a. Lovastatin will raise liver enzymes, especially when the drug is first started. Although this elevation is not normally serious, it is important to monitor the enzymes carefully to verify that liver function is not being impaired. Photosensitivity may occur from lovastatin, and patients should minimize their sun exposure until they know how the drug will affect them. Serious skeletal muscle effects (rhabdomyolysis) may result from lovastatin. Although this is rare, it may be fatal. The patient should report muscle pain or weakness immediately. Constipation is not a common adverse effect of lovastatin; it can be serious with cholestyramine, a bile acid sequestrant.

CASE STUDY

1. The lovastatin was showing therapeutic effect because the LDL cholesterol level had dropped. Although the liver enzymes (AST and ALT) are elevated, they are not considered significantly elevated at this time.
2. He needs to return so the effect of the drug on the LDL levels and liver enzymes may be further evaluated.

CRITICAL THINKING CHALLENGE

The nurse should contact the physician or nurse practitioner and inform them of the elevated liver enzymes. At this point, the enzymes are more than three times the upper range for normal and may indicate liver damage. Consult with the prescriber about decreasing the dose. It is also possible that the drug will be discontinued, but, because Mr Chilcoat has no other noted complications from the drug therapy, this is not as likely. If the dose is decreased, Mr Chilcoat should return in 6 more weeks for further evaluation. If the dose is not decreased, he will also need to return for further evaluation, but the interval may be longer, as decided by the physician or nurse practitioner.

Chapter 35

KEY TERMS

True/false

1.	False	antitussives
2.	False	histamine
3.	True	
4.	False	decongestants
5.	False	cilia
6.	False	expectorants
7.	False	common cold
8.	False	pharyngitis
9.	False	sinus
10.	True	
11.	True	
12.	False	laryngitis

PHYSIOLOGY AND PATHOPHYSIOLOGY: THE BODY HUMAN

Essay

1. Nose, mouth, pharynx, larynx, trachea, and bronchial tree
2. Produce mucus and entrap dust, foreign substances, or microorganisms
3. Particles are projected toward the throat by cilia
4. Cough, sneeze

CORE DRUG KNOWLEDGE: JUST THE FACTS

Multiple choice

1. a   2. c   3. b   4. a   5. c
6. a   7. d   8. b   9. b   10. a

CORE PATIENT VARIABLES: PATIENTS, PLEASE

Multiple choice

1. d   2. d   3. c   4. d   5. a
6. a   7. c

NURSING MANAGEMENT: EVERY GOOD NURSE SHOULD . . .

Multiple choice

1. d. Because dextromethorphan may cause drowsiness, driving and operating machinery that requires alertness should be avoided until it is known if drowsiness will occur. Alcohol and other CNS depressants may increase sedative effects and should be avoided. It is not recommended for use in children and should be kept out of their reach to prevent accidental overdosage or poisoning.
2. b. Drinking plenty of fluids will keep mucous membranes moist. Dietary fiber has no effect on pseudoephedrine. Hot, steamy showers will have a similar effect as using a humidifier and will also keep mucous membranes moist, which would be beneficial. To minimize adverse effects, do not take for more than 4 days; 14 days is too long.
3. c. GI distress is a common adverse effect and is minimized if the drug is taken with food. There is no indication the patient should stop taking the drug. Decreasing the dose will prevent full therapeutic effect from being

achieved and may not relieve GI upset. The use of other antihistamines should be avoided while on this drug.
4. d. Both dextromethorphan and guaifenesin are not to be used if the patient has chronic asthma or emphysema, or if the cough is from smoking. Dextromethorphan interacts with several other drugs, whereas guaifenesin does not. This information may indicate which preparation would be preferred for this patient.

CASE STUDY

LIFESTYLE, DIET, AND HABITS

Do you drive? Do you do other skills/activities that require concentration?

ENVIRONMENT

Do you have stairs in your house? Do you have railings on your stairways? Do you have loose rugs in the halls?

Due to Mr Fox's age, he is at increased risk of drowsiness from fexofenadine. If he drives or does other activities that require concentration and alertness, such as using power tools and saws or using a riding lawn mower on hills, he should limit these activities until he knows how he will respond to the fexofenadine.

If he does become drowsy, he may be at increased risk of falling. Stairs without railings and scatter rugs increase his risk of a fall.

CRITICAL THINKING CHALLENGE

1. Mr. Fox has likely taken another antihistamine, such as diphenhydramine (Benadryl). Mr. Fox is likely having drowsiness as an adverse effect from drug therapy.
2. Taking two antihistamines together has likely intensified the CNS depression, causing drowsiness. Diphenhydramine is readily available over the counter and is commonly used for itching. As a first-generation antihistamine, diphenhydramine causes considerable sedation. Because Mr. Fox is an older adult, he is more sensitive to this adverse effect.

Chapter 36

KEY TERMS

Multiple choice

1. c   2. e   3. i   4. f   5. d
6. h   7. a   8. g   9. b

PHYSIOLOGY AND PATHOPHYSIOLOGY: THE BODY HUMAN

Essay

1. Paired lungs, bronchi, alveoli, blood vessels
2. No. The act of breathing in and out is actually ventilation. The passage of gas across the alveolar membrane is respiration.
3. The vagus nerve stimulates diaphragm contraction and inspiration. It also induces bronchoconstriction.
4. In the respiratory system, stimulation of the sympathetic nervous system results in bronchodilation.

CORE DRUG KNOWLEDGE: JUST THE FACTS

Multiple choice

1. c	2. b	3. a	4. a	5. d
6. b	7. d	8. a	9. b	10. c
11. a	12. c	13. b	14. d	15. b
16. a	17. b	18. c	19. b	20. d

CORE PATIENT VARIABLES: PATIENTS, PLEASE

Multiple choice

1. a	2. c	3. b	4. d	5. c
6. d	7. b	8. b	9. a	10. c
11. d	12. b			

NURSING MANAGEMENT: EVERY GOOD NURSE SHOULD . . .

Multiple choice

1. d. A sticky residue may form on the patient's face. This should be removed with water after drug administration. Diluted acetylcysteine should be refrigerated, not left at room temperature. Nebulization of acetylcysteine causes an unpleasant, transient smell. The purpose of the therapy is to loosen thick secretions so that they may be coughed up. Therefore, coughing is expected and to be encouraged, not discouraged.

2. d. Breath sounds should clear if therapy is effective; assessment throughout therapy is important. Insomnia, tachycardia, and irritability are signs of adverse effects and should be assessed. Blood will need to be drawn so blood levels of theophylline can be measured to determine if therapeutic or toxic levels have been achieved.

3. d. All of the above are true and should be included in patient education.

4. a. Because Martha has a history of lactose intolerance, she may have the same type of problems from the use of cromolyn sodium. She needs to contact the prescriber if she has any of these symptoms of lactose intolerance. Cromolyn sodium is used as prophylaxis, not to treat an acute episode of asthma. Metered-dose inhalers require the patient to exhale, trigger the release of medication, and then inhale. (Irregular menstrual periods pose no additional risk for adverse effects from cromolyn sodium, and no special teaching is required.)

5. c. Iced tea contains caffeine. Caffeine is a xanthine like theophylline. Adverse effects from the theophylline are more likely if caffeine is taken also. If he drinks several glasses a day, he needs to avoid it, although an occasional glass would be acceptable. Sprite soda does not contain caffeine. Although lemon meringue pie and fettucine alfredo are high in carbohydrates, eating these occasionally is acceptable, as long as his protein intake is normal. Overall, he should avoid a high-carbohydrate, low-protein diet because this can decrease urinary elimination of theophylline. One particular food item does not alter the overall dietary pattern. Cheerios cereal would have no effect on theophylline.

6. c. A yellowing of the whites of the eyes is a sign of jaundice and may indicate that hepatitis or hepatic failure is developing. These are serious adverse effects of zafirlukast. Absence of wheezing is a positive effect from the drug, indicating that the therapeutic effect is being achieved. A mild headache and an upset stomach can be common adverse effects from zafirlukast, not signs of serious problems.

CASE STUDY

1. Mr. March is showing symptoms of theophylline toxicity. His blood levels are elevated above the therapeutic range, and he is showing CNS excitation as an adverse effect. Cigarette smoking increases the metabolism of theophylline. Because Mr. March has ceased smoking after the dose of theophylline has been adjusted, the metabolism of theophylline was no longer stimulated. Thus, the metabolism rate of theophylline slowed, allowing more theophylline to circulate in the bloodstream and be active.

2. Contact the physician or nurse practitioner who had prescribed the theophylline. Inform him or her of the current blood levels, adverse effects, and that Mr. March was no longer smoking cigarettes. A dose adjustment of theophylline is needed.

CRITICAL THINKING CHALLENGE

1. Mr. March appears to be having toxicity from the theophylline, most likely due to a drug interaction with the ciprofloxacin.

2. To confirm this assessment, a blood level of theophylline is needed. If he is in a toxic range, the theophylline either needs to be decreased or the ciprofloxacin needs to be changed to another antibiotic (this is the more probable action).

Chapter 37

KEY TERMS

Matching

1. g	2. a	3. e	4. k	5. f
6. m	7. b	8. d	9. c	10. i
11. l	12. j	13. h		

PHYSIOLOGY AND PATHOPHYSIOLOGY: THE BODY HUMAN

Essay

1. mouth, oropharynx, esophagus, stomach, duodenum

2. *mucosa:* forms folds and projections that increase the surface area of the intestine
   submucosa: contains blood vessels that provide nutrients and oxygen to the tissues and remove the products of digestion
   muscularis externa: contains muscles that are responsible for peristalsis
   serosa: contains secretory cells that keep the outer surface of the tract moist and lubricated

3. mucous, chief, and parietal

4. parasympathetic

5. *amylase:* splits starch or glycogen into disaccharide
   lipase: hydrolyzes fats to fatty acids
   trypsin, chymotrypsin, and carboxypeptidase: split proteins into amino acids

CORE DRUG KNOWLEDGE: JUST THE FACTS

Multiple choice

1. c	2. b	3. a	4. d	5. c
6. c	7. d	8. d	9. a	10. d
11. b	12. b	13. c	14. c	15. c
16. b	17. a	18. c	19. d	20. b
21. d	22. b			

CORE PATIENT VARIABLES: PATIENTS, PLEASE

Multiple choice

1. d	2. c	3. a	4. b	5. d
6. a	7. b	8. a	9. c	10. c
11. c	12. a	13. d	14. b	15. b
16. b	17. a	18. d		

NURSING MANAGEMENT: EVERY GOOD NURSE SHOULD . . .

Multiple choice

1. a. Shaking the bottle will disperse the drug evenly in the suspension. Administer the drug 1 hour after meal for maximum effectiveness. Do not mix the drug with water. When aluminum hydroxide and magnesium hydroxide are given as tablets, they should be chewed and then followed with water to promote dissolving.

2. a. It is necessary to stagger oral aluminum hydroxide with magnesium hydroxide and oral cimetidine because the antacid will decrease the absorption of the cimetidine. Giving the cimetidine immediately before a meal and the antacid immediately after the meal will not separate the ingestion of the two drugs enough to prevent alterations of the absorption of cimetidine. Also, if three meals are taken, this is not the proper dose for either drug.

3. d. Administering metoclopramide 30 minutes before each meal will allow time for the drug to become effective before eating. Depression may be a serious adverse effect of metoclopramide and should be assessed. Drowsiness and fatigue are common adverse effects of metoclopramide, and patients should be warned of this.

4. b. Asthma attacks can occur after sniffing pancrelipase powder. Pancrelipase is administered with every meal and snack. Steatorrhea stools are a sign that insufficient digestive enzymes are present. Steatorrhea stools should greatly diminish, if not disappear, while on pancrelipase if the dosage is sufficient.

5. c. *H pylori* organisms are normally responsible for gastric ulcers; the antibiotics will eradicate the organisms, and the omeprazole will decrease gastric acid, relieving pain and helping to eradicate the *H pylori* organisms. Eradication of *H pylori* is needed to prevent or minimize recurrence of the gastric ulcer. Bismuth therapy is not used in this patient due to his allergy to salicylates.

6. b. For orlistat to be most effective the total daily fat intake should be evenly divided throughout the day at different meals. Orlistat needs to be taken with meals that contain fat. Because Samantha often skips breakfast, telling her to take the drug in the morning (as opposed to with meals) may cause her to take the drug on an empty stomach and lose effectiveness of the drug. She might need to take the dose with her snack, if it contains fat, or she should skip a dose if she doesn't eat breakfast that day. A diet to promote weight loss and promote health should have no more than 30% of its calories from fat. Orlistat does not replace the need to exercise or modify the diet.

7. a. Ondansetron should be administered 30 minutes before starting chemotherapy. The drug is not administered IV push though, but should be infused over 15 minutes. Additional doses should be used after treatment.

CASE STUDY

In addition to general teaching about the drug (what it does, how it works, what is proper dose, when to take the drug, adverse effects), other points for education include:

Take the drug exactly as prescribed for the entire prescribed length of therapy, even if symptoms disappear.

The effects smoking, drinking alcohol, drinking caffeinated drinks, eating spicy food, and taking products with aspirin or ibuprofen have on the effectiveness of cimetidine

Counseling on stopping smoking

CRITICAL THINKING CHALLENGE

1. Have you stopped smoking? Because smoking antagonizes the effect of cimetidine, if Mr. Bernstein had stopped smoking, this would have a similar effect to increasing the cimetidine dose. Are you taking OTC medications that treat excess acid? If Mr. Bernstein has been taking an OTC form of cimetidine or other H2 receptor antagonist in addition to his prescription drug, he may have caused an overdosage.

2. What is his SGOT and SGPT? These tests will show functioning of the liver. History of chronic alcohol use may have affected liver function, placing Mr. Bernstein more at risk of developing adverse effects from the cimetidine.

   What is the serum trough (low point) of the drug? The patient may be having adverse effects because the blood levels are above therapeutic range. This may be because of impaired liver function.

Chapter 38

KEY TERMS
Unscrambling Exercise

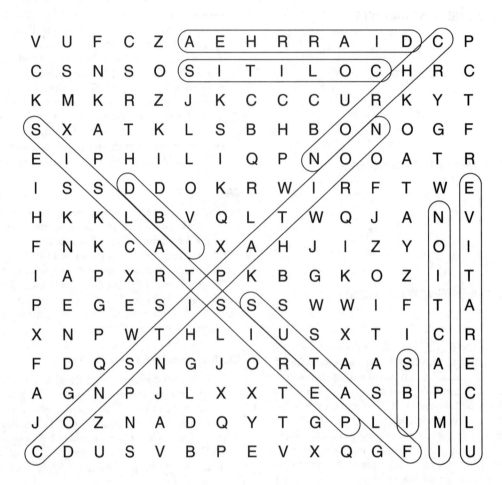

PHYSIOLOGY AND PATHOPHYSIOLOGY: THE BODY HUMAN
Essay

1. cecum, appendix, colon, rectum, and anal canal
2. ascending, transverse, descending, and sigmoid
3. relaxation of the internal and external sphincters
4. dead bacteria, fat, inorganic matter, protein, dried digestive juices, and indigestible components of food
5. vitamin K, vitamin B_{12}, riboflavin, and thiamine

CORE DRUG KNOWLEDGE: JUST THE FACTS
Multiple choice

1. b	2. a	3. a	4. c	5. b
6. d	7. c	8. c	9. b	10. c

CORE PATIENT VARIABLES: PATIENTS, PLEASE
Multiple choice

1. b	2. a	3. b	4. b	5. c
6. d	7. a	8. c		

NURSING MANAGEMENT: EVERY GOOD NURSE SHOULD . . .

Multiple choice

1. a.   This promotes dispersion of the drug in the intestine. Simethicone should be administered after meals and at bedtime. Cabbage, cucumbers, and onions are gas-forming foods and should be avoided. Increased belching will occur as a mechanism of passing the gas bubbles.
2. d.   Sue is showing signs of atropine toxicity. This can be very serious. No further drug should be given at this time, and the doctor needs to be notified.
3. c.   The magnesium may be retained in a patient with renal failure, causing hypermagnesemia. As multiple doses are expected to be needed, this becomes a greater risk.
4. c.   Fluid and electrolyte imbalances may occur if given in large doses over a prolonged period of time. Additionally, chronic use of laxatives leads to dependency on laxatives for a bowel movement to occur. The use of magnesium sulfate is not intended as a dietary source of magnesium. Magnesium sulfate has both antacid and laxative effects.
5. b.   PEG-ES is used to clean the GI tract of stool so the GI tract can be clearly visualized during x-ray and other types of GI examinations. It induces diarrhea to do this. It does not prevent constipation. It has no effect on blood ammonia levels, unlike lactulose.

CASE STUDY

HEALTH STATUS

Postmyocardial infarction (don't want patient constipated)

LIFE SPAN AND GENDER

Older adult increases risk of constipation

LIFESTYLE, DIET, AND HABITS

On bed rest, decreased activity decreases peristalsis, thereby increasing the risk of constipation
Bland diet, post-GI bleeding may contribute to constipation

ENVIRONMENT

Hospitalized, out of normal environment, may influence elimination patterns, especially as on bed rest (unable to use toilet)

CRITICAL THINKING CHALLENGE

A Valsalva maneuver (pushing against a closed glottis) is necessary to expel a bowel movement. Straining that occurs with constipation causes an extended Valsalva maneuver and stimulates the vagal nerve. Vagal stimulation causes bradycardia, which is usually undesirable after a myocardial infarction. Stool softeners such as ducosate help trap water in the stool to keep it soft, prevent constipation, and promote ease of having a bowel movement.

Chapter 39

KEY TERMS

Matching

1. h   2. n   3. g   4. c   5. j
6. m   7. e   8. d   9. f   10. i
11. a   12. k   13. l   14. o   15. b

PHYSIOLOGY AND PATHOPHYSIOLOGY: THE BODY HUMAN

Essay

1. Hypothalamus
2. Temperature, perspiration, GI activity, appetite and thirst regulation, blood pressure, respiration, regulation of basic body rhythms, and complex behavioral and emotional reactions
3. Growth hormone-releasing factor, thyrotropin-releasing factor, gonadotropin-releasing factor, and corticotropin-releasing factor
4. Growth hormone, thyrotropin, adrenocorticotropin, follicle-stimulating hormone, luteinizing hormone, and prolactin
5. Antidiuretic hormone and oxytocin
6. Iodine
7. The half-life of T_4 is approximately 1 week compared to 12 hours for T_3, and T_4 is converted to T_3 (a more active hormone) at the cellular level.
8. Heat production and body temperature; oxygen consumption and cardiac output; blood volume; enzyme system activity; metabolism of carbohydrates, fats, and proteins; and regulation of growth and development
9. Parathormone
10. Membrane transport processes, nerve impulse conduction, muscle contraction, and blood clotting

CORE DRUG KNOWLEDGE: JUST THE FACTS

Multiple choice

1. b   2. c   3. d   4. c   5. a
6. a   7. d   8. b   9. d   10. a
11. b   12. c   13. d   14. b   15. b
16. d   17. d   18. a   19. b   20. d

CORE PATIENT VARIABLES: PATIENTS, PLEASE

Multiple choice

1. d   2. b   3. b   4. a   5. c
6. d   7. d   8. b   9. a   10. d
11. b   12. c   13. b   14. b   15. a
16. b   17. a   18. c

NURSING MANAGEMENT: EVERY GOOD NURSE SHOULD . . .

Multiple choice

1. a.   How to administer an SC injection. Somatropin is administered by SC and IM routes only. Patients and families need to learn how to safely administer the drug. Proper storage is in the refrigerator after it has been diluted. Limping and hip or knee pain are possible signs of slipped capital femoral epipheses or avascular necrosis of the femoral head, a serious complication that should be reported at once by the patient.

2. d.   All of the above. Ms. Wiggins will now have hypothyroidism because she no longer has a thyroid gland. If the replacement hormone dose is too high, she will have signs of hyperthyroidism (tachycardia, hypertension, increased sweating, and intolerance to heat, among others). If the replacement dose is too low, she will show signs of hypothyroidism (bradycardia, decreased blood pressure, decreased sweating, and intolerance to cold, among others).

3. b.   Take small, frequent meals. Nausea, vomiting, and GI distress may be minimized if the patient does not eat three large meals a day but eats small, frequent meals (such as six meals a day). Taking the drug on an empty stomach will aggravate the nausea and abdominal pain. Propylthiouracil must be taken in evenly spaced intervals throughout the 24-hour period. All daily doses cannot be taken in the evening. The patient should not be taken off the drug. The drug must be used for a prolonged period of time to induce the desired effect. Techniques to minimize adverse effects should be tried instead.

4. b.   Calcium. Calcitrol is designed to raise blood calcium levels. Calcium levels should be monitored to determine that they have reached normal but are not elevated above normal levels. Potassium, BUN (an indication of kidney function), and SGOT (an indication of liver function) levels are not directly related to drug therapy.

5. c.   Perform a skin test with calcitonin, salmon. Calcitonin, salmon carries the risk of allergic reaction to the salmon antigen in this calcitonin; therefore, a skin test with 0.1 mL of a 10-IU/mL solution is given SC. If no reaction is seen in 15 minutes, the drug may be given. Calcium levels are already elevated; you would not want to give more calcium. Vitamin D is needed for calcium absorption and is not needed here. Acute severe hypercalcemia needs to be treated as an emergency. Bone deformity, which might be seen in Paget disease, is not a critical assessment at this time.

CASE STUDY

Propylthioracil is given to treat hyperthyroidism in preparation for subtotal thyroidectomy. By decreasing the activity of the thyroid gland before surgery, there is less chance of a serious adverse effect from sudden changes in thyroid level. Propylthiouracil inhibits peripheral conversion of T_4 to T_3, but it does not have an effect on existing T_4 and T_3, which are stored or circulating. Thus, it takes 3 to 4 weeks to cause a depletion of T_4 levels.

CRITICAL THINKING CHALLENGE

1. An increased anticoagulant effect may have occurred from a drug interaction of propylthiouracil and warfarin as propylthiouracil has an anti-vitamin K effect.
2. Prothrombin (PT) levels should be checked to determine if the bleeding time is excessively lengthened.

Chapter 40

KEY TERMS

Fill in the blanks

1. mineralocorticoid
2. Addison's disease
3. gluconeogenesis
4. salt-losing adrenogenital syndrome
5. corticosteroid
6. hyperaldosteronism
7. glucocorticoid
8. circadian rhythms
9. Cushing's syndrome

PHYSIOLOGY AND PATHOPHYSIOLOGY: THE BODY HUMAN

Essay

1. epinephrine and norepinephrine
2. glucocorticoids and mineralocorticoids
3. regulation of potassium, sodium, and water balance
4. circulating cortisol levels, stress, circadian rhythms
5. suppression of HPA-axis resulting in adrenocortical atrophy and impaired glucocorticoid biosynthesis
6. aldosterone
7. cortisol and cortisone

CORE DRUG KNOWLEDGE: JUST THE FACTS

Multiple choice

1. b   2. b   3. c   4. d   5. b
6. d   7. b   8. a   9. c   10. b
11. a   12. c   13. b   14. c

CORE PATIENT VARIABLES: PATIENTS, PLEASE

Multiple choice

1. d   2. b   3. c   4. a   5. b
6. d   7. a   8. a   9. c   10. a
11. d   12. b

NURSING MANAGEMENT: EVERY GOOD NURSE SHOULD . . .

Multiple choice

1. b.   Administer the drug with milk or food. Prednisone is irritating to the GI tract and can cause peptic ulcer, which may hemorrhage or perforate. Milk or food given with the drug will decrease the gastric irritation from the prednisone. Proton pump inhibitors and H2 antagonists also are used to decrease the risk of ulcer development. Administering prednisone on an empty stomach would increase the risk of ulcer formation. Additional prednisone may be needed in times of physical stress, such as illness, injury, or surgery, to prevent adrenal crisis.

2. a.   Take the drug early in the morning. Intrinsic cortisol secretion is highest early in the morning. Taking prednisone at this time will stimulate this intrinsic cycling of cortisol levels and allow the body to use the drug in the most physiologic manner.

3. e.   None of the above. Hypokalemia, hypertension, and weight gain are signs of excessive fludrocortisone dosing.

4. d.   Wear or carry a Medic-Alert bracelet or card. Information as to whether the patient is taking corticosteroids is important if emergency care is needed. This information can also help emergency personnel in determining whether an adrenal crisis is occurring. Potassium intake should be increased somewhat and sodium intake decreased somewhat to offset the mineralocorticosteroid effects of the fludrocortisone. Drug therapy should not be stopped during illness; this may induce an adrenal crisis. Dosage may need to be increased during illness to meet the increased need for glucocorticoids.

5. d.   All of the above. Thyroid function may be decreased (hypothyroidism) during aminoglutethimide therapy. Blood pressure may drop due to suppression of aldosterone release secondary to aminoglutethimide use. Although used for hypercortisolism (excess production of corticosteroids by the adrenals), adrenal insufficiency may occur if the dose is too high or if the need for corticosteroids is increased due to stress or illness.

CASE STUDY

1. A glucocorticosteroid was ordered for its anti-inflammatory effect to counteract the inflammation of the respiratory tract, which occurs in chronic asthma.

2. Ms. Sommers needs to learn what the drug is for, how it will work, when she should take it, how much she should take as a dose, and possible adverse effects. She also needs to be instructed in how to use a metered-dose inhaler properly and the importance of rinsing her mouth after use of the inhaler to prevent oral candidiasis.

CRITICAL THINKING CHALLENGE

1. It appears that Ms. Sommers is experiencing adrenal crisis.

2. Some stressor placed on the body may have increased the need for glucocorticosteroids. Due to drug-induced suppression of the adrenals, she was not able to produce additional glucocorticosteroids on her own, and the dose from the prednisone was inadequate to meet her current, elevated needs. Alternately, she may have stopped taking the prednisone abruptly, and this precipitated the adrenal crisis. When the crisis is passed and Ms. Sommers is stabilized, she can be questioned about discontinuing the drug. Alternately, her family members may know this information now. Knowing about her limited income, be sure to explore whether financial reasons contributed to her stopping the drug, if she did indeed stop taking the drug suddenly.

Chapter 41

KEY TERMS

Crossword puzzle

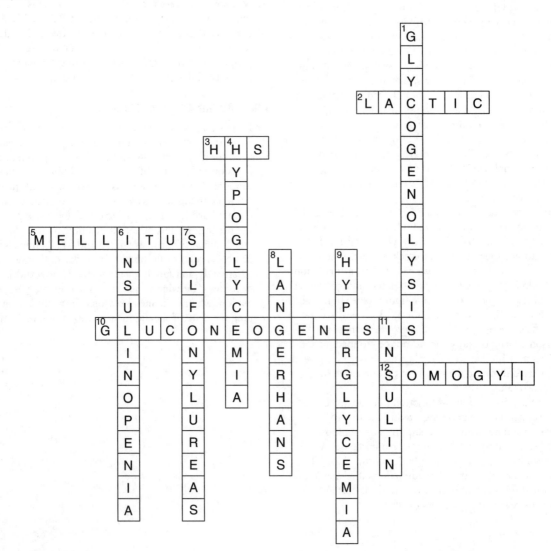

PHYSIOLOGY AND PATHOPHYSIOLOGY: THE BODY HUMAN

Essay

1. insulin and glucagon
2. beta cells: insulin
   alpha cells: glucagon
   delta cells: somatostatin
   F cells: pancreatic polypeptide used in digestion
3. promotes the uptake and storage of glucose in the form of glycogen; promotes the conversion of excess glucose into fat; suppresses the production of glucose and the breakdown of glycogen to glucose; promotes the uptake and metabolism of glucose in muscle cells
4. plasma glucose level
5. stress or illness; secretion of insulin-antagonistic hormones; the rate of gluconeogenesis or glycogenolysis, insulin antibodies; use of glucose by peripheral cells or tissues; and number of cellular insulin receptors.

CORE DRUG KNOWLEDGE: JUST THE FACTS

Multiple choice

1. b	2. b	3. a	4. a	5. c
6. b	7. c	8. d	9. b	10. c
11. d	12. d	13. a	14. c	15. b
16. a	17. b	18. d	19. c	

Matching

1. c	2. b	3. a	4. d	5. c
6. b	7. d	8. a	9. b	

Matching

1. b	2. d	3. e	4. a	5. a
6. d	7. a	8. e	9. c	10. c

CORE PATIENT VARIABLES: PATIENTS, PLEASE

Multiple choice

1. b   2. c   3. c   4. a   5. c

6. a   7. c   8. d   9. a   10. d

NURSING MANAGEMENT: EVERY GOOD NURSE SHOULD...

Decision tree

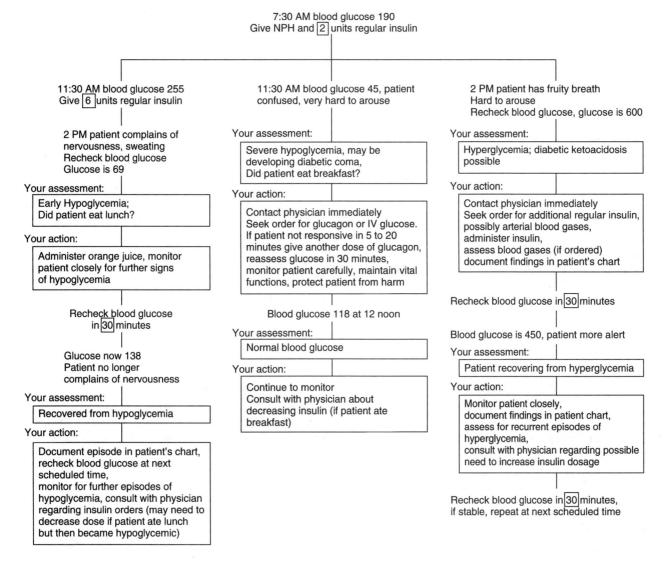

CASE STUDY

1. Ms. Parsons was not started on insulin initially because insulin is only used in patients with type 2 diabetes whose disease cannot be controlled with diet, weight loss, exercise, and oral antihyperglycemics.

2. Ms. Parsons was not started on glyburide, because it is chemically related to sulfa antibiotics, to which she is allergic.

3. Teach Ms. Parsons what metformin is, how it works, the proper dose, when to take the drug, and its adverse effects. Teaching for Ms. Parsons should also include information about diabetes, diet instruction, and the importance of weight control and exercise.

CRITICAL THINKING CHALLENGE

You would expect to see that Ms. Parsons is started on regular insulin, most likely on a sliding-scale basis. The insulin may be in addition to the metformin or in place of it. Elevated blood glucose levels occur with physical stress such as infection or illness. Insulin needs are therefore greatly increased. Administration of regular insulin will help control the elevated glucose. Sliding-scale administration of insulin is aimed at controlling blood glucose on an as-needed basis to prevent hypoglycemia from occurring from too much insulin or the combination of insulin and metformin. As the infection is controlled and blood sugar returns to normal, the sliding-scale insulin will be stopped.

Chapter 42

KEY TERMS

True/false

1. False androgens
2. False follicle-stimulating hormone (FSH) and luteinizing hormone (LH).
3. False erectile dysfunction
4. False benign prostatic hypertrophy
5. True

PHYSIOLOGY AND PATHOPHYSIOLOGY: THE BODY HUMAN

Essay

1. Testosterone
2. Retention of sodium, potassium and phosphorus; decreases urinary excretion of calcium; stimulates skeletal muscle tissue; enhances growth of long bone in prepubescence; ossification process of the epiphyseal growth plates; stimulates production of RBCs
3. The parasympathetic system innervates the penile arteries. Normal erection involves the release of nitric oxide, secondary to sexual stimulation, in the erectile tissue of the penis. The nitric oxide activates an intermediary enzyme that boosts cyclic guanosine monophosphate (cGMP), a substance that mediates the action of certain hormones. By some unknown mechanism, cGMP stimulates smooth muscle, producing relaxation and an inflow of blood into the erectile tissue.

CORE DRUG KNOWLEDGE: JUST THE FACTS

Multiple choice

1. b 2. d 3. c 4. b 5. a
6. a 7. c 8. d 9. d 10. c
11. d 12. d

CORE PATIENT VARIABLES: PATIENTS, PLEASE

Multiple choice

1. a 2. d 3. c 4. b 5. a
6. c 7. a 8. c 9. b 10. c

NURSING MANAGEMENT: EVERY GOOD NURSE SHOULD . . .

Multiple choice

1. b. Verify that x-rays are taken every 6 months. X-ray films will help to document the long bone maturation and the effect of testosterone on the epiphyseal centers. Early closure of the epiphysis is to be avoided. Testosterone (short acting) is never administered IV but always by the IM route into a deep gluteal muscle. BUN and creatinine are not affected by testosterone (short acting). Liver function tests, however, should be monitored.
2. c. Testoderm TTS is applied to arm, back or upper buttocks, unlike some other testosterone products applied to the scrotum. It should be applied to dry skin that is NOT irritated or damaged. It is left on the skin and changed every 24 hours. The adhesive on the patch should keep the patch in place if the system is firmly pressed into place with the palm of the hand for about 10 seconds.
3. d. All of the above. Sexual activity places additional stress on the heart. Information on the signs of cardiac problems such as angina or MI is important to teach, especially to patients who have risk factors for cardiovascular disease. Frank has two risk factors: family history and elevated cholesterol levels.
4. c. A woman in childbearing years should not handle crushed or broken finasteride pills because the risk for absorption through the skin is greatest then. Finasteride is a pregnancy category X drug. If Robert has difficulty swallowing pills, forcing him to swallow all medication may lead to choking. Patients should not be forced to do anything. Finasteride must be administered orally; it cannot be administered by way of the urethra. Administering the drug just before urination has no relevancy to drug efficacy.
5. b. Fine, soft colorless hair may grow first; this will later be replaced by hair of the same color and texture as on the rest of the head. Minoxidil is available topically over the counter; no prescription is required. Topical minoxidil has no effect on blood pressure. Oral minoxidil will decrease, not raise, blood pressure. Hair growth is not seen until minoxidil has been applied topically twice a day for at least 4 months.

CASE STUDY

Electrolyte values should be monitored, especially sodium, calcium, potassium, chloride, and phosphates, as these can be elevated from testosterone administration. Blood cholesterol levels should also be assessed as increases in cholesterol levels are also possible, and this is especially problematic for Eduardo due to his history of coronary artery disease.

CRITICAL THINKING CHALLENGE

Eduardo may have developed edema, and possibly CHF, from testosterone's effect on fluid levels. (Increased sodium retention leads to increased water retention also.) His diabetes may have narrowed vessels to his kidneys as well as his heart, placing him at increased risk of developing edema secondary to testosterone use.

Chapter 43

KEY TERMS

True/false

1. False estrogens
2. False progestin
3. False gonadotropin-releasing hormone (GRH); follicle-stimulating hormone (FSH), and luteinizing hormone (LH)
4. True
5. False osteoporosis
6. False secretory phase
7. False proliferative phase
8. True
9. False Paget disease

PHYSIOLOGY AND PATHOPHYSIOLOGY: THE BODY HUMAN

Essay

1. estrogen and progestin
2. estradiol
3. Affect release of pituitary gonadotropins; cause capillary dilation; promote fluid retention; enhance protein anabolism; thin cervical mucus; inhibit or facilitate ovulation; prevent postpartum breast pain; strengthen the skeleton by conserving calcium and phosphorus; encourage bone formation; maintain tone and elasticity of urogenital structures; promote growth during the adolescent growth spurt; stimulate closure of epiphyseal growth plates of long bones
4. Hypothalamus secretes gonadotropin-releasing hormone → release of FSH and LH → stimulate development of ovarian follicles → release of the ovum from mature follicle → production of estrogen → increases the vascularity of uterine lining → stimulation of GRH → more LH → rupture of mature follicle and ovulation occurs. After ovulation, follicle becomes corpus luteum → produces progesterone and estrogen → prepares uterine lining for implantation → if none occurs, corpus luteum disintegrates → estrogen and progestin levels decrease → menses

CORE DRUG KNOWLEDGE: JUST THE FACTS

Multiple choice

1. b	2. c	3. a	4. d	5. b
6. a	7. b	8. b	9. d	10. c
11. a	12. a	13. d	14. c	15. d

CORE PATIENT VARIABLES: PATIENTS, PLEASE

Multiple choice

1. c	2. b	3. c	4. c	5. b
6. d	7. b	8. a	9. c	10. c

NURSING MANAGEMENT: EVERY GOOD NURSE SHOULD . . .

Multiple choice

1. d. All of the above. Estrogen is used as hormone replacement with primary ovarian failure, loss of ovaries due to surgery, and to manage the discomforts of menopause.
2. a. Take the drug for 3 weeks, then stay off the drug for 1 week. This cyclic approach to drug therapy will mimic the natural cycling of estrogen. Photosensitivity may result from estrogen replacement; patients should avoid prolonged sun exposure. X-rays are taken when estrogen is given for hypogonadism before the adolescent growth spurt; they are not needed when estrogen is used after the final growth spurt has occurred. Sudden, severe headaches are signs of serious adverse effects. If they occur, they need to be reported to the physician at once.
3. d. Do all of the above. Progesterone is avoided in patients with thrombophlebitis because this is an adverse effect of the drug. If thrombophlebitis occurs during drug therapy, the progesterone should be discontinued. Progesterone is avoided in the first 4 months of pregnancy because it is a pregnancy Category D drug. For appropriate blood levels to be obtained, progesterone needs to be administered on a regular basis for 6 to 8 days.
4. e. None of the above. Levonorgestrel implants prevent pregnancy for up to 5 years. Intrauterine progesterone inserts may have serious adverse effects, including septic abortion or congenital anomalies (if pregnancy occurs), pelvic inflammatory disease, and perforation of the uterine wall or cervix. Oral contraceptives should be avoided in women over 35 who smoke because these women have the highest risk for serious cardiovascular adverse effects.
5. d. All of the above are necessary. Because mifepristone may cause serious harm, the patient must be aware of the potential complications and her role in reducing complications. This is the purpose of the Medication Guide. Two follow-up visits are necessary to confirm that pregnancy was completely terminated. If bleeding hasn't started by Day 3 (the first visit), the patient will be given a different drug, misoprostol, which induces uterine contractions. Day 1 is the day that the mifepristone tablets are taken. Because this drug is not distributed to pharmacies, but only to approved prescribers, the drug is taken in the prescriber's office in his or her presence.

CASE STUDY

Lorinda may resume birth control even though she has not yet had a menstrual period. She may resume the Ortho-Novum 7/7/7 as birth control if she wishes. She should begin the oral contraceptives after she stops breast-feeding.

CRITICAL THINKING CHALLENGE

Tell me about how you take this oral contraceptive. Everyday? At a certain time? Did you miss any days? How many days in a cycle did you miss? What did you do when you missed a day?

Although pregnancy is possible with the correct use of oral birth control pills, pregnancy is normally prevented with correct use. Therefore, it is likely that Lorinda has not been taking the drug as prescribed or that she has not used appropriate measures if she misses a pill.

Chapter 44

KEY TERMS

Anagrams

1. antepartum
2. tocolytics
3. postpartum
4. uterine tetany
5. oxytocics
6. intrapartum

PHYSIOLOGY AND PATHOPHYSIOLOGY: THE BODY HUMAN

Essay

1. weeks 38 to 42
2. vascular constriction, and increased water reabsorption from the glomerular filtrate
3. oxytocin, cAMP, calcium, and prostaglandins
4. fluctuations of cardiac output, heart rate, and blood pressure
5. hyperventilation with resultant respiratory alkalosis; muscular contraction induces metabolic acidosis uncompensated by respiratory alkalosis
6. leukocytosis
7. concentrated urine with a trace of protein
8. cessation of gastric motility and increase in gastric acidity

CORE DRUG KNOWLEDGE: JUST THE FACTS

Multiple choice

1. c   2. a   3. b   4. c   5. c
6. d   7. c   8. a   9. c   10. d

CORE PATIENT VARIABLES: PATIENTS, PLEASE

Multiple choice

1. b   2. d   3. c   4. b   5. c
6. d   7. b   8. a   9. c

NURSING MANAGEMENT: EVERY GOOD NURSE SHOULD . . .

Multiple choice

1. c.   Assess that cervical ripening is favorable through Bishop's scoring. A Bishop's score of 5 or better should be present before beginning induction. Otherwise, the cervix needs to be primed with prostaglandin E_2 gel. Contraindication to vaginal delivery, significant cephalopelvic disproportion, and fetal distress when delivery is not imminent are all contraindications to the use of oxytocin.
2. a.   5% dextrose in lactated Ringer's. A solution of 0.9% sodium chloride could also be used. Solutions of 20% glucose in water are hypertonic and would not be used. Solutions of 0.2% sodium chloride are hypotonic and would not be used. Oxytocin is never given IV undiluted.
3. c.   Shut off the oxytocin. Contractions occurring more frequently than every 2 minutes, lasting longer than 90 seconds, or having resting tone greater than 15 mmHg pressure indicate a hypercontractile labor pattern from the oxytocin. Additional oxytocin is contraindicated. Increased IV mainline fluids are indicated.
4. d.   5% dextrose and water. Because of the risk of pulmonary edema, solutions with saline are not used.
5. a.   Use an IV pump. This will regulate the rate to prevent overdosage. Patients should be positioned on their left side to prevent hypotension and to promote circulation to the fetus. High fluid intake is contraindicated due to risk of pulmonary edema.

CASE STUDY

1. Yes, these are appropriate orders. Oxytocin is indicated to augment labor that is not progressing as long as cervical ripening, as measured by 5 or more on the Bishop's scale, is present. Oxytocin should be started at 0.5 to 1 mU/minute and then increased by this amount every 30 to 60 minutes. This dosing pattern allows the drug to reach steady state, and full therapeutic effect to occur, before the dose is increased. It also mimics the natural release of oxytocin.
2. The nurse should dilute the oxytocin in 0.9% normal saline or 5% dextrose in lactated Ringer's solution. The drug should be piggybacked onto mainline fluids, and a pump or controller should regulate the infusion of the oxytocin. The nurse should monitor the patient and fetus carefully throughout drug infusion. Assess maternal vital signs, fetal heart rate, contractile rate, and fetal movement. These must be checked before increasing the infusion rate. If hypertension or other significant maternal vital sign changes occur, fetal heart rate decreases, or fetal movement stops, the nurse must notify the physician or nurse midwife immediately. If a hypercontractile pattern occurs, the oxytocin infusion should be stopped and the health care provider notified. The nurse should also assess intake and output and encourage the patient to urinate every 2 hours.

CRITICAL THINKING CHALLENGE

1. The oxytocin has been effective, and Jenny has progressed through labor. She is ready to deliver and has the urge to push.
2. The nurse should have the physician or nurse midwife present, prepare for delivery of the baby, and coach or assist Jenny with pushing effectively to deliver the baby.

Chapter 45

KEY TERMS

Crossword puzzle

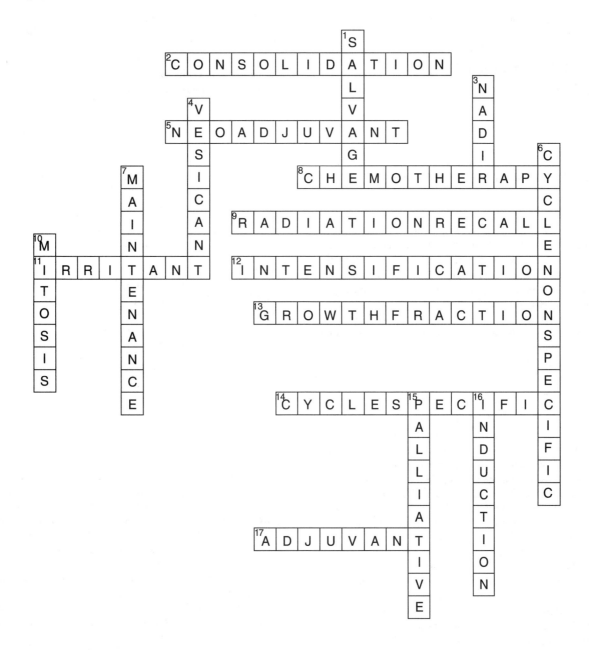

PHYSIOLOGY AND PATHOPHYSIOLOGY: THE BODY HUMAN

Multiple choice

1. d   2. b   3. e   4. c   5. a

Essay

1. prophase, metaphase, anaphase, and telophase
2. actual division of the cytoplasm into new daughter cells
3. the length of time needed to complete the cell cycle
4. uncontrolled cell proliferation; decreased cellular differentiation; inappropriate ability to invade surrounding tissue; ability to establish new growth at ectopic sites
5. The number of tumor cells killed by an antineoplastic drug is proportional to the dose used.

CORE DRUG KNOWLEDGE: JUST THE FACTS

Multiple choice

1. d   2. d   3. b   4. c   5. c
6. b   7. a   8. b   9. d   10. b
11. d   12. a   13. a   14. a   15. d
16. b   17. c   18. d

CORE PATIENT VARIABLES: PATIENTS, PLEASE

Multiple choice

1. c   2. b   3. a   4. b   5. c
6. a   7. b   8. d   9. c   10. c
11. d   12. c

NURSING MANAGEMENT: EVERY GOOD NURSE SHOULD . . .

Multiple choice

1. c.   Eat more gelatin and pudding. Soft, cool, bland foods such as these will be less irritating. Hot beverages are usually too irritating. Commercial mouthwash is too astringent and will irritate mouth sores. Aspirin should be avoided because it may promote bleeding as the platelet count is decreased from the 5-FU.

2. d.   Report immediately if IV site is burning or looks red. This is a sign of infiltration and extravasation. An antidote is needed immediately to prevent serious tissue damage. Hair should be brushed carefully because hair and skin become weak from the drug therapy, although this doesn't occur until 2 or 3 weeks after treatment. Patients need a high-fiber diet with plenty of fluids to prevent constipation. Heart rate is not significantly affected by vincristine.

3. a.   Turn off the infusion. It appears that the IV line has infiltrated and that the vincristine has extravasated. Shutting off the infusion will minimize the amount of drug that enters the tissues and the damage that may occur. Hyaluronidase is the antidote for vincristine extravasation, not isotonic sodium thiosulfate. Warm compresses should be used to the extravasation site after vincristine extravasation.

4. b.   Administer the drug slowly over at least 30 to 60 minutes. Hypersensitivity reactions to etoposide are related to infusing the drug too rapidly. The drug is administered by IV infusion, not IV push, which would be an extremely concentrated and rapid delivery rate. The nurse should stay with the patient during the infusion due to the severe consequences of hypersensitivity reaction. It is not appropriate to leave the patient alone or to expect family members to be responsible for the patient.

5. b.   Yes, hair loss may occur and may be severe. Support the patient emotionally on this issue and discuss the use of wigs, hats, and scarves to cover her head during the period of alopecia. Hair loss may be severe and include eyebrows, eyelashes, axillary hair, and pubic hair. Although myelosuppression, neurotoxicity, and hypersensitivity reactions pose more significant risks to the patient's physical health, hair loss is what concerns the patient, and the nurse should not minimize the patient's feelings.

6. d.   Do all of the above. CBC should be checked for presence of anemia, leukopenia, and low platelet counts. Drug therapy should begin before radiation therapy, but then may continue throughout therapy. BUN and creatinine levels may increase due to deterioration of renal function secondary to drug therapy.

7. c.   To prevent accidental skin exposure to a hazardous drug, you should use a sterile gauze pad around the connecting site connect when disconnecting IV tubing. Also use a gauze over the tip of the syringe when purging air from a chemotherapy-filled syringe, when opening chemotherapy vials and ampules, when removing syringes from IV lines after IV push administration, and, finally, when removing empty chemotherapy bags or bottles from IV spikes. IV tubings should be purged with normal saline, not the antineoplastic drug. All chemotherapy waste should be disposed of in an impervious, leakproof container, not open trash cans. Avoid all eating, drinking, smoking, chewing gum, and applying makeup when preparing hazardous drugs. You should wash your hands before and after working with antineoplastic drugs.

CASE STUDY

1. 5-Fluorouracil (5-FU) interferes with the synthesis of DNA and RNA. It is clinically effective in treating solid tumors, including colorectal cancers. Levamisole is a T/B cell modulator that restores depressed immune function, stimulates antibody formation, enhances T cell response, and potentiates monocyte and macrophage activity. Levamisole is adjunct therapy in the treatment of colorectal cancers. Because it stimulates the immune function of the body, it is helpful in preventing adverse effects from the antineoplastic drug 5-FU.

2. Mr. Meyers' CBC count needs to be monitored before, during, and after therapy. 5-FU should not be given if the WBC is less than $3500/mm^3$ because this indicates leukopenia. Bone marrow depression from levamisole is rare but potentially serious. Also monitor for nausea, vomiting, stomatitis, and diarrhea because these can be adverse effects from both drugs. GI ulceration and hemorrhage can occur from 5-FU use. Headache can be an adverse effect from either drug therapy. However, if from levamisole, other CNS effects of dizziness, depression, and paresthesia may also be present. If the headache is related to 5-FU use, it indicates the development of acute cerebellar syndrome. This syndrome would also have disorientation and nystagmus as symptoms; photophobia and ocular changes may also be present.

CRITICAL THINKING CHALLENGE

1. Dark, tar-colored stools are a sign of old GI bleeding. GI bleeding is a serious complication of 5-FU therapy. Report these findings to the physician at once. Consult with physician regarding decreasing dose of 5-FU. Assess for bright red bleeding, which would indicate active bleeding. Assess patient's hematocrit and hemoglobin for information regarding severity of bleeding. Monitor patient closely.

Chapter 46

KEY TERMS

Fill in the blanks

1. radiomimetic
2. hormones and antihormones
3. combination therapy
4. alkylator
5. nitrosureas
6. antitumor antibiotics
7. disease flare
8. cell cycle-nonspecific
9. anthracycline
10. acute emesis
11. delayed emesis
12. tumor burden
13. emetogenic

CORE DRUG KNOWLEDGE: JUST THE FACTS

Multiple choice

1. d   2. d   3. a   4. c   5. b
6. b   7. b   8. d   9. d   10. a
11. b   12. d   13. c   14. a

CORE PATIENT VARIABLES: PATIENTS, PLEASE

Multiple choice

1. b   2. c   3. a   4. b   5. d
6. c   7. c   8. b   9. a   10. a

NURSING MANAGEMENT: EVERY GOOD NURSE SHOULD . . .

Multiple choice

1. b.   Prehydrate with 1 to 2 L of normal saline with potassium and magnesium. Prehydration is important to flush the kidneys well during and after therapy to minimize renal toxicities. Oral prehydration may also be used. Diuretic drugs cause dehydration and would not be appropriate. Limiting potassium and magnesium is not relevant. Aminoglycoside antibiotics also cause nephrotoxicity like cyclophosphamide, and should be avoided due to additive effects.
2. d.   All of the above are possible adverse effects and should be included in patient education.
3. c.   Monitor for rales and dyspnea. These are signs of congestive heart failure. As doxorubicin is a vesicant, a large vein should be used. Aspirin should be avoided, as it may induce bleeding when platelet counts are low. Reddish-colored urine is a normal effect from doxorubicin and is not an adverse effect.
4. c.   Administer the next dose of tamoxifen as ordered. Bone pain and pain at the site of the tumor are signs of disease flare, which occurs with tamoxifen therapy. They are actually signs of tumor response to the drug. Although the physician should be aware of disease flare, there is no need to contact him or her immediately, as a problem does not exist.
5. c.   Platelets. Thrombocytopenia can occur at 6 weeks after carmustine treatment. Adequate platelet function needs to be determined before administering another dose of carmustine. Weight, blood pressure, and BUN are not critical measurements that must be assessed before a dose of carmustine can be given.

6. a.   As doxorubicin is a vesicant, it is important to prevent extravasation. Verifying that the IV is patent and running well is one important step in this process. Although ice might be applied after an extravasation has occurred, it is not done before drug administration. Use of a tourniquet would likely cause extravasation as it would impede circulation. Massaging the vein is not helpful or indicated.

CASE STUDY

1. Although both doxorubicin and cyclophosphamide are cell cycle-nonspecific drugs, using two drugs, or combination therapy, has advantages. Combination therapy maximizes cell kill, has a broader range of kill, and minimizes emergence of cancer cells resistant to chemotherapy. Dosage of each drug can be kept to a minimum, thus decreasing serious toxicities from each drug.
2. Selma may have nausea and vomiting, an adverse effect from doxorubicin, and the same may also occur with cyclophosphamide. Abnormal blood cell levels are also possible as cyclophosphamide causes leukopenia and doxorubicin causes bone marrow depression. Cardiotoxicity is a significant risk as both drugs cause this adverse effect. Alopecia also may occur with either drug. Hemorrhagic cystitis, syndrome of inappropriate antidiuretic hormone, hypersensitivity, reproductive effects, cutaneous problems, mucositis, extravasation injury, and radiation recall are all possible, although the risk is minimized due to combination drug therapy that minimizes the dose of each drug used.

CRITICAL THINKING CHALLENGE

1. The combined chemotherapy has been effective so far, and there are no adverse effects from the drug therapy as of today. All blood work is within normal ranges, and the ECG is normal.
2. Yes, you should administer the next prescribed doses of cyclophosphamide and doxorubicin.

Chapter 48

KEY TERMS

Matching

1. a   2. d   3. f   4. e   5. b
6. c

CORE DRUG KNOWLEDGE: JUST THE FACTS

Multiple choice

1. c   2. a   3. b   4. b   5. d
6. b   7. a   8. c   9. c   10. b
11. d   12. b   13. a   14. d   15. c
16. b

CORE PATIENT VARIABLES: PATIENTS, PLEASE

Multiple choice

1. d	2. b	3. a	4. b	5. d
6. d	7. b	8. c	9. c	10. d
11. b	12. a			

NURSING MANAGEMENT: EVERY GOOD NURSE SHOULD . . .

Multiple choice

1. d.   Administer the drug for at least 2 days after patient feels better. This helps to ensure that all of the organisms have been killed, so that a reinfection does not occur. Administer oral penicillin G on an empty stomach. Doses should be evenly spaced throughout the 24-hour period. Take IV forms of penicillin G out of the refrigerator for 15 minutes before administering.

2. d.   All of the above. Alcoholic beverages and products containing alcohol should be avoided because a disulfiramlike reaction (or alcohol intolerance) may occur, making the patient feel quite ill. Elixirs always have alcohol in them, and over-the-counter cough medicines frequently have alcohol in them.

3. b.   Slow IV infusion. Vancomycin should be administered over at least 60 minutes to decrease risk of ototoxicity and red-man syndrome. IV push would be too concentrated and too fast, and would produce adverse effects. Vancomycin is extremely irritating to the tissues and should never be given SC. Poor absorption occurs from the oral route; this route is seldom used and is not appropriate for serious infections outside of the GI tract.

4. d.   Do all of the above. Before beginning antibiotic therapy, a culture and sensitivity should be obtained, if at all possible, to determine the exact organism present and which drug therapy will be effective in eradicating the organism. A sputum culture would be appropriate for pneumonia. It is important to always verify with patients that they are not allergic to a medication when you administer the first dose. This is especially true with penicillins as anaphylactic reactions are possible drug allergy responses. Because of possible drug allergies, observe the patient closely during the first 30 minutes of drug administration for signs of adverse effects.

5. c.   Procaine penicillin is administered by IM injection. Like all penicillins, it is important to identify an injection site accurately to prevent accidental administration into a vein or nerve. Procaine penicillin, like all penicillins, should be administered deep into a large muscle. The deltoid is too small to be appropriate. As procaine penicillin is thick and viscous, it is administered more easily if it is removed from the refrigerator about 15 minutes before administration.

6. c.   BUN (blood urea nitrogen) is a measurement of kidney function. Nephrotoxicity is more likely to occur when the patient takes more than one drug that may cause nephrotoxicity, in this case, cefazolin and gentamicin. The nurse should also monitor creatinine levels to assess renal function. Hematocrit is not affected by cefazolin therapy. Blood coagulation time, aPTT (active partial thromboplastin time) is only altered if the patient is receiving oral anticoagulants, such as warfarin, and cefazolin. Cefazolin is not a drug that the blood levels indicate a therapeutic or toxic level, and cefazolin levels are not measured. Gentamicin levels are, however, monitored.

CASE STUDY

1. It appears that Ms. Maraglia is demonstrating signs of ototoxicity from the vancomycin. Her fall and the comment about being tipsy indicate ataxia, or possibly vertigo. The cricket sound may be the onset of tinnitus.

2. The nurse should check the peak and trough levels of the drug. If they have not been done recently, and order should be sought for one, and the physician should be informed of these adverse events.

CRITICAL THINKING CHALLENGE

1. The peak and trough are both higher than the normal therapeutic range and support your assessment that ototoxicity is occurring. The trough should be below 10 µg/mL, and the peak should be below 60 µg/mL.

2. Contact the physician regarding these results; consult with the physician regarding decreasing dose or discontinuing drug. An audiogram may also be indicated.

Chapter 49

KEY TERMS

Matching

1. f	2. d	3. h	4. b	5. i
6. c	7. j	8. a	9. e	10. g

CORE DRUG KNOWLEDGE: JUST THE FACTS

Multiple choice

1. b	2. d	3. a	4. a	5. c
6. c	7. b	8. b	9. d	10. a
11. c	12. b	13. c	14. d	15. c
16. a	17. a	18. b	19. d	20. c
21. a	22. d			

CORE PATIENT VARIABLES: PATIENTS, PLEASE

Multiple choice

1. b	2. a	3. a	4. c	5. d
6. c	7. a	8. c	9. d	10. c
11. a	12. b	13. a	14. c	15. a

NURSING MANAGEMENT: EVERY GOOD NURSE SHOULD ...

Multiple choice

1. d.   Do all of the above. Gentamicin has adverse effects of nephrotoxicity and ototoxicity. Output will decrease with nephrotoxicity. Tinnitus demonstrates damage to the cochlear branch of the 8th cranial nerve. Loss of balance demonstrates damage to the vestibular branch of the 8th cranial nerve.

2. c.   Slow down the rate of the infusion. Burning and irritation to the vein are common with erythromycin administration. Slowing the rate will help to minimize the discomfort. Iced compresses may be used if pain persists. Burning is not a sign of drug allergy with erythromycin. Unless the IV is infiltrated or not patent, it should not be removed due to the burning sensation.

3. b.   Obtain order for laboratory examination of the stool specimen. Anna may be experiencing pseudomembranous colitis, a serious adverse effect of clindamycin. The stool should be examined for WBCs, mucus, and blood. Antidiarrheals may treat the symptom; however, if pseudomembranous colitis is present, antidiarrheals may mistakenly lead the nurse and doctor to believe that the diarrhea is not serious, thus delaying needed diagnosis and treatment of the disorder. A high-roughage diet will further irritate the inflamed bowel and is not appropriate.

4. d.   Keep this drug secured and out of reach of children. Tetracycline causes mottling and discoloration of teeth in children. Tetracycline should be taken with water, not milk, as milk chelates with tetracycline, preventing absorption. Tetracycline, like all antibiotics, should be taken for the full course of therapy to prevent recurrence of the infection. Tetracycline causes photosensitivity, placing the patient at increased risk for sunburn. Patients should avoid direct sun exposure.

5. d.   All of the above. Bruising and fatigue are signs of anemia and bone marrow depression. Elevated hepatic enzymes are signs of liver damage. These are all serious adverse effects of chloramphenicol.

6. b.   Quinupristin/dalfopristin must be flushed with D_5W as it is incompatible with both normal saline and heparin. Quinupristin/dalfopristin can only be administered IV. It is preferable that quinupristin/dalfopristin be administered either through a PICC line (peripherally inserted central catheter) or a central line. Although diazepam will have a drug interaction with quinupristin/dalfopristin due to P450 inhibition, and diazepam levels will rise, drugs that are needed for seizure control cannot be easily discontinued. Administer the drug, but monitor the patient for signs of adverse effects from the diazepam. It is possible that a lower dose of diazepam will need to be ordered.

7. a.   Blue cheese is an aged cheese that is high in tyramine. As linezolid is a nonselective MAO inhibitor, a hypertensive crisis can occur if foods with high tyramine content are eaten. Strawberries, graham crackers, and carrots do not have high tyramine levels. (Hint: Need help? See Chapter 18 for a discussion of MAO inhibitors used as antidepressants.)

CASE STUDY

1. *Health status:* Mr. Pearson's diabetes may have contributed to his renal dysfunction. The renal impairment puts him more at risk of developing nephrotoxicity from the gentamicin. Additionally, diabetes impairs circulation throughout the body, and blood supply to the infection may be hindered, making it more difficult to treat the infection.

2. Trough levels are ordered to determine whether therapeutic levels are maintained by the dosing schedule. Peak levels are ordered to determine whether blood levels are too high, placing the patient at risk for adverse effects. Pharmacists frequently monitor these blood reports, as they have the most knowledge of pharmacokinetics and pharmacodynamics of drugs such as gentamicin. The nurse should see that the trough is drawn 30 minutes before the next dose. It is important to administer the drug on time after the trough has been drawn. The peak should be drawn 30 to 45 minutes after the infusion is completed. Monitor the infusion carefully and note the exact time the infusion is complete.

CRITICAL THINKING CHALLENGE

1. It is important to give the antibiotics on time and to document the exact time of each dose. This information will be needed for accurate laboratory interpretation of the peak and trough levels.

2. Additionally, as Mr. Pearson's wound is infected with bacteria that are resistant to many antibiotics, it is important to place him on wound and skin isolation and to wash your hands thoroughly after providing care to him to prevent the spread of these difficult-to-treat bacteria.

Chapter 50

KEY TERMS

Fill in the blanks

1. fluoroquinolone
2. postantibiotic effect
3. arthropathy

CORE DRUG KNOWLEDGE: JUST THE FACTS

Multiple choice

1. b   2. d   3. c   4. a

5. a   6. b   7. a   8. d

CORE PATIENT VARIABLES: PATIENTS, PLEASE

Multiple choice

1. c   2. a   3. b   4. d   5. c

NURSING MANAGEMENT: EVERY GOOD NURSE SHOULD . . .

Multiple choice

1. a.   Ciprofloxacin may cause photosensitivity. Sunscreen will help prevent serious burns if the patient must be outdoors. Fluid intake should be increased to help offset complications from GI effects. Small meals will minimize GI upset. A dose may be taken late if it is forgotten, but a double dose should not be taken.
2. b.   Ciprofloxacin inhibits the hepatic metabolism of theophylline and may result in elevated theophylline levels. Tachycardia and insomnia are adverse effects of theophylline. New onset of these problems may indicate theophylline toxicity. Insomnia may also be an adverse effect of ciprofloxacin. The patient has a severe infection plus has respiratory compromise; exercise is most likely not desirable at this time and may not be tolerated well. Ciprofloxacin may cause photosensitivity so the patient should not be exposed to excessive sunlight. Both theophylline and ciprofloxacin need to be administered regularly throughout the day for optimum effectiveness.
3. d.   GI distress is a frequent adverse effect of ciprofloxacin. Eating small, frequent meals may help to manage these effects. Nausea and abdominal pain are not signs of drug allergies. Dairy products, such as yogurt, contain a large amount of calcium, and impair the absorption of ciprofloxacin. Avoid taking these at the same time.

CASE STUDY

Teach her to take the drug on an empty stomach every 12 hours. Teach her what the drug is for, and possible adverse effects. Instruct her what to do if she has possible adverse effects. Verify that she is not pregnant before starting the drug therapy. If she uses oral contraceptives, teach her to also use a backup method of contraception while on ciprofloxacin. Teach the importance of taking the full prescription, and not to stop if she feels better.

CRITICAL THINKING CHALLENGE

Ask when she takes her medicine in relationship to eating. Is she taking it on an empty stomach as she should? Does she take it on an empty stomach but then immediately eats so that the drug is not broken down or absorbed before food is placed in the stomach? This would also decrease the absorption of the ciprofloxacin. Does she take dairy products near the time of her medicine? Does she use antacids? Does she take a vitamin supplement at the same time that she takes her ciprofloxacin? All of these things may decrease the absorption of the ciprofloxacin.

Chapter 51

KEY TERMS

Anagrams

1. reinfection
2. cystitis
3. urethritis
4. pyelonephritis
5. relapse
6. recurrent
7. prostatitis
8. crystalluria
9. sulfonamides
10. PABA

PHYSIOLOGY AND PATHOPHYSIOLOGY: THE BODY HUMAN

Essay

1. kidney, ureter, bladder, and urethra
2. mucin layer of the urinary bladder; washout phenomenon; immunoglobulin A; phagocytic blood cells
3. Most UTIs occur because of ascending bacteria from the outside of the body up through the urethra. Protective mechanisms of the body have more ability to abate the ascension of bacteria due to the length of the urethra in men.

CORE DRUG KNOWLEDGE: JUST THE FACTS

Multiple choice

1. c   2. b   3. d   4. a   5. a
6. c   7. a   8. c   9. a   10. b

CORE PATIENT VARIABLES: PATIENTS, PLEASE

Multiple choice

1. c   2. a   3. c   4. d
5. b   6. a   7. c   8. a

NURSING MANAGEMENT: EVERY GOOD NURSE SHOULD . . .

Multiple choice

1. d.   All of the above are correct. Although this drug is normally recommended to be taken on an empty stomach, GI upset is common, and patients may need to take the drug with food to minimize this discomfort. Extra water should be encouraged to dilute the urine and decrease the risk of crystalluria and bacterial multiplication. Sulfamethoxazole-trimethoprim causes photosensitivity, and patients need to protect themselves from ultraviolet light.
2. a.   A CBC should be monitored because blood dyscrasias are possible from SMZ-TMP. These adverse effects are more likely to occur if the patient has a folate deficiency or is immunocompromised. As an older adult, Ms. Coombs is more likely to be both immunocompromised and folate deficient. None of the other factors are adverse effects related to sulfamethoxazole-trimethoprim use.
3. d.   Do all of the above. Patients who are immunocompromised, such as patients with AIDS, are more at risk of adverse effects, and long-term therapy also places the patient more at risk of crystalluria. Assessing intake and output provides some knowledge as to how well the kidney is functioning. Acidic acid increases the risk of crystalluria. Presence of crystals would indicate the formation of crystalluria.
4. e.   None of the above. SMZ-TMP should be infused slowly over 60 to 90 minutes. It is never given rapidly, as a bolus, or as an IM injection. All lines should be flushed to remove residual drug. Once reconstituted in preparation for IV infusion it should not be refrigerated.

CASE STUDY

An allergic reaction has occurred. Pruritus (itching) and maculopapular rashes (reddened areas with some raised spots) are types of cutaneous allergic reactions to SMZ-TMP.

CRITICAL THINKING CHALLENGE

The nurse failed to consider that an allergy to hydrochlorothiazide may produce cross allergies to SMZ-TMP. This is because hydrochlorothiazide, like all thiazides, has a chemical structure that is similar to sulfa. This similarity in chemical structure allows for cross allergies.

Chapter 52

KEY TERMS

True/false

1. True
2. False   *M tuberculosis*
3. False   Ghon complex
4. False   chemoprophylaxis
5. True
6. False   *M avium*
7. False   leprosy
8. False   *Mycobacterium avium* complex
9. False   *M leprae*

CORE DRUG KNOWLEDGE: JUST THE FACTS

Multiple choice

1. c   2. b   3. d   4. c   5. b

6. a   7. c   8. c   9. b   10. c

11. c   12. a

CORE PATIENT VARIABLES: PATIENTS, PLEASE

Multiple choice

1. c   2. a   3. b   4. d   5. a

6. b   7. c   8. c

NURSING MANAGEMENT: EVERY GOOD NURSE SHOULD . . .

Multiple choice

1. d.   Explain the rationale for triple-drug therapy. Triple-drug therapy is the standard for TB treatment, as the TB bacillus can become easily resistant to one drug. Thus, using multiple drugs helps to eradicate the disease and prevent relapse with strains of bacteria that are resistant to common antitubercular drugs. Information about the reason behind therapy and the importance of multidrug therapy should help to gain patient acceptance toward therapy. Due to the concerns with multidrug-resistant TB, the nurse should never administer the drugs sporadically, or only give one of the ordered drugs. The nurse cannot force the patient to take ordered drug therapy, as patients have the right to refuse therapy.

2. d.   All of the above. Avocados and chocolate are high in tyramine and may cause hypertension. Tuna fish is high in histamine and may cause headache, palpitations, hypotension, or other reactions.

3. a.   SGOT and SGPT are liver enzymes and indicate liver functioning. As hepatitis and other liver problems are frequent adverse effects of INH, these enzymes should be monitored closely. Creatinine clearance and BUN indicate renal function and are not a major concern with INH. Vital capacity is not altered by INH.

4. c.   Giving patients all of their pills and watching them swallow them is an important aspect of direct observational therapy short course. (DOTS). This confirms that patients are taking all of their medicine, eliminates TB in the patient, and helps prevent multidrug-resistant TB from developing in the patient due to not taking all of the medicines for the full course of treatment. Although the patient needs encouragement to adhere with therapy, this is not the most effective way to achieve adherence. All drugs need to be taken in multidrug therapy, not just one, to help prevent resistance. Although most patients may be a reliable source as to whether they have taken their medication, some will not be reliable.

CASE STUDY

1. Because of his age, his drinking, and prescribed drug therapy, he is at increased risk of liver damage and hepatitis.

2. Mr. Bowen will need to be seen regularly and checked for elevated liver enzymes or symptoms of liver disease. He should be encouraged to stop drinking alcohol. Referral to Alcoholics Anonymous might be appropriate. Visits to him at the shelter where he often stays might be appropriate to assess him for liver problems if he doesn't come to the clinic daily.

CRITICAL THINKING CHALLENGE

1. Disulfiram and isoniazid have a drug interaction that induces excess dopaminergic activity. Impulsivity, affective instability, and anxiety are characteristics of excessive dopaminergic activity. Individuals with a tendency toward impulsivity tend to externalize their problems and overreact to environmental events. Individuals with affective instability are characterized by rapidly occurring shifts in affect, changing from anger to disappointment to excitement in a matter of hours or minutes. They are also sensitive to shifts in the environment, such as separation or frustration. Individuals with high anxiety have a greater readiness to anticipate punishment or aversive consequences of their behavior and often show concomitant autonomic arousal associated with their fearfulness.

2. The physician needs to be notified at once of these changes.

Chapter 53

KEY TERMS

Crossword puzzle

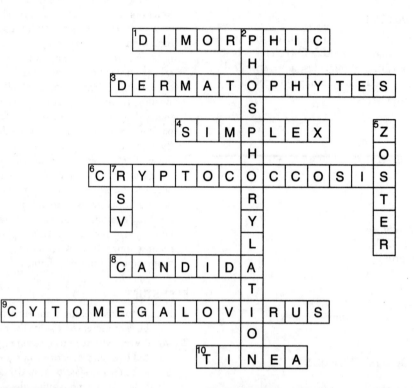

PHYSIOLOGY AND PATHOPHYSIOLOGY: THE BODY HUMAN

Essay

1. Adsorption, penetration, uncoating, replication and transcription, assembly and release
2. Budding from the parent cell into identical daughter cells
3. Long, hollow, branching filaments of a mold
4. Cutaneous level of the body
5. A dermatophyte cannot grow at the body's core temperature. A systemic mycosis is a serious, deep tissue infection by a fungus capable of growth at the body's core temperature.

CORE DRUG KNOWLEDGE: JUST THE FACTS

Multiple choice

1. b	2. c	3. b	4. a	5. d
6. d	7. c	8. a	9. d	10. c
11. b	12. d	13. a	14. b	15. c
16. d				

CORE PATIENT VARIABLES: PATIENTS, PLEASE

Multiple choice

1. c	2. d	3. a	4. a	5. c
6. b	7. c	8. b	9. c	10. c
11. b				

NURSING MANAGEMENT: EVERY GOOD NURSE SHOULD...

Multiple choice

1. c. Come in to the health center to be examined. Jerry may have a secondary infection from the acyclovir. He needs to be seen to be properly assessed and treated. Taking aspirin may mask the symptoms and allow the infection to become worse. Soaking in a bathtub may spread the infection to other areas, such as areas with broken skin or mucous membranes of the rectum. Stopping the acyclovir will cause the viral infection to become worse and could possibly lead to resistance of the virus to the acyclovir.

2. d. Do all of the above. Amphotericin may cause infusion reactions. The vital signs should be monitored first to serve as a baseline. A test dose should be given to assess for an infusion reaction. Antipyretics, such as ibuprofen or acetaminophen, are helpful in preventing or minimizing the infusion reaction. Other drugs that might be given are corticosteroids, antihistamines, meperidine, and possibly dantrolene.

3. e. Do none of the above. Ashley is demonstrating signs of infusion reaction. The infusion should be stopped and the physician notified. Increasing the infusion rate would worsen the reaction. Amphotericin B should be administered through a large vein, preferably a central vein due to its irritant properties. Slowing the infusion has not been demonstrated to decrease the infusion reaction.

4. b. Seek an order for an antidiarrheal. Diarrhea is common but not a serious adverse effect of fluconazole. The fluconazole should not be discontinued, as the patient needs this drug therapy to prevent potentially fatal infections. The diarrhea is not a sign of infection; no culture is needed.

5. c. Have the patient swish the suspension in her mouth before swallowing it. This will provide topical application of the antifungal to the affected area. The suspension should be shaken, but it should not be applied to the hip wound, mixed with water, or administered to the back of the throat.

CASE STUDY

1. His medications digoxin and hydrochlorothiazide, a thiazide diuretic, are both risk factors. The amphotericin B may induce hypokalemia, which increases the risk of digitalis toxicity. The thiazide diuretic also increases potassium loss, so the effect of hypokalemia may be intensified. Again, this places the patient at increased risk of digoxin toxicity and for the adverse effects associated with hypokalemia (such as possibly fatal arrhythmias).

2. The nurse should check his potassium level before and then throughout the therapy. If he is hypokalemic before start of therapy, he should receive a potassium supplement. Hydrate as much as possible, but do not push excessive fluids, as this may precipitate CHF. Monitor for signs of fluid overload.

CRITICAL THINKING CHALLENGE

1. The oral corticosteroid, prednisone, made Mr. March immunocompromised. This allowed him to develop aspergillus without his normal ability to ward off the infec-

tion or keep it as a minor infection that the body could eradicate.

2. Yes, you should give the amphotericin B. Although amphotericin B is not recommended to be given with digoxin or thiazide diuretics, amphotericin B appears to be the only drug of choice to treat an infection that could be fatal. This is the traditional "rock and a hard place." Because the risk of not receiving the drug could be death, the drug should be given. Monitor very carefully. Nephrotoxicity can easily send this patient into acute CHF. The dose may need to be decreased from a standard dose due to his other pathologies. Possibly the other drugs could be withdrawn or their dosage decreased, but this might also precipitate acute CHF.

Chapter 54

KEY TERMS

True/false

1.	T	
2.	F	enzyme immunoassay (EIA) and enzyme-linked immunosorbent assay (ELISA)
3.	F	progression of the disease
4.	F	CD4+ T cells
5.	F	HIV RNA
6.	F	polymerase chain reaction (PCR)
7.	F	Western Blot
8.	F	protease inhibitors
9.	F	HAART (highly active antiretroviral therapy)
10.	T	

PHYSIOLOGY AND PATHOPHYSIOLOGY: THE BODY HUMAN

Essay

1. control of viral replication and mutation, reduction of viral burden, prevention of progressive immunodeficiency, maintenance of a normal immune system, delay progression to AIDS, prolongation of life, decreased risk of selection of resistant virus, decreased risk of drug toxicity

2. reduced quality of life from adverse effects, earlier development of drug resistance, limited future choices of antiretroviral agents, risk of dissemination of drug-resistant virus, unknown long-term toxicity of certain drugs, unknown duration of effectiveness of current antiretroviral therapies

3. After multiple clinical trials, the outcome of treatment has been proven to be improved by triple- or quadruple-drug therapy. Monotherapy has extremely limited benefits for the patient.

CORE DRUG KNOWLEDGE: JUST THE FACTS

Multiple choice

1. d	2. a	3. d	4. c	5. b
6. a	7. c	8. a	9. c	10. d
11. d	12. b	13. c	14. b	

CORE PATIENT VARIABLES: PATIENTS, PLEASE

Multiple choice

1. b 2. a 3. b 4. d 5. b
6. a 7. b 8. d

NURSING MANAGEMENT: EVERY GOOD NURSE SHOULD . . .

Multiple choice

1 c. Instruct the patient to avoid fatty foods. High fat intake impairs absorption. Zidovudine should be given 1 hour before meals. The daily dose should be divided into two or three doses.

2 a. Administer 30 minutes after meals. Taking on a full stomach will help to decrease GI effects and promote absorption, especially if there is fat in the meal and the meal is high calorie. Skipping even a single dose may increase viral load and have a negative effect on the disease suppression.

3. d. Administer therapeutic dose gradually by dose escalation. Increasing the dose to therapeutic dosing in steps helps to minimize the onset of rash, which is a common adverse effect. Nevirapine may be given regardless of food intake. Food has neither a positive nor negative effect on nevirapine. The dose should be divided into two daily doses.

4. d. Sulfamethoxazole-trimethoprim. Anthony is at risk of developing PCP pneumonia and should be treated prophylactically with sulfamethoxazole-trimethoprim (Bactrim). Isoniazid and rifampin are used to treat TB. Amphotericin B is used to treat serious systemic fungal infections.

5. d. All of the above. Zidovudine should be taken on an empty stomach, saquinavir should be taken on a full stomach. GI upset can occur from both of these drugs. The patient may accommodate to these adverse effects with time, but not always. The viruses may develop resistance to the drugs if the drugs are not taken regularly as prescribed. This is important for the patient is understand. When drug resistance develops, the pharmacotherapy for HIV is very limited.

CASE STUDY

Lisa may need to be taught the importance of the drug therapy for treating her infection and preventing worsening of her disease or relapses of PCP. She should know what each drug is for, why it is prescribed, and exactly when and how to take it. This is especially true of the SMZ-TMP, which will be an additional drug therapy for her at home. It is also important for her to understand what drug resistance is and how the virus becomes drug resistant with inconsistent dosing.

Additionally, Lisa needs to be encouraged to live a healthier lifestyle to maintain her health. She should be encouraged to refrain from substance abuse. Counseling or support groups, if available, may be helpful. She may have used substances as a coping mechanism and now will need to learn other coping skills. If she does continue with drug abuse, she should be taught to use clean needles and never share her needles with anyone else to prevent spread of infection. She also needs to receive information regarding having her partner use a condom to prevent spread of disease.

CRITICAL THINKING CHALLENGE

1. Why are you refusing to take your medications?
   How do the medications make you feel?
   What is the hardest part about taking these medications for you?
   What is the easiest part about taking these medications for you?
   Who are you close to? Who helps you cope?

2. The regimen of drug therapy for HIV is demanding and difficult for every patient, no matter what their background or lifestyle. Drug therapy may cause people to feel sick a good bit of the day. The intensity of the regimen and the severity of the illness may make them feel overwhelmed. It is important to talk with Lisa, not just to her, to understand what her concerns are so that, together, you can address these concerns. The other nurse's comments that Lisa is expected to be noncompliant because of her history of IV drug abuse devalue Lisa as a person and an individual. It is not a therapeutic response of the nurse. Taking the time to ask a few more questions and to be empathetic creates a therapeutic nurse–patient relationship. When Lisa believes her feelings are valued by the nurse, she may be more likely to accept teaching the nurse offers.

   You might learn from these questions that Lisa doesn't want to take the drugs because they make her nauseous all the time or cause diarrhea. A prescription for an antimetic or antidiarrheal might then help her to adhere to her drug therapy. Maybe Lisa tells you that she can't remember to take the pills at different times. A drug time schedule could then be made up by the nurse and Lisa to help her remember exactly what to taken when, based on her normal eating schedule and other daily routines. Maybe she doesn't want to take any medication during the middle of the day because she doesn't want her friends or family to know she has HIV.

   Based on the knowledge you learn, your teaching plan can then be tailored to be specific for Lisa and her needs. Thus, Lisa sees that what you are offering is helpful for her, as opposed to being "your agenda." Patient education is most effective when it begins by addressing what the patient wants to know, as opposed to what you believe the patient needs to know.

Chapter 55

KEY TERMS

Crossword puzzle

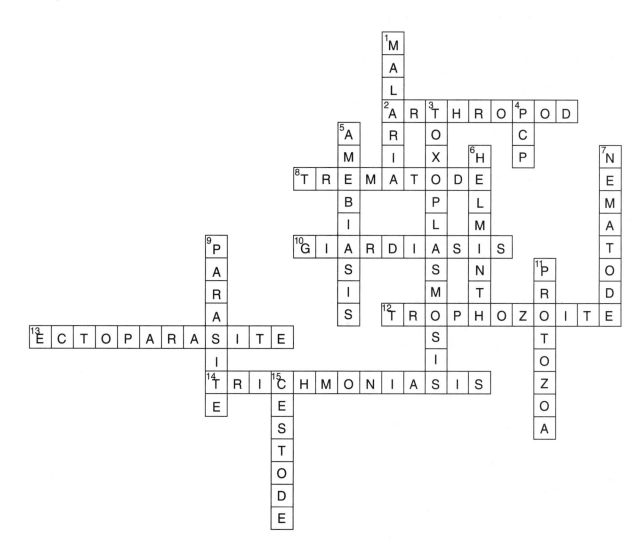

CORE DRUG KNOWLEDGE: JUST THE FACTS

Multiple choice

1. c 2. c 3. d 4. c 5. a
6. d 7. a 8. b 9. b 10. d
11. d 12. a 13. c 14. d 15. b
16. d 17. a 18. c

CORE PATIENT VARIABLES: PATIENTS, PLEASE

Multiple choice

1. b 2. d 3. d 4. a 5. c
6. d 7. a 8. c 9. b 10. a

NURSING MANAGEMENT: EVERY GOOD NURSE SHOULD . . .

Multiple choice

1. a. Begin drug therapy 2 weeks before the planned travel schedule. This will allow the drug to become effective before risk of exposure. The drug should be continued until 4 weeks after the patient has left the malarial area. The drug should be taken weekly, on the same day. Taking the drug with food will minimize GI upset.

2. b. OTC liquid cold medicines. These preparations often contain alcohol. Metronidazole has a disulfiramlike reaction when taken with alcohol. Milk, rice, and antipyretics have no interaction with metronidazole.

3. d. All of the above. If she has a current sexual partner, that person also needs to be treated with metronidazole. He likely has the infection also, and this will prevent reinfection of Brenda after the metronidazole treatment. The drug is not recommended in the first trimester as risk is unknown. Anticoagulants interact with metronidazole, producing greater anticoagulant effects.

4. e. Do none of the above. Dilute pentamidine in 5% dextrose and water. Saline solutions will form a precipitate with the pentamidine. Blood pressure should be monitored throughout the infusion, not temperature. IM injections should not be used due to risk of thrombocytopenia from pentamidine.

5. d. All of the above. Chewing the tablets will best promote effectiveness. Taking with something fatty, such as milk, cheese, or ice cream, will also promote effectiveness. Other family members are likely to be infected as well and should be treated at the same time to prevent reinfection.

CASE STUDY

1. The nurse should monitor the blood pressure carefully while administering the drug. The other vital signs should also be monitored. A set of vital signs should have been taken just before the infusion for a baseline comparison.

2. The patient's respiratory status should be assessed throughout therapy for evidence of bronchospasm. The patient should be kept in bed during the transfusion. Emergency resuscitation equipment should be handy.

CRITICAL THINKING CHALLENGE

Aaron may be having a hypoglycemic attack related to the pentamidine. The nurse should check his blood glucose with a blood glucose monitor. The nurse should also check his vital signs.

INSTALLING THE STUDENT QUIZ BANK

The installation program should automatically start a few seconds after you have inserted the CD-ROM into your CD-ROM drive. Follow the directions on the screen to complete the installation. If the installation program does *not* automatically start, follow these steps:

1. Open the Start menu and select Run.
2. In Open box, type d:\setup, where d is the letter representing your CD-ROM drive, and press Enter. (If your CD-ROM drive is a letter other than d, substitute that letter.)
3. Follow the directions on the screen to complete the installation.
4. The program will add a shortcut to your Desktop.
5. To launch the program, double click on the icon on the Desktop.

SYSTEM REQUIREMENTS

This program will run on any IBM-PC or compatible computer that *minimally* includes:

a Pentium 100 CPU;
32 MB RAM (64 recommended);
Windows;
SVGA display supporting 256 colors (16 bit recommended);
12X CD-ROM drive;
800x600 monitor resolution;
mouse;
5 MB of hard-disk space

Note: In order to run this program, you must have Macromedia Flashplayer installed on your PC. If you do not currently have this program installed, it is a free download available at: http://www.macromedia.com/software/flashplayer/.